Hearing Conservation in Industry

Hearing Conservation in Industry

ALAN S. FELDMAN, Ph.D.

President
Environmental Hearing and Vision Consultants
E. Syracuse, New York
    and
Professor Emeritus
State University of New York
Upstate Medical Center
Syracuse, New York

CHARLES T. GRIMES, Ph.D.

Associate Professor
Department of Otolaryngology
Director, Communication Disorder Unit
State University of New York
Upstate Medical Center
Syracuse, New York

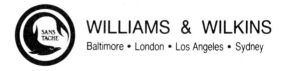

WILLIAMS & WILKINS
Baltimore • London • Los Angeles • Sydney

Editor: John P. Butler
Associate Editor: Victoria M. Vaughn
Copy Editor: Caral Shields Nolley
Design: JoAnne Janowiak
Illustration Planning: Lorraine Wrzosek
Production: Raymond E. Reter

Printed in the United States of America

Library of Congress Cataloging in Publication Data

Main entry under title:

Hearing conservation in industry.

  Bibliography: p.
  Includes index.
  1. Deafness, Noise induced—Prevention. 2. Industrial noise—Physiological effect. I. Feldman, Alan S. II. Grimes, Charles T.
RF293.5.H4 1985   363.7′4   84-20958
ISBN 0-683-03112-0

Composed and printed at the
Waverly Press, Inc.

85 86 87 88 89
1 2 3 4 5 6 7 8 9 10

Preface

The past decade has been seen a proliferation of activity in the area of occupational noise and industrial hearing conservation programs (HCPs). Prior to 1970, relatively few companies provided protection of the worker from noise, either through noise reduction at the source or with personal hearing protective devices (HPDs). Preemployment hearing testing, when it was performed, was usually done because of concerns about worker compensation regulations rather than as a first step in monitoring the effects of noise on hearing.

Increased attention to the problem of industrial noise-induced hearing loss was generated when the Occupational Safety and Health Administration (OSHA) began its rule-making process in the early 1970s. A number of professionals, primarily audiologists, began to offer services to industry that were designed to assist companies in the development of HCPs. Others who have been involved with HCPs and other facets of occupational noise within industry include physicians, industrial hygienists, occupational nurses, and safety personnel. The backgrounds of these varied professionals are quite different, as are their roles.

Since 1983, a federal noise standard has been in place. Millions of workers are included in hearing conservation programs. This book has as its primary purpose, the objective of serving as a reference for those persons whose primary or tangential interests impact on the problems of occupational noise, its effect on hearing and the prevention of damaging exposure of industrial workers. This would include not only audiologists who could be directly involved in the development of HCPs in industry, but also the variety of other personnel who relate to, or have responsibility for, occupational noise related programs, either in whole or in part.

Any one who has been involved in the area is well aware that no single program can stand as a model for all others. The problems in industry vary and any number of approaches may be utilized to achieve the desired goal of the prevention of hearing loss due to exposure to hazardous noise. This book, as a consequence, does not offer a singular approach to the problem. Instead, it has as its intention an identification of the challenge and a consideration of the methods one may utilize to achieve the goal of prevention of hearing loss.

At the onset, an overview of the problem is set forth and this is followed by a consideration of the physiological and engineering factors of noise. In either case, it is recognized that the primary purpose of this book is not to serve either as an engineering text or as an exhaustive physiological manual of noise and its effects on the ear. Instead, these topics are covered in terms of their relevence to the entire picture. Dr. Nábělek has provided an extensive list of applicable standards in Appendix II.

The background of regulations leading up to the present OSHA noise standard and a discussion of that standard follows in Chapter 4. The approach to the review of the standard is from the perspective of how it can lead to a comprehensive noise control and hearing conservation program. This review is followed by Chapter

5, dealing with the various approaches that may be utilized to implement programs. The options of in-house and consultative services, including on-site mobile hearing testing, are considered along with a discussion of the components that are essential to all programs.

A fundamental premise of the OSHA noise standard is that the prevention of hearing loss due to noise exposure may be achieved through the proper use of HPDs. Chapter 6 provides a superb examination of the breadth of topics pertinent to HPDs and affords insight into the contribution of HPDs to effective HCPs.

Many audiologists and other professionals are regularly engaged in providing courses intended to prepare people as occupational hearing conservationists (or industrial audiometric technicians). Chapter 7 offers an opportunity to study the background and objectives of the standard course for this purpose. It is based on the outline of the course developed by the Council for Accreditation in Occupational Hearing Conservation (CAOHC). Another facet of education, the training and motivating of workers included in HCPs, is highlighted in Chapter 8. This topic is included because of the requirement of the noise standard that workers exposed to hazardous noise receive an annual training program.

An essential component of the audiometric testing program is the professional review of the audiometric data. Chapter 9 explores this very important topic in conjunction with the subsequent recommended course of action. Referral and follow-up criteria are subjects handled by the interdisciplinary team of authors of this chapter.

Too often, evaluation of the effectiveness of a HCP is overlooked. It is not correct to assume that, simply because a HCP contains all the required components, it will be effective. Chapter 10 specifically examines the questions of what contributes to, and how to evaluate the effectiveness of, HCPs.

Although not a part of OSHA's occupational noise standard, the topic of Workers' Compensation as it relates to occupational hearing loss is essential in any textbook on this subject. Chapter 11 provides the reader with a clear and detailed review of this topic.

The final two chapters offer rather pertinent, but novel, topics for a textbook in occupational hearing conservation. Legal considerations are very real issues for practitioners in the public domain. Licensure constraints, liability potential and forensics are rather new considerations for many audiologists as are the pragmatics of marketing one's services. While hardly constituting a comprehensive coverage, their inclusion within this textbook will provide the reader with an appreciation of their importance and, hopefully, a motivation to explore them in greater depth.

An extensive set of references is supplemented by detailed appendicies including the current noise standard and other citations. The OSHA Regulation (Appendix I) is referred to frequently throughout this text. The reader may find it helpful to become familiar with the material in Appendix I beforehand. Doing so will greatly facilitate the appreciation of the topics covered in this book.

Finally, the selection of contributing authors for this text was accomplished with a specific goal in mind. That was to have the topics presented by people who were knowledgeable and experienced in their respective areas. Five of the authors contributing to this textbook, Melnick, Feldman, Thomas, Joseph and Grimes, have served as members of CAOHC. There probably have been no more prolific authors in the area of HPDs than the Royster's. All of the contributors have been actively engaged in some facet of consultation with industry in noise and hearing conservation. Melnick coauthored a United States Department of Labor sponsored investigation of the handicap of occupational hearing loss and disability compensation. Feldman and

Grimes were involved with the establishment of a company that pioneered mobile audiometric testing services to industry in the Northeast. Thomas and Royster were among those focusing on studies of the effectiveness of HCPs. Morrill has been successful in marketing full range hearing conservation services to industry on a national basis and Muraski has combined his legal and audiologic education to provide pertinent consultation services.

This wide range of experience has allowed the contributing authors to generate a text that is both practical and theoretical at the same time.

Coincidental with the submission of this manuscript for publication, the United States Court of Appeals for the Fourth Circuit arrived at a three-judge split decision on a petition by the Forging Industry Association. The petition contended that the regulation exceeded the scope of OSHA's statutory authorization by triggering action by the employer even though the employee's hearing loss may have occurred off the job. The effect of this decision was to vacate the Hearing Conservation Amendment to the occupational noise exposure standard, 29CFR 1910.95 (see Appendix I). The decision was handed down on November 7, 1984 and OSHA has submitted an appeal to the full court.

The basic premise of the decision dealt with the trigger effect of a standard threshold shift (STS) and the fact that such a STS could have arisen from off-the-job exposure. Rather than vacate a portion of the rule, the court dismissed the entire amendment. This leaves the standard as it was prior to March 1983. As a result, a hearing conservation program (HCP) is mandated, but there are no specifics in regulation concerning the HCP. The reader must understand that the hearing conservation regulatory mandates alluded to throughout this text refer to 29CFR 1910.95 prior to November 7, 1984, pending the outcome of appeal or a rewriting of the rule.

A. S. FELDMAN
C. T. GRIMES

Contributors

Jeffrey E. Copeland, M.B.A.
Director of Marketing
Impact Hearing Conservation, Inc.
Kansas City, Kansas

Alan S. Feldman, Ph.D.
President
Environmental Hearing and Vision
 Consultants
E. Syracuse, New York
 and
Professor Emeritus
State University of New York
Upstate Medical Center
Syracuse, New York

Charles T. Grimes, Ph.D.
Associate Professor
Department of Otolaryngology
Director of Communication Disorder
 Unit
State University of New York
Upstate Medical Center
Syracuse, New York

Donald Henderson, Ph.D.
Acting Dean/Director
Callier Center for Communication
 Disorders
University of Texas
Dallas, Texas

Donald Joseph, M.D.
Professor of Otolaryngology
University of Missouri
School of Medicine
Columbia, Missouri

William Melnick, Ph.D.
Professor
Department of Otolaryngology
Ohio State University
Columbus, Ohio

Jeffrey C. Morrill, M.S.
President
Impact Hearing Conservation, Inc.
Kansas City, Kansas

Anthony A. Muraski, J.D., Ph.D.
Associate Professor
Detroit College of Law
Detroit, Michigan

Igor V. Nábělek, Ph.D.
Professor
Department of Audiology & Speech
 Pathology
University of Tennessee
Knoxville, Tennessee

Julia Doswell Royster, Ph.D.
President
Environmental Noise Consultants, Inc.
Cary, North Carolina

Larry H. Royster, Ph.D.
Professor
Department of Mechanical and Aerospace
 Engineering
North Carolina State University
Raleigh, North Carolina

William G. Thomas, Ph.D.
Associate Professor
Division of Otolaryngology
Director of Audiology
University of North Carolina
School of Medicine
Chapel Hill, North Carolina

Contents

CHAPTER 1

An Overview of Noise Exposure and Hearing Conservation in Industry

ALAN S. FELDMAN and CHARLES T. GRIMES

Exposure to loud, distracting and possibly hazardous noise is a common experience for everyone. Whether to allow such exposure to be hazardous to one's hearing is often a personal choice. Personal portable stereo equipment exemplifies this choice. For example, in one study the average user intensity level of such equipment has been measured at between 106–113 dB at the ear, with more than 66% of the sample exceeding an 8-hr 90 dB exposure (1). Such exposure to hazardous noise levels is no longer condoned in the workplace.

Occupational noise exposure was limited until the early 1900s. After the time, noise levels in the workplace increased in direct relation to advances in technology and industrialization and exposure or nonexposure was not really an option available to the worker (2); instead, exposure to industral noise was often considered a normal aspect of one's work. Over 3 decades ago Carhart (3) referred to noise as the most frequent threat to the ears in industry. The option of personal ear protection was seldom exercised, even in those rare instances when it was made available. As a consequence, over the years, exposure of industrial workers to hazardous noise has resulted in hearing loss for millions of employees. Occupational hearing loss continues to be one of the most prevalent occupational diseases, with an estimated prevalence in excess of 10 million workers (4).

By the 1950s hearing loss secondary to noise exposure on the job was beginning to be accepted among the various states as a compensable occupational disease under worker's compensation legislation (5, 6). This, however, did not provide much impetus for the development of hearing conservation programs. Likewise, the inclusion of noise exposure standards in the 1969 revision of the Walsh-Healy Public Contracts Act (7) failed to create much interest in the implementation of hearing conservation efforts. The major thrust toward the development of hearing conservation in industry has come as a result of the Hearing Conservation Amendment to the Occupational Safety and Health Administration's (OSHA) regulation FR1910.95 (8). Delays in implementing occupational hearing conservation programs have not really been a consequence of denial of the hazard posed by exposure to high levels of noise. Rather, they would appear to have been motivated more by economic factors as well as by public ignorance about the impact of hearing loss.

It is perhaps unfortunate that the hearing loss one sustains from exposure to noise is painless and insidious. Were that not the case, it is likely that priorities attached to this industrial hazard by both employee and employer would be substantially elevated. Considerable research, both in the laboratory and in the field, has provided us with a good deal of information about noise exposure as an industrial health problem.

Some facts about noise and the effects of noise exposure are:

Noise exposure can produce a permanent hearing loss, known as noise-induced permanent threshold shift (NIPTS)

Noise-induced hearing loss may be transient (temporary) or permanent—or a combination of these

Noise exposure may also cause tinnitus

Noise-induced hearing loss is insidious in its development and is unaccompanied by pain or other physical discomfort

The amount of hearing loss sustained by exposure to noise varies from person-to-person and is dependent upon prior hearing level, duration of exposure and level of the noise

Noise-induced hearing loss has serious impact on the understanding of speech. People with NIPTS frequently attribute their problem to unclear speech production by the speaker, rather than to poor hearing.

Noise-induced hearing loss can be prevented

Noise exposure may also result in nonauditory effects such as fatigue, vascular changes and voice disorders

NOISE AND NOISE EXPOSURE

All sound has the potential to be described as noise. Classically, the distinction is not its level that categorizes sound as a noise as much as whether or not it is desired. To the rock music enthusiast good is often synonomous with loud, while, to some of us, that experience would be classified as a noisy one. At the same time, an extraneous but soft signal introduced into a sound field during some threshold experiments would have the effect of introducing a noisy variable. Though considered a noise, the latter could hardly be classified as a hazard to hearing, while the damaging effects of the former have long been identified (9–12).

Within the context of this book, the term, noise, is generally used to describe an aperiodic signal occurring as a by-product of some process or mechanical activity, usually in the workplace. Its intensity level is great enough that it poses a potential hazard to one's hearing and it may also constitute a hazard to other anatomic structures or physiologic systems if exposure were to continue over time.

AUDITORY EFFECTS OF NOISE

It is a well established fact that exposure to noise can damage one's hearing. While one may debate certain aspects of damage risk criteria, there is general agreement that given sufficient intensity and duration of exposure, hearing loss will occur (12, 13). The extent of a noise-induced hearing loss does vary according to individual susceptibility and extent and duration of exposure (13, 14).

The initial result of exposure to noise in laboratory animals and humans is similar. Exposed ears exhibit a temporary threshold shift (TTS). The threshold will shift gradually over time of exposure, ultimately reaching a plateau after about 8–12 hr (15). The level of this plateau or asymptote will also be dependent upon the stimulus level and frequency characteristics.

As time away from exposure increases, the ear will recover, usually within a period that can be measured in hours up to several days. With repeated exposure, recovery diminishes and a permanent threshold shift (PTS) or noise-induced permanent threshold shift (NIPTS) is exhibited. At any one time in the early years of exposure it is likely that measured hearing loss could be a combination of TTS and PTS. Ultimately, however, recovery fails to occur and the entire loss becomes permanent.

The tinnitus that occurs in ears exposed to noise is usually a persistent ringing and is often a bigger complaint than is the hearing loss. Tinnitus may occur in the absence of measurable hearing loss but is usually accompanied by some impairment in hearing. The effects of the hearing loss on communication are frequently projected as a consequence of someone else's "mumbling" rather than the listener's poor hearing. Unlike the hearing loss, the ringing in the ear cannot readily be externalized.

NONAUDITORY EFFECTS OF NOISE

While not as well documented as are auditory effects of noise exposure, there are a number of other physiologic functions that may be compromised with noise exposure (16, 17). The specificity of damage risk criteria in this domain has yet to be established. Reports persist that vascular effects such as vasoconstriction of small blood vessels of the extremities and decreased systolic and increased diastolic blood pressures have been observed in noise-exposed workers.

Studies in industrial settings as well as laboratories have been cited (18) which document a higher rate of heart disease, high blood pressure and higher blood cholesterol levels when there is exposure to high noise levels.

In general, the types of physiologic effects that have been reported are those mediated by the autonomic nervous system and are the same functional changes associated with stress situations.

Other nonauditory effects may include:

1. Interference with sleep
2. Decrease of work performance
3. Disturbances of equilibrium
4. Psychological disturbances. e.g. headache, mood changes, anxiety

ACCEPTANCE OF NOISE IN INDUSTRY

As has often been observed in studies of human behavior, changes in one's environment serve to modify behavior but adaptation will generally be observed. It was observed by Kryter (12) some time ago that subjective tolerance to noise is quite substantial and adaptation is a normal course of events. This is quite consistent with the usual comment of industrial workers who report initial discomfort when exposed to workplace noise but then pronounce they "got used to it." Despite the psychologic adaptation and acceptance of noise, it is well documented that prolonged exposure to noise impairs hearing. Whether damage risk criteria for physiologic effects other than hearing loss will ultimately be documented is not known at this time.

It is unquestionably true that workers have not been outspoken about the need to reduce the noise, or at least exposure to it. Labor has been slow to accept occupational noise as a serious health hazard, partially because acceptance could place demands on the worker that the employee is not yet ready to assume. For example, mandated use of hearing protective devices (HPDs) places some responsibility for compliance on the worker.

As a consequence, the thrust of labor leadership has been to demand a reduction of noise level as the preferred way to prevent noise-induced hearing loss. The negative side of this is that all hazardous noise cannot be engineered out, regardless of cost. The positive side is that labor has now begun to accept the principle that noise exposure is hazardous.

COST OF ELIMINATION OF NOISE

Management, for the most part, has not been any more aggressive in moving to prevent exposure to noise. The cost of engineering sound reduction is a consideration, but so is the cost of implementing a full scale hearing conservation program (HCP). However, compensation claims for occupational hearing loss could be the most expensive feature of all if HCPs are not implemented.

The magnitude of the problem is hard to understate. Conservative estimates range from 5–10 million employees with potential exposure to hazardous noise (4, 19). These employees are located in some 300,000 businesses. Both worker's compensation and earlier federal regulations should have been a stimulus leading to protection of the hearing of these workers. It is clear from the record that such has not been the case. It was estimated that barely $15.7 million, or $3/exposed worker, was being spent in 1981 on industrial hearing conservation (19). Not considering the cost of engineering noise reduction, OSHA estimated the cost of protecting the entire workforce at $254.3

million, or about $53/yr/employee. Considering the $15.7 million expenditure for hearing conservation prior to 1981, one would have to conclude that barely 6% of the work force that was exposed to noise was being protected against material impairment prior to the promulgation of OSHA's hearing conservation amendment.

It should be evident that, while it is difficult to place a price on the impact a hearing loss has on the quality of life, the cost of implementing HCPs in industry is sizable. This is particularly relevant when the affected party, the worker exposed to noise, is not highly motivated to prevent a hearing loss from developing.

CONTROL OF THE PROBLEM

The problem of occupational noise exposure and the prevention of noise-induced permanent threshold shift is not readily resolved. It requires more than a decision by the employer to develop programs that include either reduction of noise or reduction of exposure along with a monitoring of effectiveness. It also requires acceptance of, and cooperation with, that program by the employee.

The first step in controlling the problem involves the identification of both the noise levels that contitute a hazard and the employees who are exposed to the noise. When engineering the noise out is not feasible, then an ongoing HCP must be implemented (4).

In Chapter 3, the breadth of the topic of noise, noise exposure measurement and control of noise is comprehensively explored. Many of us, regardless of our individual disciplines, can participate in measurement of noise levels and noise exposure. It is only mentioned briefly here to reinforce the concept that the bulk of the expertise in this area is within the domain of the engineer.

SOCIAL AND LEGISLATIVE FORCES

As we have moved into the latter part of the 20th century, society has begun to exhibit a greater social consciousness.

Along with this has come a broadening acceptance of handicaps. Although the gap is far from closed, there is a better appreciation of hearing loss and increased insight into the effect a loss of hearing has on one's social interaction in general, and communication specifically. Thus, worker acceptance of HCPs is on the upswing. The task of motivating workers to use HPDs becomes easier the longer such programs are in effect. One is less likely today to see a stigma attached to the use of personal hearing protection.

At the same time, the historical failure of industry to effectively prevent occupational disease and injury has led to a promulgation of regulations designed to protect the worker. Although we may witness some pulling back from excessive over-regulation with more conservative administrations, there is little reason to doubt that those hazards posing life-threatening and otherwise significant health and safety hazards will continue to be the subject of regulation. Occupational noise exposure and hearing loss fall into this category.

ELIMINATION OF NOISE VERSUS PERSONAL HEARING PROTECTION

Much of the delay prior to the March 1983 promulgation of the hearing conservation amendment to CRF 1910.95 was a consequence of a debate about whether or not the use of HPDs offers a viable alternative to the elimination of noise via an engineering approach (20). In the period between 1972 and 1981 several industries challenged OSHA's insistence on engineering as the required methodology of noise (exposure) reduction. OSHA had insisted that only when engineering and administrative controls were not feasible would the alternative of personal HPDs be permissable. The issue tested was partially related to cost-benefit factors and, repeatedly, decisions were made in favor of industry's contention that alternatives to engineering controls should be allowed when a cost-benefit analysis shows HCPs to be less costly than engineering or administrative control of noise. For example, as a consequence of a 1982 ruling by the U.S. Court of Appeals for the Ninth Circuit (21), OSHA instructed its field inspectors to permit reliance on hearing protectors and HCPs rather than engineering and administrative controls when noise levels were below 100 dB (22).

The current regulation permits the use of personal hearing protective devices as the primary means of preventing exposure and stipulates monitoring audiometry as a means of validating the program effectiveness. Theoretically, as industries develop effective HCPs, the annual incidence of significant hearing threshold shift should decline to the same level as would be measured in a nonexposed, but otherwise similar, population.

HEARING LOSS AS A COMPENSIBLE OCCUPATIONAL DISEASE

In the past decade rather significant changes have been occurring in the realm of worker's compensation for occupational hearing loss. This issue is discussed in considerable detail in Chapter 11. For now it is enough to identify that, by far, the greatest potential cost to industry is in worker's compensation claims for damage already done. Sataloff (23) estimates the potential direct compensation costs for occupational hearing loss to be in excess of 20 billion dollars. Interestingly, this threat traditionally has been one of the major *deterrents* to an early implementation of HCPs. Management is quite understandably timid about testing workers' hearing and then advising them of the existence of hearing losses. It has been described as a fear of opening Pandora's box.

Confrontation with this fear should not be further delayed. The longer HCP implementation is delayed, the greater the number of potential compensation claims becomes. This increase occurs not only because workers are sustaining greater hearing loss, but also as a consequence of changing definitions about what constitutes a hearing handicap (24).

The rather archaic "speech frequency" designation of 500 Hz, 1000 Hz and 2000 Hz is being replaced by more realistic inclusion of higher frequencies. The professional has been aware for a long time that the contribution of high frequencies to speech intelligibility is very important. The real-life communication experience demands very little from frequencies below 1000 Hz but is very dependent upon those up to 4000 Hz.

As formulas change and other restrictions about filing compensation claims (e.g. long waiting periods, termination of employment) are eased, the impetus for these claims will not stem from the existence of hearing conservation programs. Rather, they will occur regardless of their existence.

TYPES OF HEARING CONSERVATION PROGRAMS

The diversity of industrial settings dictates that there be no single type of HCP (25, 26). Large employers with substantial health and safety personnel may elect to provide the complete program in-house. This would necessitate the purchase of audiometer(s), booth(s) and the training of personnel as occupational hearing conservationists. Some larger companies employ audiologists to coordinate and supervise these programs, others may use staff physicians while still others employ outside consultants to review and interpret test results.

Mobile testing services are usually engaged by smaller industries or large, but scattered, ones. However, even some very large employers elect to uses mobile consulting services for their entire program— the advantage to this being that it gets the job done in a shorter and finite period of time. Fig. 1.1 illustrates a mobile unit that can both test the hearing and provide an educational program for more than 175 employees in an 8-hour shift.

Any and all combinations are possible. Regardless of the approach, the intent is to develop a program that meets all standards and which is cost effective. The fun-

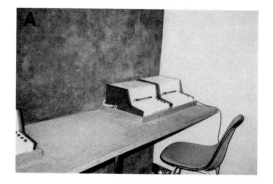
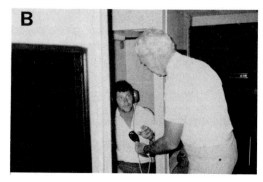
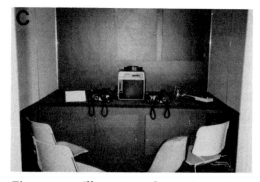
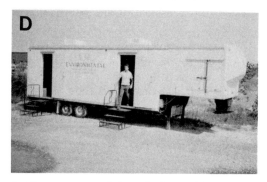

Figure 1.1. Illustration of an industrial hearing testing van containing: *A*, four self-recording audiometers; *B*, four minibooths for individual employee testing; *C*, four locations for an audiovisual presentation to employees prior to their hearing test; *D*, Employee leaving the mobile unit after receiving the annual hearing test and annual training program. (Reproduced by courtesy of Environmental Hearing and Vision Consultants, LTD, E. Syracuse, NY)

damental goal is to develop a program that protects the employees from developing hearing loss as a consequence of exposure to noise in the workplace.

While inclusion of all necessary components does not insure that a program will be effective, management's first step is to see that all facets of a comprehensive HCP are in place. Table 1.1 is an example of an approach used by one hearing conservation service company to alert management to the necessary components of an HCP. It also represents a tool for the marketing of hearing conservation services to industry. Marketing principles and approaches are considered at greater length in Chapter 13.

WHAT CONSTITUTES AN EFFECTIVE PROGRAM

The features of comprehensive HCPs were identified in Table 1.1. However, it is safe to say that the evaluation of the effectiveness of a HCP is not determined by a detailing of its components, but rather can be assessed either by the study of the individual worker, subgroups of workers or on a company-wide or perhaps even an industry-wide basis and other characteristics (26, 27). The characteristics common to effective HCPs have been identified by Royster et al. (26). They emphasize that no ingredient is of greater importance than is the genuine support of top management. Further, they note that strict enforcement of the HPD program is essential, and such enforcement should include a four-step procedure: (*a*) verbal warning; (*b*) written warning; (*c*) brief suspension (no pay); and, finally, (*d*) termination.

There also needs to be a key individual committed and personally responsible for the program. With the responsibility must

Table 1.1[a]

---

proView®

MANAGEMENT'S HEARING CONSERVATION PROGRAM COORDINATOR

Let Environmental Hearing and Vision Consultants' **experience** work for you. The OSHA-mandated program for Occupational Hearing Conservation involves many features that require coordination for effective management control. proView® is a time-tested service that achieves this objective.

DOES YOUR PROGRAM HAVE:

Comprehensive records of workplace noise levels and Time Weighted Average **(TWA) exposures?**

A **plan** for reducing employee exposure to hazardous noise?

Valid baseline and annual **audiograms?**

Professional **review** and documented **recommendations** for appropriate course of action?

Systematic records of equipment **calibration** and test area sound level certification?

Qualified hearing **testers** and supervising **professionals?**

An ongoing Hearing Protective Device **(HPD)** program for exposed employees?

An annual **training program** for employees exposed to hazardous occupational noise?

An efficient **record keeping** system that coordinates the data from the multiple features of a comprehensive hearing conservation program?

A worker's **compensation** analysis?

A procedure for evaluation of the **effectiveness** of your program?

If your answer is **YES** to all of the above then you don't need proView®.

If your answer is **NO** to any of the above, let Environmental Hearing and Vision Consultants use its experience to **help your program conform with regulations.**

For an analysis of how you shape up and assistance in improving your program contact:

ENVIRONMENTAL HEARING AND VISION CONSULTANTS

19 Corporate Circle
East Syracuse, New York 13057

---

[a] Reproduced by courtesy of Environmental Hearing and Vision Consultants, Ltd.

---

also reside the authority to implement the program. Active communication lines must be open between all levels of management. Finally, the HPDs that are provided must be effective, comfortable, durable, and easy to use.

SUMMARY

The problem of occupational noise and the development and implementation of HCPs in industry no longer relies on the goodwill of management. Realistic regulations are in place and progress is being made toward the goal of prevention of occupational hearing loss. As a greater awareness of the hazard of noise and increased social concerns about hearing loss become a reality, so too will increased management and worker compliance with the elements that are so essential to effective HCPs.

References

1. Bienvenue GR: *Personal Stereo Systems: Can They Be Used Safely?* Paper presented at the 24th Annual Convention, New York State Speech-Language Hearing Association, April 1984.
2. Ward WD: Noise-induced hearing loss. In Northern J (ed): *Hearing Disorders*, Boston, Little Brown, 1976, p 161.
3. Carhart R: The ears of industry. *Arch Ind Hyg Occup Med* 2:534–541, 1950.
4. Snow JB, Jr: Otological considerations in noise-induced hearing loss, in Henderson D et al. (eds): *Effects of Noise on Hearing.* New York, Raven Press, 1976, p 467.
5. *Slawinski vs Williams & Co.*, 298 N.Y. 546, 81 N.E. 2d 93, aff'g 273 App. Div. 826,76 N.Y.S. id. 888, 1948.
6. *Wojeik vs. Green Bay Drop Forge*, 265 Wis. 38, 60 N.W. 2d. 409, rehearing denied, 61 N.W. 2d 847, 1953.
7. Walsh-Healy Public Contracts Act, Title 41 C.F.R., Chapt. 50 Washington, D.C., Superintendent of Documents, U.S. Government Printing Office.
8. Occupational Safety & Health Administration: Occupational Noises Exposure; Hearing Conser-

vation Amendment, Final Rule. *Federal Register*, 48:9738–9785, 1983.

9. Lebo CP, Oliphant KS, Garritt J: Acoustic trauma from rock and roll music. *Calif Med* 107:378–380, 1967.

10. Rintlemann WF, Borus JF: noise-induced hearing loss and rock and roll music. *Arch Otolaryngol* 88:377–385, 1968.

11. Speaks C, Nelson D, Ward WD: Hearing loss in rock and roll musicians, *J Occup Med* 12:216–219, 1970.

12. Kryter KD: *The Effects of Noise On Man*, New York, Academic Press, 1970.

13. Glorig, A, Ward, WD, Nixon, J: Damage risk criteria and noise-induced hearing loss. *Arch Otolaryngol* 74:413, 1961.

14. Henderson D, Hammernick R, Dosanjh DS, Mills JH (eds): *Effects of Noise on Hearing*. New York, Raven Press, 1976.

15. Melnick W: Human asymptotic threshold shift. In Henderson D, et al. (eds): *Effects of Noise on Hearing*. New York, Raven Press, 1976, p 277.

16. Anticaglia JR, Cohen A: Extra-auditory effects of noise as a health hazard. *Am Ind Hyg Assoc* 5:31, 277–281, 1970.

17. Cohen, A: Extra-auditory effects of noise. In Olishifski JB, Harford ER (eds): *Industrial Noise and Hearing Conservation*. Chicago, National Safety Council, 1975, p 259.

18. *Noise: A Health Problem*: Office of Noise Abatement and Control. U.S. Environmental Protection Agency, Washington, D.C., 1978.

19. Occupational Safety and Health Administration: *Occupational Noise Noise Exposure: Hearing Conservation Amendment. Federal Register* 46: 4078–4179, 1981.

20. Miller JC III, and Walton TF: Protecting workers' hearing: an economic test for OSHA initiative. *Regulation* Sept–Oct: 31–37, 1980.

21. Donovan vs Castle and Cooke Foods and OSAHRC (No. 77-2565): U.S. Court of Appeals for the Ninth Circuit, 1982.

22. OSHA Instruction CPL 2-2.35: Office of Health Compliance Assistance, November 9, 1983.

23. Sataloff J: W.C. Hearing loss claims should be handled with care. *Occup Health Saf* March: 35, 1984.

24. Suter AH: Calculations of impairment or handicap. In Kramer MB, Armbruster JM (eds): *Forensic Audiology*, University Park Press, Baltimore, 1982, p 259.

25. Feldman AS: Industrial Hearing Conservation Programs. In Henderson D et al. (eds): *Effects of Noise on Hearing*. Raven Press, New York, 1976, p 525.

26. Royster LH, Royster JD, Berger EH: Guidelines for developing an effective hearing conservation program. *Sound Vibration* 16:6, 1982.

27. Royster LH, Lilley DT, Thomas WG: Recommended criteria for evaluating the effectiveness of hearing conservation program. *Am Ind Hyg Assoc J* 41:40–48, 1980.

CHAPTER 2

Effects of Noise on Hearing

DONALD HENDERSON

INTRODUCTION

For hundreds of years we have known that exposure to loud noise can produce hearing loss. However, the recent expansion of the industrial sector of society has increased the number of people exposed to dangerous noise and made the problem of noise-induced hearing loss (NIHL) more acute. Furthermore, there has been a change in the mores of society and it is no longer acceptable to develop a handicapping condition as a consequence of an individual's occupation.

The Department of Labor estimated that of the 14.3 million production workers in the United States, 26% were exposed to noise levels of 90 dBA or above for 8 hr/day and 57% were exposed to levels of 85 dBA or greater (1). The actual total number of people exposed to dangerous noise is far greater when military and general environmental noise are included. The more severely affected individuals live with hearing losses that greatly degrade the quality of their life and contribute to a life-style of isolation.

Given that noise can produce serious health effects in a large segment of the population, it would seem to be a simple matter to avoid the problem by protecting individuals from dangerous noise. However, what constitutes "dangerous noise" and how much of a given noise is too much are difficult scientific and political questions. When setting noise standards, if we overestimate the hazards of noise, the noise standards will be an unnecessary constraint to the industrial process; if we err by making the noise standards too lax, we introduce serious health risks to larger segments of the population. Thus, an accurate description of the relationship between the acoustic parameters of noise and changes in hearing is an essential first step in establishing an effective and fair noise standard. However, the actual criterion levels for acceptable noise exposure then become an ethical decision that is most properly made by labor, management and government.

This chapter is focused on two questions. First, what is the relationship between the physical parameters of a noise exposure and the ensuing hearing loss? Such an understanding is an essential first step in creating a scientifically based noise standard. Second, how does noise actually disrupt the process of auditory sensations? An understanding of the biological changes in the auditory system associated with exposure to noise will eventually lead to better management of individuals with hearing losses and possibly lead to ways to identify individuals with particular sensitivity to noise-induced hearing loss.

APPROACHES TO STUDYING THE EFFECTS OF NOISE

The effects of noise can be studied using: (a) the demographic approach where one correlates the noise exposure in the workplace with the hearing levels of the worker, (b) the laboratory approach where temporary hearing loss is studied in human subjects and (c) the animal model where hearing loss is manipulated in appropriate experimental animal models. Each approach has strengths and weaknesses. Collectively, data from each approach is necessary for eventually understanding NIHL.

Demographic Approach

The demographic approach to learning the relationship between noise and hearing loss is conceptually the simplest, but practically the most difficult. Basically, if one is interested in the effects of a given noise on people, then it would seem to be an easy matter to correlate the amount of hearing loss with exposure to the noise of a given level and duration. The problems that arise include: the difficulty in establishing accurate histories of individual exposures, the separation of NIHL from hearing losses of other causes (i.e. aging, drugs, diseases, and other undocumented noise exposure) and large intersubject variability in susceptibility to NIHL.

Taylor et al. (2) provide a very instructive example of the problems associated with the demographic approach. Figure 2.1 comes from a careful study of Scottish weavers where the noise was measured precisely, the work conditions (and presumably, the noise levels) were stable over many years and the subjects were screened for complicating otological histories. The data show the relationships between the amount of noise exposure at the workplace and the amount of hearing loss. However, even with the care taken by Taylor, there still is a very large degree of variability. The variability seen in Figure 2.1 is typical of other demographic studies (3, 4).

Thus, even though the demographic approach is conceptually the most parsimonious approach to defining the relationship between noise exposure and hearing loss, it is complicated by the problem of controlling individual noise exposure, extraneous causes of hearing loss and other sources of poorly understood intersubject variability.

Laboratory Studies of Temporary Threshold Shifts

A second approach to establishing the relationship between noise and hearing loss is to study transient or temporary threshold shifts (TTS) of auditory threshold in response to controlled exposure to noise. Laboratory studies of TTS in humans played a major role in establishing noise guidelines (5).

Because the temporary loss of sensitivity following noise exposure is accompanied by the same set of aural symptoms seen in the condition of permanent threshold shifts (PTS), (i.e. ringing in the ear or tinnitus, rapid growth of loudness, loss of frequency selectivity (6) and breakdown of temporal integration (7)), it has been assumed that the two phenomena, TTS and PTS, share a common etiology. The Committee on Hearing and Bioacoustics (CHABA) of The National Research Council has formalized the relationship between TTS and PTS by developing three hypotheses:

1. Temporary threshold shift 2 min after a noise exposure (TTS_2) is a measure of the potential hazard of a noise exposure
2. All exposures that produce the same TTS_2 are equally hazardous
3. The TTS_2 after an 8-hr exposure is equal to the noise-induced permanent threshold shift after 10-yr exposure to that noise

Obviously, it is difficult to test these hypotheses in humans because the tests would require monitoring hearing functions over many years and controlling other variables. There is, however, the possibility of directly testing the relationship between TTS and PTS in animal experiments. For example, Henderson et al. (8) exposed chinchillas to impulse noise of various levels and correlated the amount of TTS found immediately after noise exposure with the eventual PTS. The amount of TTS immediately after the exposure had almost no correlation with the amount of PTS found 30 days postexposure. A second experiment also confirmed that a knowledge of TTS following an exposure is not predictive of the eventual PTS (9).

If one is interested in understanding the rules governing PTS there are two serious limitations to using TTS as a model. First, for ethical reasons, laboratory studies of TTS are limited to exposures that produce

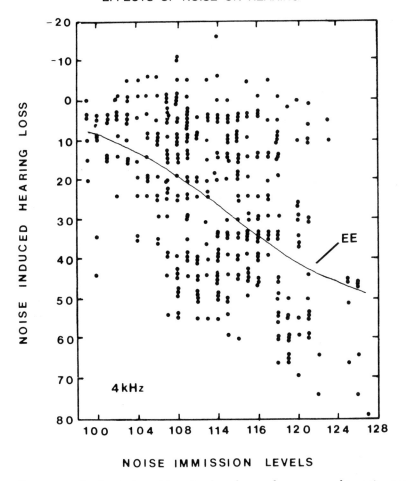

Figure 2.1. The range of noise-induced hearing loss for workers exposed to noise ranging from 100–128 dB. *Points* refer to individual auditory thresholds at 4 kHz.

10–30 dB shifts in sensitivity, while our clinical interest is in PTS levels of 30–40 dB or more. Second, in the few studies that actually measured TTS and PTS in the same subject, there was not a strong correlation between the two measures. This suggests there are partially different processes underlying TTS and PTS. Thus, because of the limited range of TTS that can be safely produced in the laboratory, as well as the likelihood that different morphological and physiological changes underlie TTS and PTS, laboratory studies of TTS have limited value in our understanding of the rules and processes governing PTS.

Animal Models in Noise Research

The logic supporting animal models of NIHL is that the mammalian inner ear is similar morphologically, physiologically and psychophysically across a wide range of species. In fact, there are certain common laboratory animals which have hearing capabilities similar to man, e.g. the cat (10), and the chinchilla (11). Thus, given the similarities in normal audition between man and certain animals, it is logical to postulate that these animals respond to traumatic noise as does man.

The animal model used for most of the recent research in noise has been the chinchilla. The chinchilla offers a number of advantages: its auditory capabilities are very similar to man's; its cochlea is located in a large auditory bulla where it is easily accessible to experimental manipulation; it tolerates anesthesia; it is easily conditioned for behavioral evaluation; and it seems to be immune to many of the infections that occur in the middle ears of guinea pigs, cats and rats. Given these advantages, the general strategy in many of the experiments that will be discussed in this chapter is to first establish baseline hearing sensitivity by either behavioral or physiological procedures, expose the animal to a well controlled noise environment, reevaluate its hearing ability at intervals of several hours to several months, and kill the animal and analyze its cochlear tissue.

The eventual constraint that is applied when one is using such studies to establish noise standards for humans is that there are differences in the susceptibility of man and most of the experimental animals. However, the results from the animal experiments provide important insights into the parameters of noise exposure that are critical for producing the hearing loss. Furthermore, the correlation of anatomical changes in the cochlea with the hearing loss provides an important perspective on the mechanism of the hearing loss.

All three of these approaches do provide useful information concerning the conditions leading to NIHL. In the next sections we will discuss the response of the auditory system to traumatic levels of noise.

MECHANISM OF NOISE-INDUCED HEARING LOSS

It is clear from experimental animal data and the few relevant human temporal bones, that exposure to noise permanently destroys the delicate tissue and functioning of the inner ear. The damage is pervasive and involves the sensory cells, nerve cells, vascular supply, and supporting cells.

To appreciate the range of effects seen in the cochlea, it is useful to review the basic anatomy and physiology of the inner ear. Figure 2.2 shows a schematic of the auditory mechanism and how the cochlea changes the pattern of acoustic vibrations into a neural code. The normal sequence of events starts with the transmission of sound waves through the external auditory meatus (EAM), the action of the ossicles, the piston movement of the stapes (Fig. 2.2A), the traveling wave of activity from the stapes down the basilar membrane (Fig. 2.2 B) and, finally, a shearing action at the tectorial membrane stereocilia junction (Fig. 2.2 C). The movement of the stereocilia is the site of transduction where acoustic vibrations are encoded as neural messages (Fig. 2.2 D) which lead to the sensation of "hearing." One should bear in mind that excessive noise is not a pollutant, per se, but rather a harmful level of a form of energy that the ear is designed to transmit.

NIHL is typically considered a form of sensorineural hearing loss. However, the anatomical basis for the loss includes changes throughout all the major cellular subsystems of the cochlea. At low levels of exposure, excessively high levels of metabolism are probably responsible for damaging the hair cells and afferent dendrites. At a higher level of exposure it is possible to rupture tight cell junctions, thereby allowing the mixing of endolymph and perilymph. At still higher levels of continuous noise (greater than 120 dBA) or impulse noise, the cochlea can be damaged by mechanical processes. Not only are the sensorineural elements damaged by noise but it is obvious that changes in the sensory cells are accompanied by changes in the vascular elements of the basilar membrane and the lateral wall of scala media, as well as in the supporting cells of the organ of Corti.

In Figure 2.3, representative samples of the different classes of pathologies are shown. The *top* two panels show a surface view of the same area of the organ of Corti, but photographed in different focal planes. The *left* photo shows a relatively normal region of inner and outer hair cells. However, three cells are missing in the first row of hair cells. The *right* photo, which is focused at a lower plane of the same area, shows the corresponding outer

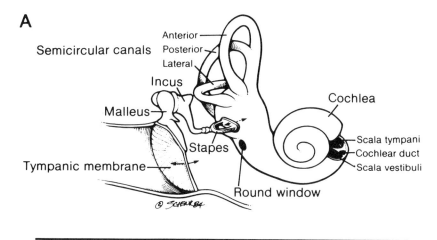

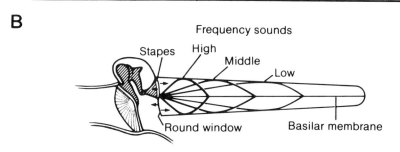

Figure 2.2 A and B.   A, the left outer, middle and inner ear. The cut-out of the cochlea shows the relationship of the perilymph-filled *scala tympani* and *vestibuli* and endolymph-filled *scala media*. B, the cochlea has been uncoiled and the envelope of basilar vibration is shown for stimulation by high, medium and low frequency sounds. This pattern of vibration is referred to as a travelling wave.

pillar cells that have become detached from the basilar membrane. Not only is this defect of supporting cells closely related to the loss of a few hair cells but, perhaps more significantly, it is indicative of a possible change in the mechanical properties of the cochlea in that area.

The *middle* micrographs of Figure 2.3 illustrate some of the changes in the vascular supply to the area of the spiral ligament following a severe noise exposure. The *left* photo illustrates a nonpatent capillary; the lumen is occluded by the enlargement of the endothelial cell nucleus. To the left of the *arrow*, the vessel has entirely collapsed. The *right* photo shows the terminal stage in the degenerative process started in the left plate. All that remains of the capillary is a strand of debris in the perivascular space (*arrow*). While such vascular changes are seen in

normal, non-noise-exposed animals such changes in a noise-exposed animal are more often more extensive.

The *bottom* two micrographs were taken from an animal killed immediately following the exposure, and are both of the same area of the organ of Corti but are focused at two different levels. This pair of micrographs illustrate the more typical appearance of a noise-induced lesion on the organ of Corti, i.e. the *left* plate shows mechanical alterations such as loss of inner and outer pillar cells and tears in the reticular lamina; the *right* plate shows what are thought to be metabolic components to the damage such as extensive swelling of the sensory cell bodies.

Circumstantial evidence to support the idea of a damagingly high level of metabolism comes from laboratory studies of

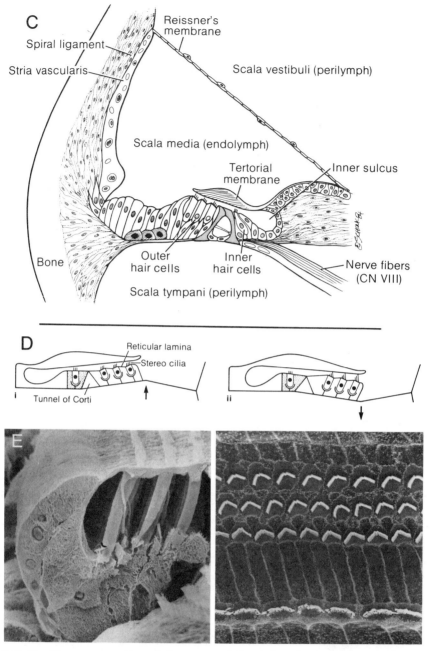

Figure 2.2 C–D. C, a cross-section of the organ of Corti showing vascular supply of the stria vascularis and the spiral ligament. D, a schematic of the shearing motion between the tectorial membrane and top of the organ of Corti. It should be noted that the outer hair cells are probably attached to the underside of the tectorial membrane by the stereocilla of the outer hair cells and are stimulated by direct mechanical action, while the inner hair cells are probably not attached to the tectorial membrane and are probably stimulated by viscous drag caused by fluid motion. E, a scanning electromicrograph of the organ of Corti.

TTS. Drescher (12) measured the amount of temporary hearing loss produced by noise exposure in guinea pigs when the guinea pigs' body temperature was sys-

tematically raised and lowered. The animals with higher temperatures rapidly developed larger amounts of TTS than animals with normal temperatures; con-

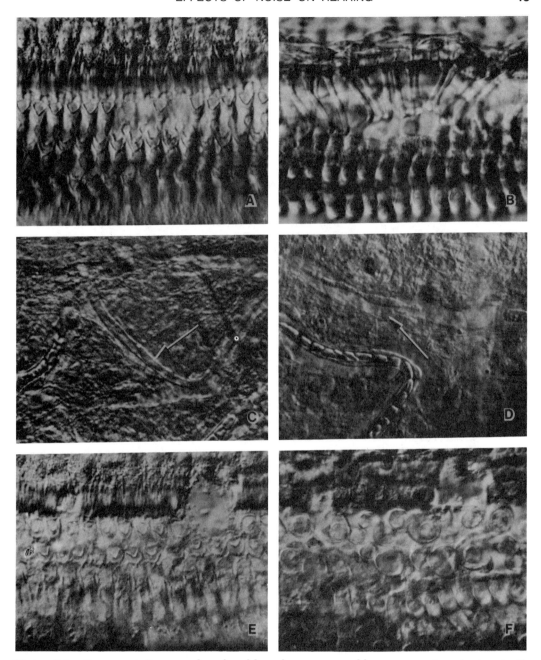

Figure 2.3.   Representative samples of cochlear damage caused by exposure to noise (see text).

versely, animals with lower temperatures were much more resistant to TTS from the noise. The assumption is that the controlling of the animal's temperature also controls the rate of metabolism in the cochlea. There are other kinds of evidence supporting the idea of dangerous rates of metabolism being responsible for NIHL (13).

With high levels of noise [>140 dB sound pressure level (SPL)] it is clear the cochlea can be damaged by direct mechanical destruction. A graphic example of mechanical damage in the cochlea is given in Figure 2.4. The animal was exposed to impulse noise (155 dB SPL) and killed ½ hr after exposure. It appears that the whole organ of Corti is ripped off the

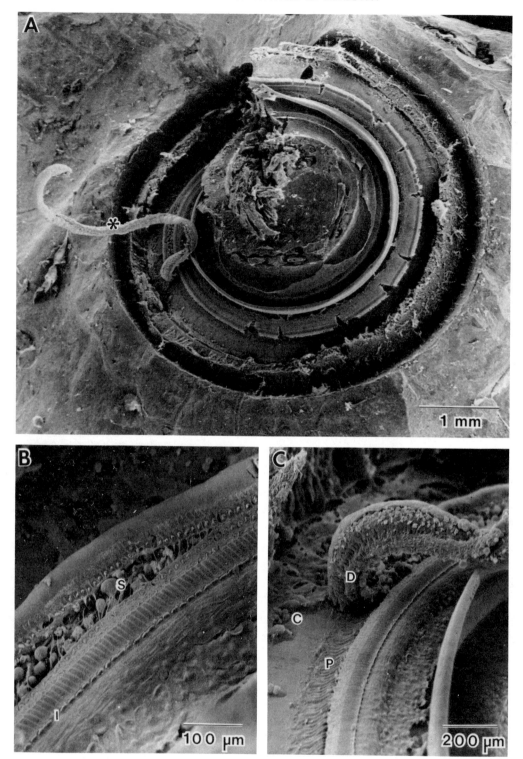

Figure 2.4. Scanning electromicrographs of the cochlea following exposure to high level impulse noise. *A*, the cochlea was viewed ½ hr after the exposure and the organ of Corti (∗) is ripped off the basilar membrane. *B*, a more apical region of the cochlea shows a longitudinal fracture (s) between the pillar cells and outer hair cells. *C*, higher power of the ripped organ of Corti (D), outer sulcus (C) and outer pillars (P).

basilar membrane. Other animals exposed to the same noise, but sacrificed at later periods, showed the same pathology, but with various stages of absorption of the damaged tissue.

Whether the ear is damaged by metabolic or mechanical factors, the changes, if severe enough, are permanent. Furthermore, there does not seem to be a primary therapy to prevent serious TTS resolving into PTS or reversing PTS. There is a large body of literature describing the biological basis of hearing loss, which has been summarized in two volumes (14, 15).

One of the most important, enduring questions is what are the relevant variables in determining an individual's susceptibility? This is a key question for managing workers exposed to noises of different characteristics. We will now discuss the relationship between the parameters of noise exposure and the pattern of hearing loss.

PHYSICAL PARAMETERS OF NOISE EXPOSURE

Any given noise exposure can be described by its level (dB re some standard), bandwidth, spectral distribution, duration and temporal pattern. For impulse noise, the process is even more complicated and to adequately describe an exposure it is necessary to measure the rise time, level, duration, rate, number of impulses, and background level. The following discussion attempts to identify the contributions of these variables to the production of a hearing loss.

Frequency

The auditory system is more susceptible to high frequency sound than to sound of low frequency. The difference is obvious in the results of demographic studies of NIPTS. Figure 2.5 shows the growth of hearing loss in a population of workers exposed to an average level of 95 dBA for 40 yr. We can assume that most exposures are broadband. The loss of sensitivity happens rapidly at 3 and 4 kHz and plateaus

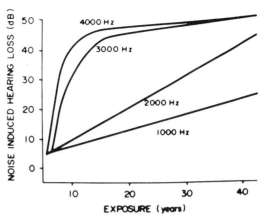

Figure 2.5. Growth of permanent hearing loss from exposure to average industrial levels of 95 dBA for 0–40 yr.

at a 45 dB loss after approximately 15 years. With 15 yr exposure, there is essentially no hearing loss at 1 and 2 kHz, but as time passes, sensitivity is reduced to the point that after 40 yr of exposure the loss at 2 kHz is almost as large as the loss at 3 and 4 kHz.

The differential susceptibility across frequencies is probably the result of two factors, i.e. the acoustic reflex and the transmission characteristics of the external meatus. The resonance characteristics of the outer ear are shown in Figure 2.6. The external meatus can be modeled as a resonator, closed at one end, with an approximate length of 2.3 cm and a resonant frequency of about 2800 Hz.

The fact that the peak of the transmission curve shown in Figure 2.6 is broader than a typical resonance curve is the consequence of a less-than-rigid tympanic membrane. The implication of the resonance curve is clear. If the environmental noise is broadband, then the resonance properties of the EAM act to enhance the "effective level" of mid- and high frequency sounds when they are transmitted through the EAM.

The action of the middle ear muscles also contribute to the protection of the low frequency region of hearing. When an individual is exposed to a broadband noise that activates the acoustic reflex, the low frequency components of the

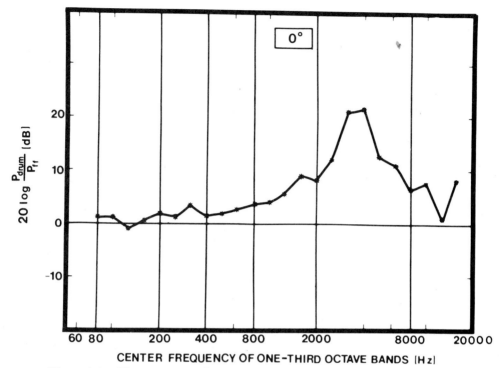

Figure 2.6.   The resonance characteristics of the external auditory meatus.

noise are significantly more attenuated in their transmission path to the cochlea. The net effect of both the EAM resonance characteristics and the attenuation characteristics of the acoustic reflex is to significantly shape the input characteristics to the cochlea, i.e. when the stimulus at the entrance to the EAM has a broad spectrum, the EAM enhances the mid- and high frequencies while the acoustic reflex attenuates the low frequencies. Returning to the original point, the fact that high frequencies are more damaging than low frequencies may simply be a reflection of the physical transformation that occurs in the external and middle ear.

The range of audiometric frequencies affected by a noise exposure is often higher than the frequency distribution of the damaging noise. Davis et al. (6) first reported that exposure to pure tones or a narrow band noise produced a maximum threshold shift which occurs ½–1 octave above the frequency of the stimulating tone or center frequency of the band of

noise. Figure 2.7 illustrates data from one of the exposures reported by Davis et al. The results are for TTS in human subjects, but there are countless examples of the ½-octave shift in experimental animals for exposures that produce both TTS and PTS. The "4 kHz" notch that is so characteristic of NIPTS from industrial noise may be explained by the resonance of the EAM. If most industrial noise has a broad spectrum, then the EAM resonance transforms the broad-spectrum to a band pass noise with a peak at 3 kHz and thus the maximum hearing loss appears at approximately 4 kHz, i.e. ½ octave above the traumatizing sound. The anatomical/physiological basis for the "½-octave" shift can be traced directly to the pattern of lesion in the cochlea. Salvi et al. (16) exposed chinchillas for 5 days to an octave band of noise centered at 4 kHz at a level of 95 SPL. Fig. 2.8 shows that the ½-octave shift is seen in the pattern of TTS, PTS and distribution of VIIIth nerve response characteristics (*lower graph*) but,

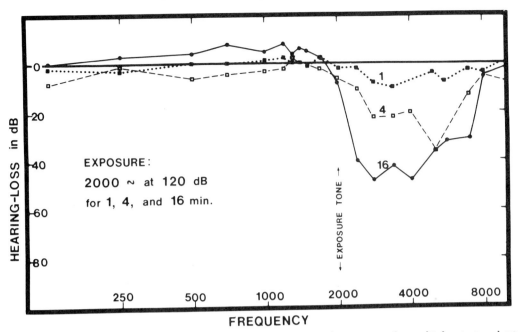

Figure 2.7. Pattern of TTS in an individual exposed to a 2 kHz noise of 120 dB for 1, 4 and 16 min. The maximal hearing loss approximately 1 octave above the frequency of the stimulating time.

most importantly, the location of the lesion in the cochlea is centered at 8 kHz, rather than 4 kHz which is the center frequency of the noise.

The mechanism responsible for the ½-octave shift is not clear, but the shift may be related to the hydrodynamics of the cochlea. The cochlea is tonotopically organized and for a given frequency there is a unique traveling wave with a point of maximum displacement (see Fig. 2.2B). However, the point of maximum pressure is basal to the point of maximum displacement and perhaps the ½-octave shift is the consequence of the location of the point of the maximum pressures rather than maximum displacement (17).

Level of Noise

The current standards for acceptable noise levels for 8-hr exposures are 90 dBA (Table 2.1). The decision to establish 90 dBA as the lowest level of acceptable noise is principally a political decision and reflects the trade-off of minimizing the extent of the population exposed to

dangerous noise and the inconvenience to the industrial process.

The basic issue of what is the lowest level of noise that will cause hearing loss is very difficult to answer. The threshold of damage varies with the frequency of the exposure, the index used (i.e. quiet threshold), damage to the inner ear, and a host of little understood variables such as impedance of the ear, eye color, smoking, thyroid function, presence of other ototraumatic agents, etc. (14, 15). Adding to these agents, the process of aging produces a steady decline in hearing that adds to the noise-induced hearing loss. Kryter et al. (18), using demographic data argued that the threshold for damage was 60 dBA. Kryter's position may be extreme. Others (3, 4) have argued that noise levels above 85 dBA are required to produce hearing loss. The data for such positions come from demographic studies which show a systematic elevation of hearing above the 85 dB level (Fig. 2.9). Given the host of complicating factors, 85 dBA would appear to be reasonable.

If we can agree that 85 dBA is the

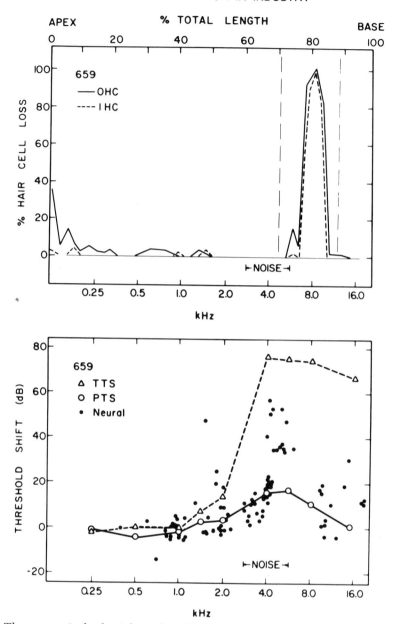

Figure 2.8. The anatomical, physiological and behavioral effects of exposure to a 4 kHz band of noise. The *top* figure shows the distribution of missing inner and outer hair cells. The horizontal axis is stated in terms of millimeters along cochlea and frequency locations. The *bottom* figure gives the distribution of the tips of individual VIIIth nerve neurons (●), the amount of TTS (△) and the amount of PTS (○).

threshold for producing hearing loss, how does hearing loss grow with increasing levels of noise? Again, a precise answer is difficult because there are too many relevant, but not fully understood, variables. The data base from Passchier-Vermeer (4) or Burns and Robinson (3) (Fig. 2.9) show a mildly accelerating function at the lower range (85–110 dBA), and at higher levels (115–130 dBA) the rate of growth of PTS is greater. The different slope in the function of Figure 2.9 is probably a reflection of different pathological processes occurring at different intensities.

An alternative perspective on the relationship between the level of noise exposure and the degree of hearing loss comes from animal studies using the paradigm

Table 2.1
Permissible contributors of noise level and duration

90 dBA or less	8 hr
95 dBA	4 hr
100 dBA	2 hr
105 dBA	1 hr
110 dBA	30 min
115 dBA	15 min

for producing asymptotic threshold shift (ATS). When the auditory system is exposed to noise for long periods (8 hr to 200+ days), auditory sensitivity is reduced steadily over the first 6–48 hr, then the loss of sensitivity remains constant or at an asymptotic level for the duration of the exposure. Theoretically, the phenomenon of ATS is potentially very important because it has been suggested that the ATS level for a given noise may be that PTS which can be expected from that noise after years of exposure. Practically, ATS is important because its condition is

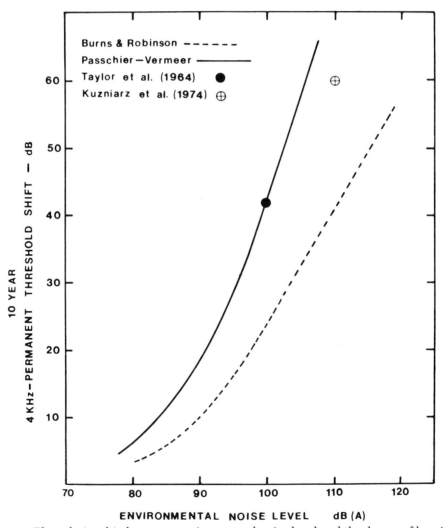

Figure 2.9. The relationship between environmental noise level and the degree of hearing loss after 10 yr. One possible reason for the differences between Burns and Robinson, 1970 (3) and Passchier-Vermeer, 1973 (4) is that the noise conditions of the latter study included combinations of continuous and impulse noise.

usually associated with minimal variability and the level of threshold seems to be independent of preexposure variation in sensitivity.

Mills (19) has systematically studied the ATS placement and compiled results from several species and several exposure paradigms. Given the species difference, the striking trend of the data is the consistent pattern of growth of ATS across species and frequencies tested. Mills postulates that ATS for a given audiometric frequency is predicted by: ATS (dB) = 1.7 OBL-C where (C) is a constant that is related to the specific sensitivity of a species for that particular frequency, (OBL) is the octave band level of the noise around the test frequency and (ATS) is the threshold at the test frequency.

The results of experiments using animal models, laboratory studies of TTS and demographic studies of workers exposed to noise all suggest a complicated relationship between the level of a noise exposure and the loss in the auditory sensitivity. At low levels, below 70–85 dBA, exposures produce only a mild hearing loss of 5–15 dB regardless of the duration of the exposure. At higher levels (85–120 dBA) TTS, and probably PTS, increases approximately 1.6 dB for each dB of noise. Above 120 dBA, the function relating hearing loss to the noise level accelerates and the mechanism underlying cochlear damage is probably different.

IMPULSE AND IMPACT NOISE

While the definitions are not definitive, impact noise is the acoustic phenomena produced by two hard objects "banging" together. The waveform of the impact noise is often described by its amplitude and duration where the amplitude is measured at the maximum peak and the duration is the time it takes for the wave to decay 20 dB from its normal level (Fig. 2.10).

Impulse noise is the acoustic phenomena associated with explosions. The waveform of impulse noise is described by the amplitude of the initial overpres-sure and the duration of time required to decay the peak overpressure to ambient pressure. It has been estimated that the range of dangerous impact noise would be above 100 dB SPL, and above 140 dB for impulse noise (Fig. 2.10).

Recent research has shown that the audiological and biological effects of impulse/impact noise may be different than the effect of continuous noise. The basis for the differences between the effects of impulse and continuous noise can be traced to the actual mode of damage in the cochlea. When the auditory system is exposed to continuous noise within moderate limits, 80–110 decibels, the actual cause of damage is not known explicitly but there is good circumstantial evidence to implicate metabolic factors underlying TTS and PTS (13). Impulse noise, however, probably damages the cochlea by direct mechanical destruction. Figure 2.4 is a photograph taken 1 hr after exposure to 155 dB impulses and it shows the organ of Corti ripped from the basilar membrane. As a secondary process to disruption of cochlear structure, the cochlear fluids will mix, leading to conditions that do not favor cell survival.

Luz and Hodge (20) suggested that impulse noise actually destroys the cochlea by a combination of metabolic and mechanical processes. The interaction of these two processes yields an unorthodox looking recovery curve for TTS. Figure 2.11 shows the Luz and Hodge model. They suggest that immediately after exposure to impulse noise, metabolic processes begin moving back to equilibrium and sensitivity begins to recover in the traditional linear fashion. However, when the noise exposure contains impulses, the large excursions of the basilar membrane cause a certain amount of concussion to the cellular elements in the cochlea producing an edematous reaction, similar to the reaction caused by trauma to soft tissue. The combination of these two processes yields a nonmonotonic recovery curve where there is initial recovery after

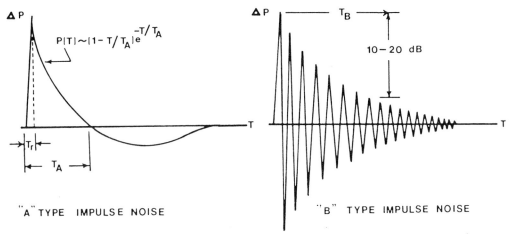

$$P(T) \sim (1 - T/T_A)e^{-T/T_A}$$

"A" TYPE IMPULSE NOISE   "B" TYPE IMPULSE NOISE

Figure 2.10. A schematic representation of the two basic impulse noise pressure-time histories. $\triangle P$ = maximum overpressure (pascals, Pa). The peak overpressure is usually referenced to 20 Pa and is referred to as dB peak SPL. T_r = rise time (seconds). The rise time is the time required for the pressure to reach $\triangle P$. As T_r becomes shorter and shorter, the wavefront becomes steeper and more "shock-like" or, conversely, less "acoustic." Shorter T_r also implies more intense high frequencies fourier components. T_A = duration of first overpressure. T_B = total duration of the "B" type impulse (seconds). The total duration is not always easy to establish, especially if the disturbances do not die out immediately. If this is the case, an arbitrary decision must be made as to how much base line fluctuation is to be accepted within T.

the noise exposure and a bounce back to high levels of TTS, and then a slower more stable recovery. The Luz and Hodge model seems to describe many of the recovery curves repeated in experimental literature on impulse noise. In Figure 2.11B, recovery of sensitivity is shown for a group of chinchillas exposed to 155-dB impulse noise. The maximum TTS occurs 8–10 hr after the noise exposure. It must be noted that most likely the animals had a larger loss immediately after the exposure.

Given the inherent interest in ATS and the differences in effect between continuous and impulse noise, it would be of interest to see if exposure to impulse noise leads to the ATS state. Henderson and Hamernik (21) approach this question by systematically exposing chinchillas to impulse noise ranging from 99–120 dB for periods lasting a week. The results showed unequivocally that impulse noise did produce a condition of ATS, but there were important differences between ATS from continuous and impulse noise. First, for a given level of ATS, if the source was

impulse noise, there would be more lasting effects, i.e. PTS and hair cell losses. Secondly, Figure 2.12 shows that the relationship between the intensity of the impulse and the level of ATS is more complicated for impulse noise. At the lower levels of exposure, the function relating ATS and noise level is shallow, while at the higher levels the function is quite steep. One interpretation of results such as these is that there appears to be a critical level of impulse noise; when impulses are below the critical level they have a minimal effect and the listener can absorb large numbers of them, but when the impulses exceed a certain critical level then damage to the cochlea accumulates rapidly with either small increases in intensity or additional impulse. It should be made clear, however, that there is no one "critical level" and each impulse profile probably has a critical level associated with it. Mills (19) has analyzed the data from ATS studies in humans, monkeys and chinchillas and reports that the major species difference is the threshold for developing a hearing

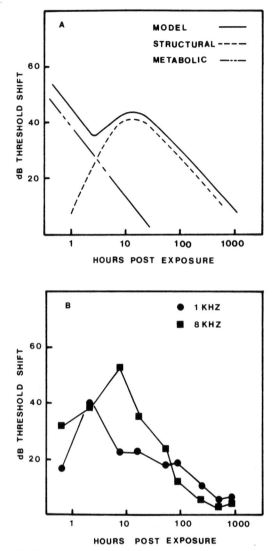

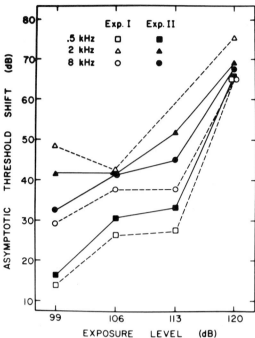

Figure 2.12. Relationship between the level of the impulse noise and the magnitude of asymptotic threshold shift.

Figure 2.11. *A*, the three curves are from a model of impulse noise TTS proposed by Luz and Hodge, 1971 (20). *B*, TTS recovery curves from exposure to 50 1-msec A-duration impulses at 155 dB, illustrating the growth of TTS.

loss, but after the threshold has been exceeded, all three species develop ATS at the rate of 1.5–1.7 dB for each dB increase in noise (19).

INTERMITTENT NOISE

Hearing loss is a function of both the intensity of a noise and also the duration of the exposure (i.e. the total energy of the exposure). What is still debatable,

however, is the amount of reduction in hearing loss that is achieved when the noise exposure is intermittent (i.e. the "on" "off" ratio). One hypothesis is that the amount of hearing loss is proportional to both the noise power and the duration of the exposure. If damage is assumed to be controlled by the total energy of the noise exposure, it follows that the 3 dB time/intensity trade-off rule should govern intermittent noise exposures of less than 8 hr (3). The Walsh-Healy Act recognizes that there is a certain amount of recovery that is possible during the quiet period of an intermittent exposure, thus the time/intensity rule was hypothesized to be 5 dB.

In practice, the debate over the 3 or 5 dB "rule" is virtually meaningless because the measurement errors in the experimental and demographic studies preclude such precise discrimination. Furthermore, as Mills (19) has pointed out, the actual trading ratio is most likely a function of the intensity of the stimulus, i.e.

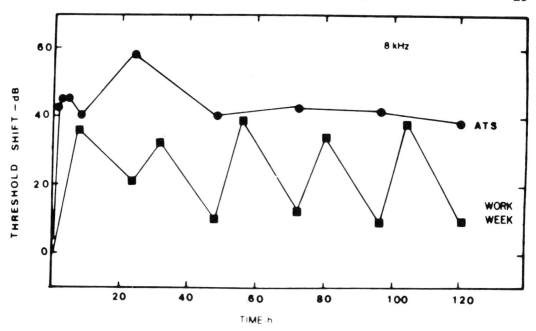

Figure 2.13. Average threshold shifts for two groups of five chinchillas exposed constantly for 5 days (•) and 8 hr/day for 5 days (■).

at low intensities one can tolerate excessively long exposures whereas at high intensities the noise is so damaging that adding 3 or 5 dB and halving the duration would significantly increase the hearing loss.

An interesting aspect of intermittent exposures has been reported (21). If one compares the patterns of TTS when chinchillas are exposed to impact noise for either 8 hr/day or 24 hr/day over a 5-day period (Fig. 2.13), the TTS at the end of an 8-hr exposure is essentially the same as the TTS for the group of animals exposed continuously for 5 days. However, when the exposure is terminated, the group exposed to the intermittent noise recovers faster, has less PTS and fewer hair cells missing. So, in one experiment, a comparison between intermittent and continuous noise exposure shows that the two exposures can produce the same level of TTS but presumably the recovery afforded during the "off" period of the intermittent exposure prevented some PTS and loss of hair cells.

NOISE STANDARDS

As we have seen in the previous sections, the frequency, intensity and temporal pattern of a noise exposure are all to play a role in NIHL. Furthermore, the effects of noise are also exacerbated by vibration, ototoxic drugs and other noises. Noise standards, to be effective, have to incorporate the most salient variables, and to facilitate their application, they should be stated simply. The federal government's solution was presented in a damage-risk criteria in the Walsh-Healy Act of 1969. The levels and duration of "permissible," or presumably safe, noise exposures are given in Table 2.1. The importance of frequency as a variable is reflected in the use of A-weighting to measure the sound, because of the A-scale discrimination against the less traumatic low frequencies. Intensity is evaluated over a limited range, i.e. noises below 90 dBA are regarded as safe and noises above 115 dBA are considered too dangerous for any period of exposure. The duration of an exposure is traded off with the intensity of the exposure. This trade-off reflects the data, showing that the damaging effects of a noise grow over at least an 8-hr period.

As a compromise strategy, the damage-risk criteria in Table 2.1 are a reasonable approach for evaluating hazardous noises in the workplace. However, it should be clear that precise predictions about the likelihood of a worker developing a hearing loss for a given noise environment are almost impossible to make using only the limited data in the criteria of Table 2.1.

SUMMARY

In this chapter we have looked at the physiological effects of noise exposure on the auditory system. Three different approaches to studying these effects have been discussed: the demographic, studies of TTS and animal models. While none of the three provides an adequate picture of how noise damages the auditory system, taken together, significant insights to the processes of NIHL are gained.

We have also surveyed the data on the relationship between NIHL and specific acoustic parameters of the noise agents. Understanding these relationships is critically important to developing the scientific basis of damage-risk criteria.

At this point in time, our understanding of the very complex relationships between noise exposure and NIHL is incomplete. It is certain, however, that there is a direct, cause-effect relationship between long-term exposure to noise and damage to the auditory system.

References

1. Bruce RD, Collen C, Fox GE, Fox HL, Swanson S: *Impact of Noise Control at the Workplace*, Report No. 2671. Boston, Bolt Beranek & Newman, 1974.
2. Taylor W, Pearson J, Mair A: Study of noise and hearing in jute weaving. *J Acoust Soc Am* 38:113–120, 1969.
3. Burns W, Robinson DW: *Hearing and Noise in Industry*. London, Her Majesty's Stationary Office, 1970.
4. Passchier-Vermeer, W: Noise-inducing hearing loss from exposure to intermittent and varying noise. In *Proceedings of the International Congress on Noise as a Public Health Problem*, EPA 550/9-73-008:169–200. Washington, DC, Environmental Protection Agency, 1973.
5. Kryter KD: Impairment to hearing from exposure to noise. *J Acoust Soc Am* 53:1211–1226, 1973.
6. Davis H, Morgan CT, Hawkins JE, Galambos R, Smith FW: Temporary deafness following exposure to loud tones and noise. *Acta Otolaryngol*, Suppl. 88, 1950.
7. Jerger JF: Influence of stimulus duration on the pure-tone threshold during recovery from auditory fatigue. *J Acoust Soc Am* 27:121–124, 1955.
8. Henderson D, Hamernik RP, Sitler RW: The audiometric and histological correlates of exposure to 1-msec noise impulse in the chinchilla. *J Acoust Soc Am* 56:1210, 1974.
9. Henderson D, Hamernik RP, Hynson K: Impulse noise-induced hearing loss from simulated work-week exposures. *J Acoust Soc Am* 65:1231, 1979.
10. Miller JD, Watson CS, Covell WP: Deafening effects of noise on the cat. *Acta Otolaryngol*, Suppl, 236:1–135, 1963.
11. Henderson D, Onishi S, Eldredge DH, Davis H: A comparison of chinchilla auditory-evoked *Percept Psychophysiol* 5:41–45, 1969.
12. Drescher DG: Noise-induced reduction of inner-ear microphonic response: dependence on body temperature. *Science*, 185:273–274, 1974.
13. Bohne, B: Mechanisms of noise damage in the inner ear. In Henderson D, Hamernik RP, Dosanjh DS, Mills J (eds): *Effects of Noise on Hearing*. New York, Raven Press, 1976, 41–68.
14. Henderson D, Hamernik, RP, Dosanjh DS, Mills J (eds): *Effects of Noise on Hearing*. New York, Raven Press, 1976.
15. Hamernik RP, Henderson D, Salvi R (eds): *New Perspectives on Noise-Induced Hearing Loss*. New York, Raven Press, 1982.
16. Salvi R, Perry J, Hamernik RP, Henderson D: Relationships between cochlear pathologies and auditory nerve and behavioral responses following acoustic trauma. In Hamernik RP, Henderson D, Salvi R (eds). *New Perspectives in Noise-Induced Hearing Loss*. New York, Raven Press, 1982, 165–188.
17. Zwislocki JJ: Micromechanics of the cochlea and possible changes caused by intense noise. In Hamernik RP, Henderson D, Salvi R (eds): *New Perspectives on Noise-Induced Hearing Loss*. New York, Raven Press, 1982, 209–226.
18. Kryter KD, Ward WD, Miller JD, Eldredge D: Hazardous exposure to intermittent and steady-state noise. *J. Acoust. Soc. Am.*, 39:451–464, 1966.
19. Mills J: Effects of noise on auditory sensitivity, psychophysical tuning curves and suppression. In Hamernik RP, Henderson D, Salvi R (eds): *New Perspectives in Noise-Induced Hearing Loss*, New York, Raven Press, 1982, 249–263.
20. Luz G, Hodge DC: The recovery from impulse noise-induced TTS in monkeys and men: a descriptive model. *J. Acoust. Soc. Am.*, 49:1770–1777, 1971.
21. Henderson D, Hamernik RP: Asymptotic threshold shift from impulse noise. In Hamernik RP, Henderson D, Salvi R (eds): *New Perspectives in Noise-Induced Hearing Loss*, New York, Raven Press, 1982, 265–281.

CHAPTER 3

Noise Measurement and Engineering Controls

IGOR V. NÁBĚLEK

Noise is an undesired sound. Sound is an audible disturbance of a medium produced by mechanical vibrations. It has physical as well as subjective or psychological dimensions which have to be understood for effective noise abatement. In this chapter only the physical and engineering aspects of the noise problems are discussed.

PHYSICAL CHARACTERISTICS OF NOISE

Dimensions of Sound

Sound Pressure

The surface of any vibrating object sets particles of the surrounding medium into motion. These particles are pushed against other adjacent particles when the surface moves outward, or are pulled toward the surface when it moves inward. Alternating compressions and rarefactions occur in the medium. The pressure variation caused by vibration is equal to the difference between the total instantaneous pressure and the atmospheric pressure. It is called the "sound pressure" (p) and is measured in pascals (Pa). The unit pascal (Pa) is equal to a newton per square meter (N/m^2); it is 10 times larger than the archaic unit dyne per square centimeter (or microbar); 1 Pa = 10 dyne/cm^2. The sound pressure of 20 micropascals (μPa) corresponds approximately to the average threshold of hearing at 1 kHz and is equal to 0 dB sound pressure level (SPL); the pressure of 20 Pa approaches the threshold of pain in the ear. The sound pressure of a gun shot is around 2000 Pa.

Speed of Sound

The particles pushed by the vibrating surface toward other particles push those particles away, and the disturbance propagates from the vibrating surface in the medium. A sound wave is produced. The velocity of propagation of the wave, measured in meters per second (m/s), is also called the "speed of sound." It is denoted by c. It depends on the physical properties of the medium and the temperature. The atmospheric pressure has small influence on c. The speed of sound in air is about 343 m/s at room temperature of 20°C.

Particle Velocity

The particles of the medium set in motion by a vibrating surface vibrate around a fixed point in space exhibiting a so-called particle velocity (v). The velocity of the air particles is very small being about 5×10^{-6} cm/s at the threshold of hearing and about 5 cm/s or 180 m/hr at the threshold of feeling. The speed of sound is obviously much greater than the particle velocity.

Types of Waves

In liquids (gases and fluids) the coupling between individual particles (molecules) of the medium is very weak and, therefore, only longitudinal waves can propagate. In these waves the particles move in the direction of the propagation of the wave. In solids, the coupling between individual molecules is very strong and, therefore, longitudinal, transversal and other waves are common. In the transversal wave, the particles move perpendicular to the direction of propagation.

Waveform

A waveform shows how a certain quantity changes in time at a certain point in space. It shows instantaneous values of the quantity as a function of time. Sound pressures and particle velocities in a sine wave are represented by waveforms shown in Figure 3.1.

Amplitude

Amplitude is the absolute value of the largest instantaneous value of the sine wave. It is a positive number. In Figure 3.1, P and V are the amplitudes in the pressure and velocity wave, respectively. The so-called effective (rms) value is equal to 0.707 of the amplitude ($P_{ef} = 0.707$ P).

Phase

In Figure 3.1, a general case is shown in which the maximal values of sound

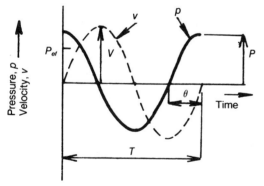

Figure 3.1. Sine waves of sound pressure (p) and particle velocity (v). P and V are amplitudes, P_{ef} is the effective (root-mean-square, rms) value of the sound pressure, T is the period, and θ the phase angle between the sound pressure and particle velocity. Small italic letters stand for instantaneous values, and capital letters for amplitudes, peak, and rms values.

pressure p and particle velocity v, or their zero crossings, do not occur at the same instant. These values occur earlier for pressure than for velocity. There is a "phase difference" between p and v. In this case the phase difference is positive.

Frequency

The number of excursions of a particle from one extreme position to the other and back to the starting position during 1 s (the number of cycles per second) is called frequency and is measured in hertz (Hz). The duration of one wave (one cycle) is called the period and is usually denoted by T. The period, measured in seconds, is equal to the inverse or reciprocal value of frequency ($T = 1/f$); it is 1 s divided by the number of cycles in a second. For example, a wave of 500-Hz frequency has the period equal to 2 ms (milliseconds). If we double a frequency, the new frequency is one octave higher than the lower one. Similarly, by halving the first frequency, a frequency one octave lower is obtained. Two frequencies, A and B, with the ratio equal to two ($f_B/f_A = 2$) form a musical interval of one octave.

Volume Velocity

Let us suppose that a surface is set into a piston-like motion. A volume V of the medium is displaced which is equal to the area of the surface S, times the excursion y of the surface: $V = S \cdot y$. The velocity u of the movement of this volume is called volume velocity:

$u = S \cdot v$, where v is the particle velocity.

Impedance

A force (F) is needed to set a surface of any object into vibration. The motion of the surface is opposed by the inertia of the mass of the surface as well as the stiffness and friction in the material. Its motion is also opposed by the reaction of the compressed and rarefied air in front of the surface. This opposition, called impedance, can be expressed in mechanical or acoustical terms. The mechanical impedance Z_m is given by the ratio of force and particle velocity:

mechanical impedance = (force)/(particle velocity).

Its magnitude is given by the ratio of the amplitudes of force and velocity:

$$Z_m = F/V,$$

and its phase by the difference of the phases:

$$\theta_Z = \theta_F - \theta_V.$$

Analogically, the acoustic impedance Z_a is given by the ratio of sound pressure p and volume velocity u. The ratio of sound pressure p and the particle velocity v is called the specific acoustic impedance, Z_s, or Z_c when representing the characteristic impedance of the medium. The magnitude of impedance is a consequence of the interaction between stiffness (negative reactance), mass (positive reactance) and friction or resistance in a system.

Resonance

If, in a system, all three components opposing the motion (friction R_a, compliance C_a, and mass M_a) are present and arranged in such a way that the volume velocity associated with all of them is the same, we speak about the "series circuit." At a certain frequency, which is called the resonance frequency, the sum of the compliance and mass effects is minimal and the impedance is equal to the resistance R_a of the circuit. The resonance frequency equals $0.159/(C_a M_a)^{1/2}$

The inverse value of impedance is called admittance, the inverse value of resistance and reactance is called conductance and susceptance, respectively. For a parallel connection of components, the negative susceptance is subtracted from the positive susceptance and, at resonance, the total susceptance is equal to 0. That means that, for a parallel circuit

at resonance, the admittance is minimal, or that the impedance is maximal.

Sound Field

Free Sound Field

Sound waves spreading from the vibrating body into the air fill out the space around the source and produce a sound field. If there are no objects that would reflect the sound, the only waves present are those propagating away from the source. The field is then called the free sound field. The front of a wave radiated from a source of small dimensions is spherical, and we speak about spherical waves (Fig. 3.2). Farther away from the source, the front of the wave can be generally regarded as plane, and we speak about a plane wave.

As mentioned before, the speed of sound in air $c = 343$ m/s at $20°C$. If, for example, the source radiates a 500-Hz tone, it produces 500 cycles in 1 s. Therefore, there will be 500 individual waves (cycles) between the source and a point 343 m from the source. A single wave will then occupy 343 m/500 = 0.686 m = 68.6 cm of the distance. This distance is called the wavelength. It is denoted by the Greek letter λ (lambda).

The product of the wavelength and of the frequency is equal to the speed of sound:

$$c = \lambda f.$$

Therefore, λ can be calculated as:

$$\lambda = c/f.$$

The same relation between the velocity of propagation, sound pressure, and frequency holds for any material. However, because the velocity of propagation depends on the properties of each particular material, the wavelengths differ for various materials. For example, speed of sound and wavelengths are larger in solids than in the air.

Obstacles

If a sound traversing a space reaches an obstacle, three things can happen: (a) part

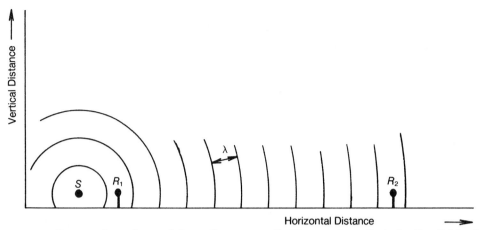

Figure 3.2. Propagation of sound from the source S. The receiver R_1 is in the field of the spherical wave, the receiver R_2 can be considered to be in the field of a plane wave. The wavelength is the distance between two consecutive maxima of the sound field.

of the impinging wave energy can penetrate into the obstacle, and either passes through it and exits on the other side of the obstacle or is absorbed and changed into heat; (b) part of the wave energy can be reflected back toward the source; and (c) part of the wave can be diffracted around the obstacle. These are shown in Figure 3.3. Which of the three possibilities prevails, depends on the acoustic similarity of the material of the obstacle and of the air, and on the size of the obstacle with respect to the wavelength. If the

specific acoustic impedance of the material of the obstacle is about equal to the characteristic impedance of the air, the wave penetrates easily into the obstacle. The larger the mismatch between the impedance of the two, the larger is the reflected portion of the wave. If the size of the obstacle is much smaller than the wavelength of the sound wave, the wave is diffracted and not reflected. The larger the ratio of the size of the obstacle ℓ to the wavelength, the more the reflection, the less the diffraction, and the larger the shadow behind the obstacle. Considerable reflection occurs if ℓ equals, or is smaller than $\lambda/4$.

Reflection

For a large mismatch between the specific acoustic impedances of the air and of the obstacle, for example a wall, a large amount of the sound power is reflected.

If Z_{S1} and Z_{S2} are the specific acoustic impedances of the air and of the wall material, respectively, and the wall is large, thick and rigid, the so called sound power reflection coefficient is equal to:

$$\alpha_r = \left(\frac{Z_{S2} - Z_{S1}}{Z_{S2} + Z_{S1}}\right)^2.$$

The reflected waves combine with the incident waves and produce standing

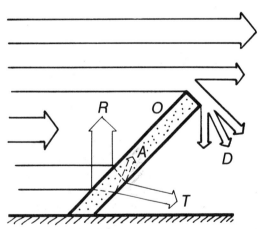

Figure 3.3. Schematic representation of sound impinging on an obstacle, O. R stands for the reflected sound, D for the diffracted sound, A for the absorbed sound and T for the sound transmitted to the space beyond the obstacle.

waves. The standing waves are characterized by maxima and minima of sound pressure. The difference between the maxima and minima is large when the reflection coefficient is large and it is small when the coefficient is small. In a general case, a sound is composed of a wave propagating from the source and of a standing wave.

In a room, the walls, ceiling and floor act as reflecting surfaces and multiple reflections take place. The waves from various directions overlap and form a diffuse sound field in which individual maxima and minima of the sound pressure usually can be detected only at low frequencies.

The direct sound from the source arrives at the listener first and is followed by a series of reflected sounds. Reflections decay in time because at each successive reflection some of the sound energy is absorbed by the walls. Decay is fast if the walls are very absorptive and slow if the walls are highly reflective. The prolonged presence of sound in the room is called reverberation and its measure is called reverberation time (RT; T is often used to denote reverberation time but T has been used for the period in this text). The RT is defined as the time during which the intensity of the sound declines from the value at the cessation of the sound production to a value 1 million times smaller. Because the sound pressure is proportional to the square root of intensity, the sound pressure declines during the RT to $1/1000$ of its original value (to −60 dB).

At a point close to the sound source, a wave coming directly from the sound source, the so-called direct sound, prevails. Because the intensity of the direct sound decreases with $1/(r^2)$ where r is the distance from the source, the direct sound becomes weak at a larger distance from the source, and the reverberated sound prevails. The distance from the source, at which the intensity of the direct sound is equal to the intensity of the reverberated sound, is called the critical distance.

Power and Intensity

The energy of sound transmitted by the source/1 s, is called the power. The power transmitted through a unit area perpendicular to the direction of the energy flow is called the sound intensity, usually denoted as I. It is measured in watt per square meter (W/m²). The sound intensity I is equal to the average value of the product of sound pressure p and particle velocity v over one or several periods.

In a free field, the sound pressure and the particle velocity are in phase for a plane wave. The intensity is equal to the product of effective values of both quantities and is expressed:

$$I = P_{ef} \cdot V_{ef}.$$

The characteristic impedance Z_c of the medium is purely resistive and the field is called active. The z_c changes with temperature and barometric pressure. At normal atmospheric conditions it equals 406 N s/m³.

The source of noise can be thought to be encircled by a sphere through which all the sound energy has to flow. The larger the distance is, the larger the sphere is (its surface increases with the square of the radius), and the more the energy is spread. Therefore, the sound intensity decreases with the square of the distance from the source.

The field that is close to the source of sound is called the near field and that in a larger distance from the source is called the far field.

In a pure standing wave there is no net flow of energy between the source of sound and the reflecting surface. The particle velocity is 90° out of phase with the sound pressure and the field is called reactive. In an ideal diffuse sound field, the energy flowing to a certain point from all directions is the same, and the net flow of energy in any direction is zero. Therefore, such a field is also purely reactive and has the total intensity flow equal to zero. However, the intensity of a diffuse sound field is considered to be equal to the power passing through a unit area from one side only. Then the formula for intensity would be:

$$I = P_{ef}^2/(4z_c).$$

Levels

The range of sound intensities over which the human ear can respond is extremely large. At the threshold of hearing the intensity is quite small. At the threshold of pain the intensity is quite large. The difference between the thresholds for hearing and pain is about 10^{14}. The use of such large numbers is inconvenient. Therefore, a logarithmic transformation of the numbers expressing ratios of intensities has been introduced. Also, the logarithmic scale corresponds more closely to our sensations than does an absolute scale. In a logarithmic scale a certain ratio is, of course, always the same number, independent of how small or how large the numerators and denominators are.

A sound is said to be at certain level L_1, if it is expressed as 10 times the logarithm with the base 10 of the ratio of the sound intensity I_1 to the reference sound intensity I_0:

$$L_1 = 10 \log (I_1/I_0) \text{dB}.$$

The "dB" stands for decibel, a unit 10 times smaller then the original "bel."

This equation can be also interpreted as the level difference $L_1 - L_0$ in which the L_0 (the level of the reference) is equal to zero.

As discussed above, the intensity is proportional to the square of the sound pressure: $I = P_{ef}^2/z_c$. Therefore, the ratio $I_1/I_0 = (P_{ef1}/P_{ef0})^2$. And L_1 can be expressed in terms of the sound pressure:

$$L_1 = 10 \log (P_{ef1}/P_{ef0})^2$$
$$= 20 \log (P_{ef1}/P_{ef0}) \text{ dB}.$$

Any value of intensity or pressure can be used as a reference. In acoustics, the reference intensity I_0 is 10^{-12} W/m^2. This intensity corresponds, approximately, to the average threshold of hearing at 1 kHz.

The corresponding reference sound pressure P_{ef0} can be calculated from the equation $I_0 = P_{ef0}^2/z_c$. Its rounded value is 20 μPa. A sound pressure level (SPL, L_p) of 94 dB corresponds to the sound pressure of 1 Pa.

Calculation of the total sound pressure level (L_t) of several sound pressure levels L_ts requires a rather complicated computation. The steps are as follows:

1. The levels are converted to the individual intensities by calculating the antilogarithm of individual levels: $I_i = I_0$ antilog $(L_i/10)$,
2. The I_ns are added together: $I_t = I_1 + I_2 + I_3 + \ldots$, or $I_t = I_0$ (antilog $(L_1/10)$ + antilog $(L_2/10)$ + antilog $(L_3/10 + \ldots)$, and,
3. The level L_t is calculated: $L_t = 10 \log \dfrac{I_t}{I_0}$.

Using sound pressure for the calculation leads to:

$$P_{eft}^2 = P_{ef1}^2 + P_{ef2}^2 + P_{ef3}^2 + \ldots$$

or

$$P_{eft}^2 = P_{ef0}^2 \text{ (antilog } (L_1/10)$$
$$+ \text{ antilog } (L_2/10) + \text{ antilog } (L_3/10) + \ldots,$$

and

$$L_t = 20 \log (P_{eft}/P_{ef0}).$$

When the intensity of the source A is equal to the intensity of the source B, $I_A = I_B$, $I_t = I_A + I_B = 2 I_A$ and $L_T = 10 \log (2I_A) = 10 \log I_A + 10 \log 2 = L_A + 10 \times 0.301 = L_A + 3$ dB. The level increase resulting from adding a weaker sound B to a strong one A is less than 3 dB. The total level can be calculated from the formula:

$$L_t = L_A + 10 \log (1 + \text{antilog } (L_B - L_A)/10)).$$

The graph representing this formula is shown in Figure 3.4 and can be used for determination of the total level of several sources by first determining the partial level from two individual levels, then determining the next partial level from the first partial level and the third individual level, and so on. So, for instance, the level of five sources with the same 100 dB sound pressure level would be: $L_t = 100$

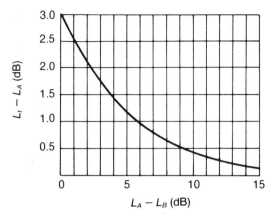

Figure 3.4. The graph representing the formula for sound level addition (see text). On the *abscissa* is the difference between two levels, on the *ordinate* is the number of decibels which have to be added to the higher level L_A to obtain the final level L_t.

dB + 3 dB + 1.75 dB + 1.3 dB + 1 dB = 107 dB.

One should remember the following:

1. A doubling/halving the intensity (1.414 times increase/decrease of sound pressure) is equivalent to a 3-dB increase/decrease of level;
2. A doubling/halving of sound pressure (quadrupling/quartering of intensity) corresponds to a 6-dB increase/decrease of level;
3. A 10 times increase/decrease of intensity (3.16 times increase/decrease of pressure) corresponds to a 10-dB increase/decrease of level;
4. A 10 times increase/decrease of sound pressure corresponds to a 20-dB increase/decrease of level; and
5. A 1-db increase/decrease of level corresponds to 12% increase/11% decrease of sound pressure or 26% increase/21% decrease of intensity.

The concept of level (in dB units) is also used in electricity for expressing power and voltage ratios. The formulas for levels are the same as in acoustics but the reference values are different. Many voltmeters have dB scales which give voltage levels relative to 0.775 V (775 mV). This voltage E_0 corresponds to a power W_0 of 1 mW dissipated in a load resistor R of 600 Ω: $W_0 = E_0^2/R$; from that $E_0 = \sqrt{(R \cdot W_0)} = \sqrt{600 \times 10^{-3}} = \sqrt{0.6} = 0.77459$ V. Other voltmeters have 1 μV, and others 1 V as reference voltages.

Types of Sound

To this point we have discussed only a pure, continuous sound with a sinusoidal waveform. The sine waves are used extensively for laboratory measurements of acoustical properties of materials, and in psychoacoustics as stimuli for percepts of hearing. Environmental sounds such as speech, music and noise usually contain many frequencies and are not always continuous and steady.

Pure Tone, Complex Tone and Harmonics

A sound that has a sinusoidal waveform is called a pure tone, or simple tone. Several simultaneous simple tones of different frequencies form a complex tone. Individual simple tones of a complex tone are called frequency components. Components which are integer multiples of a so-called fundamental frequency, are called harmonic components, or harmonics.

A complex tone with harmonic components is an example of the so-called periodic wave. The waveform in the periodic wave is repeated periodically with the period corresponding to the fundamental frequency. A waveform whose components are not harmonically related is called aperiodic. A wave which is not exactly periodic, but is close to it, is called quasiperiodic. For example, a sustained vowel represents a quasiperiodic wave.

The effective (rms) value of a complex tone with n components is equal to the square root of the sum of the squares of effective values of each component:

$$P_{ef} = \sqrt{P_{ef1}^2 + P_{ef2}^2 + P_{ef3}^2 + \ldots + P_{efn}^2}.$$

Two waves can have the same frequency content and the same effective (rms) value but different forms. The form depends on the relative phases of the components. For example, if each harmonic component starts at 90° phase we obtain a train of narrow impulses; if the components start with random phases, the impulsive character of the signal disappears. Nevertheless, both waves would have the same effective value. Therefore, for one wave, the ratio of peak-to-effective value, called the crest factor, can be large, and for another one, with the same frequency content, the crest factor can be small. (For ANSI definition of the crest factor, see the section on sound level meters.) The positive parts of complex-tone waves may have different shapes than their negative parts, and the maximal positive value (the positive peak, $+p$) may be different from the negative peak ($-p$). Therefore, the term amplitude, should be used only for sine waves (pure tones). For complex waves, a more general term—peak value—should be used. Peak-to-peak value is denoted by "p-p".

Spectrum

Sound can last for a long period of time without any change in the frequency or amplitude of its components. The components are then continuous and in a steady state. In this sense, a sustained sequence of repeated tone bursts, in which each burst starts with the same phase and ends with the same or other constant phase, is also a periodic sound and can be considered as steady or continuous. Each sustained, periodic sound can be subjected to a so-called fourier analysis to obtain the amplitude or power spectrum. The spectrum of such sound is called the line spectrum. All energy of the sound is concentrated at harmonic frequencies. If the fundamental frequency is high, the distance between individual harmonics is large, if the fundamental frequency is low, the harmonics are close together. For instance, if the repetition rate of a tone burst is 100 bursts/s, the closest distance between the components is 100 Hz. If the rate is 1 burst/s, the distance between components is only 1 Hz. The lower the repetition rate is, the more dense the components are. In the

extreme, a single burst or a single impulse has energy spread continuously over a frequency range whose width depends on the duration of the burst. Then we speak about spectrum density and spectrum level or spectrum density level. The spectrum level shows the power level per 1-Hz wide frequency band as a function of frequency.

The spectrum of a series of impulses with amplitudes randomly distributed in magnitude and time is also continuous. If the noise has energy distributed evenly across the whole auditory frequency range, it is called the white noise; its average power in each 1-Hz wide frequency band is the same. If the power decreases with frequency so that the spectrum density drops to half (spectrum level drops 3 dB) with each doubling of frequency, the noise is called pink noise.

For noise analysis, analyzers with a constant absolute frequency bandwidth (e.g. 25 Hz) over the whole frequency range can be used. The white noise spectrum obtained with such an analyzer is represented by a horizontal flat line, the pink-noise spectrum is represented by a line with a slope of -3 dB/octave. Other analyzers (such as the ⅓-octave or 1-octave frequency band spectrum analyzers) use a constant relative bandwidth over the frequency range. In these analyzers, the absolute bandwidth increases proportionally with frequency. If the frequency is doubled, the absolute bandwidth is also doubled. The spectrum level of the white noise obtained with such analyzers increases 3 dB with each doubling of frequency (or 10 dB for each 10 multiple of frequency), because, as the absolute bandwidth is doubled (increased 10 times), power is also doubled (increased 10 times). The spectrum density of the pink noise is compensated by the increase of bandwidth.

If a noise is filtered and only a band of frequencies is allowed to pass through the filter, the noise is called the band-noise.

If the duration of a pure tone is long,

for instance 10 s or more, the tone spectrum is represented by a single vertical line, whose height is equal to the amplitude or the power of the signal. At the other extreme, a very short tone burst has a continuous spectrum covering the whole frequency range. Shortening of the burst broadens the spectrum. By using the fourier transform it can be calculated that a pure-tone burst with a rectangular envelope has the amplitude spectrum as shown in Figure 3.5. The Fourier analysis is used for periodic signals while the fourier transform is used for a single burst of impulse. This spectrum has a main lobe and a number of side lobes. The maximum of the spectrum occurs at the carrier frequency, the zeros at $f_{0n} = f_c \pm n/t_b$. In this formula f_c stands for the carrier frequency, n equals 1, 2, 3 . . . , and t_b is the duration of the burst. It can be seen that by shortening of t_b the zeros move farther away from the carrier frequency, the main lobe of the spectrum becomes wider, and the energy is spread over larger range.

The spectrum shown in Figure 3.5 is continuous because it belongs to a single burst. By periodic repetition of the bursts without changing the burst duration, the continuous spectrum will become a line spectrum, but the shape of the envelope curve of the spectrum will remain the same (Fig. 3.5). Increasing the repetition rate will not change the shape of the en-

velope of the spectrum, but the distance between lines of the spectrum will increase. Finally, if we increase the repetition rate so much that the pauses disappear, the tone becomes continuous, and the individual components disappear (their frequencies coincide with the frequencies of the zeros $f_c \pm n/t_b$).

Each waveform has a particular amplitude or power spectrum. However, for reconstruction of the wave form from spectra, both amplitude and phase spectrum are required.

MEASUREMENT OF SOUND

Basic Quantities

For noise-rating determination and silencing of various devices, the power emitted by them has to be found. The power measurement, in general, has to be performed at the site of the manufacturer or institutions rating the products.

Measurement of particle velocity is difficult. It is being performed only in few laboratories, and is not practical for the field measurement of sound. Therefore, it will not be discussed here further.

Contrary to velocity, the sound pressure, can be measured rather simply and easily. For convenience, measuring devices have indicators calibrated in levels re 20 μPa, and we generally speak in terms of sound pressure levels (in dB) instead of sound pressures (in Pa). Practically all field measurements of sound are based on the determination of sound pressure levels—be it a simple measurement of the overall level, or determination of spectra, intensity or other parameters.

In the following, measurement of sound pressure level will be discussed in detail. Means to be used to provide answers to the following questions will be described: (a) how strong is the sound; what are its rms and peak values, and what is its power; (b) what is the frequency and the spectrum of the sound; (c) what is the statistical distribution of the sound pressure values; (d) what is the sound exposure dosage a person accumulates in a

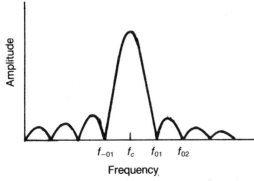

Figure 3.5. Amplitude spectrum of a sinewave burst of frequency f_c and duration t_b. The frequencies f_{0n}, at which the spectrum is equal to zero, are obtained as $f_c \pm (n/t_b)$, where $n = 1, 2, 3, \ldots$

noisy environment; and (e) how large is the vibration?

Instruments for Sound Level Determination

Sound Level Meters

A sound level meter (SLM) could be basically composed of a pressure microphone, an amplifier and an indicator. However, to serve as a SLM in its proper sense of the word, the instrument must have a particular frequency response and a calibrated attenuator. The block diagram of a SLM is in Figure 3.6.

A distinction has to be made between sound pressure level (SPL or L_p) and sound level (L_A, L_B, etc.; see below). Both have the same reference value of 20 μPa but are measured using different frequency responses. Sound pressure level is determined using the flat frequency response of the measuring system (Appendix* II A5). Intensity at each frequency has the same weight in determination of the total intensity, or of the pressure level of the sound. Sound level, on the other hand, is determined using frequency responses which are not flat. These frequency responses (A, B, C, D, or E, see Fig. 3.7) are called weighting curves, or weighting characteristics (Appendix II A2). Some components of the sound, mainly at low frequencies, are attenuated and do not contribute with the same weight to the overall sound level as other components.

In addition to summation (or integration) over frequencies, a short time averaging of sound takes place in a SLM. The averaging is exponential, which means

---

* See Appendix II.

that the contribution of the past sound to an on-going reading decreases exponentially with time. The exponential-time averaging is determined by particular time constants which influence the dynamic characteristics of the instrument; the time constants have an influence on meter reading when the pressure varies or when the sound has an impulsive character.

The ANSI (Appendix II A2) designates slow (S), fast (F) and impulse (I) exponential-time-averaging characteristics with time constants of 1000, 125, and 35 ms, respectively. The optional peak hold characteristic has an onset time constant of the order of tens of microseconds.

Various types of sound level meters have to be distinguished. The standard specifies four types of SLMs: type 0, type 1, type 2, and type S. The basic distinction between the first three types lies in the accuracy with which various sounds can be measured. Between 100 and 1250 Hz, the types 0, 1 and 2 have tolerances of ± 0.7, 1 and 1.5 dB, respectively, for sound of random incidence. At other frequencies, the tolerances are greater. The type 0 SLM, the so-called "laboratory standard," has to be accurate but does not have to satisfy requirements for usage in the field. The type 1, the so-called "precision SLM" is designed for fulfilling accurate field and laboratory sound measurements, and the type 2, general purpose SLM, is intended for measurement of environmental sounds which are not dominated by high frequencies. A typical type 1 SLM is shown in Figure 3.8.

Types 0, 1 and 2 have to have A, B and C frequency weightings and the slow and fast exponential-time-averaging charac-

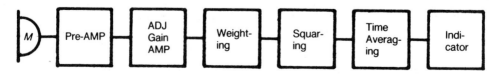

Figure 3.6. A basic block diagram of a sound level meter. M stands for microphone, AMP for amplifier.

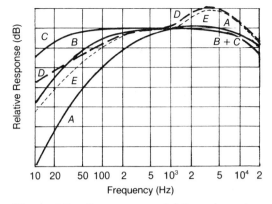

Figure 3.7. Frequency-weighting characteristics for sound level meters which produce A-, B-, C-, D-, and E-weighted sound levels.

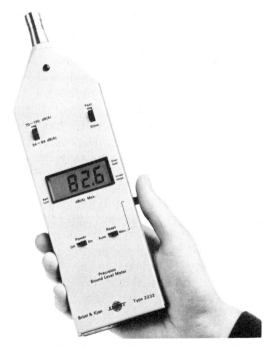

Figure 3.8. A typical type 1 sound level meter. (Reproduced by courtesy of Brüel & Kjaer Instruments.)

teristics. Type S SLM can have the accuracy of 0, 1 or 2 types, but does not have to have all three frequency weightings or both time-averaging characteristics. Type S is used for special purposes for which all characteristics of the basic types of SLMs are not needed and, therefore, the instrument can be less expensive and simpler for manipulation.

The overall accuracy of a sound level meter reading depends on the type of the instrument (0, 1 or 2), frequency content of the signal, angle of incidence of the sound on the microphone, and on the time variation of the sound pressure. The overall accuracy for all conditions can not be stated, but for some sound fields of specific types of signals a good estimate of accuracy can be made. According to the ANSI (Appendix II A2), for steady broadband noise in a reverberant sound field, the allowable error for the type 1 SLM is approximately ±1.5 dB and for the type 2 about ±2.3 dB. This accuracy is to be reached after a warm-up period specified by the manufacturer. This period should be less than 10 min.

The purpose of weighting energy of sound differently at various frequencies is to obtain a SLM reading that corresponds, at least grossly, to loudness. The A-weighting was designed for low-level intensity measurements, the B-weighting for intermediate level measurements, and the C-weighting for high level measurements. Experience has shown that the effects of sound on humans are more correlated with the A-weighted levels than with the other ones and, therefore, the A-weighting has been generally used for measuring of sound level across the whole intensity range of hearing. The flat response is to be used when subsequent spectral analysis of the sound is performed.

D- and E-weighting curves have been used for somewhat better correlation of the measured value of noise and human response. The D-weighted level (L_D, in dB) is widely used in the measurement and evaluation of aircraft noise (1) (Appendix II-C7). The E-weighted level (L_E, in dB) is closely related to the perceived level calculated according to Stevens Mark VII procedure (2). These two weighting curves are not included into standards on sound level meters. They are specified as weightings which could be used with any general sound measurement system which has a flat frequency response over the frequency range of interest (Appendix II A9).

The SLMs should be omnidirectional. Nonetheless, directional errors can not be avoided. These errors depend on frequency and direction of the sound incidence. The frequency weighting characteristics and their tolerances are stated in ANSI for random incidence of sound. The deviations from the specified frequency responses vary with the direction of incidence of the sound, however, for a given angle of incidence a frequency response approximating that for the random incidence can be obtained. This angle has to be stated by the manufacturer.

The SLM responses to short duration sounds do not generally reach the responses of long duration signals. For a tone burst of 50-ms duration, the maximum response at fast and slow averaging, should not be less than −4.8 and −13.1 dB, respectively, below the response to a continuous signal.

Various steady signals can have various crest factors. This factor is defined as the "ratio of the peak sound pressure in a stated frequency band to the square root of the 1-s exponential-time-average, squared, sound pressure in the same frequency band." For instance, the crest factor for the sine-wave is 1.4 (or 3 dB); for speech it is about 5 (12–14 dB). For the type 0 SLM, the maximum allowable error in the average rms value is ±0.5 dB when the crest factor is equal or smaller than 3, and ±1 dB when the crest factor is between 3 and 10. The corresponding values for type 1 are 0.5 and 1.5 dB. The type 2 SLM is required to handle sounds with the crest factor equal to 3 with the maximum allowable error equal to ±1 dB. The accuracy of the type 2 is not specified for crest factors larger than 3.

For type 0, 1 and impulse SLMs, overload detectors have to indicate when the crest factor capability is exceeded. In type 2 instruments, the overload detector shows the general overloading of the amplifying circuits of the SLMs.

When the crest factor is small, the reading in the upper part of the meter scale is usually more precise than in the lower part of the scale. However, if the crest factor is large, a more accurate reading of the rms value of the sound level is obtained for small deflections of the meter pointer.

Any of the types of SLMs can have additional impulse and/or peak response characteristic as options. The impulse exponential-time-averaging characteristic has time constants of 35 ms and 1500 ms for increasing and decreasing sound pressure, respectively. For types 0 and 1, a single tone burst of 5-ms duration should reach −8.8 dB (±2.0 dB) value of the continuous signal response.

The standard recommends that, in type 1 and 2 SLMs, the rise time in optional peak characteristic mode "be such that a pulse of 100 μs duration produces a deflection no more than 2 dB below the deflection produced by a pulse having a duration of 10 ms and equal peak amplitude." For type 0, the same response relations should be obtained for 50 μs and 10 ms impulse durations.

The understanding of dynamic properties of the SLM is very important for correct interpretation of the obtained reading of the meter. The values mentioned above show that it takes some time for the meter to reach the deflection corresponding to the value of the signal. The shorter the burst, the shorter the averaging time constant has to be for the meter reading to accurately display the magnitude of the signal.

The indicator can be analog or digital. It has to have a scale graduated in 1-dB intervals or less over the range of at least 15 dB. The analog indicator of type 0 and 1 SLMs should have a resolution equal or better than 0.2 dB (1 dB for type 2), and the digital indicator's resolution should be equal or better than 0.1 dB.

Integrating Sound Level Meters

Often we want to know the A-weighted level of a continuous constant sound which, over a specified time period, would contain the same acoustic energy as the actual fluctuating sound present during the same time period. That level is called equivalent sound level (L_{eq}). L_{eq} helps us to determine average noise levels in factories, around highways or airports, etc. The regular SLMs discussed above would allow us to determine L_{eq} of a fluctuating noise if a continuous graphic record or a series of readings were made. Such a procedure would be cumbersome, time consuming and possibly inaccurate because rapidly changing levels can be difficult to read. These drawbacks can be avoided by using integrating sound level meters (ISLMs) which provide L_{eq} or also SEL (sound exposure level, L_{ax}) values. The ISLMs include microprocessors which calculate and display L_{eq}s for 60 s, 8 hr or even up to 30 hr. Generally, ISLMs are type 2 instruments. A precision ISLM is shown in Figure 3.9.

The integrating sound level meters are very useful for determination of average

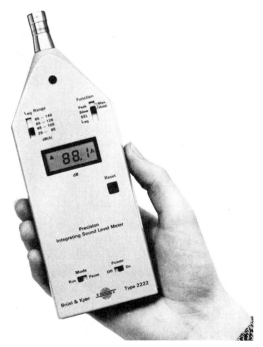

Figure 3.9. A precision integrating sound level motor. (Reproduced by courtesy of Brüel and Kjaer Instruments.)

equivalent sound levels, but for information about the dose of noise an individual worker receives during a shift, noise dosimeters have been developed.

Noise Dosimeters

Dosimeters are special purpose ISLMs. They integrate over time the A-weighted sound pressures that exceed a certain criterion level. Noise levels and durations of their occurrence are automatically monitored and daily doses are calculated.

The dose is the ratio of sound exposure and the so-called criterion sound exposure, in percentages. Sound exposure is the time integral over a stated time of the SLOW exponential-time-averaged, squared, A-weighted, sound pressure signal when the 3-dB exchange rate is used (Appendix II A8). The exchange rate is the change in sound level corresponding to a doubling or halving of the exposure duration. For the 5-dB exchange rate, the 0.6 power of the sound pressure signal (slow mode, squared, A-weighted) is used. Criterion sound exposure is "The product of the criterion duration and the mean-square sound pressure corresponding to the criterion sound level when the 3-dB exchange rate is used. The product of the criterion duration and 0.6 power of the mean-square sound pressure corresponds to the criterion sound level when the 5-dB exchange rate is used" (Appendix II A8). Criterion duration T_c is 8 hr, the criterion sound level L_c is specified by the manufacturer.

The basic block diagram of the dosimeter is shown in Fig. 3.10. The noise is picked up by a microphone, whose output is amplified and weighted in frequency. The resulting signal is squared, exponentially averaged (with the time constant equal to 1 s) and led through an exponent circuit (with the exponent equal to 1 or 0.6 according to the particular exchange rate) to a threshold circuit. This circuit allows only those parts of the signal which are equal to, or greater than, a threshold level to be integrated in an integrator. The

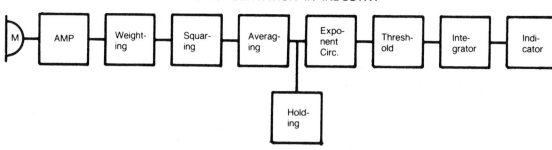

Figure 3.10. A basic block diagram of a noise dosimeter. M stands for microphone, AMP for amplifier, and *Holding* for a circuit holding the indication that the upper limit has been reached.

final result is then displayed in an indicator.

In practice, digitized dosimeters use the following simple formula for the daily dose calculation:

$$D = \sum_{i=1}^{N} (C_i/T_i), \text{ or in percentage}$$

$$D = 100 \sum_{i=1}^{N} (C_i/T_i).$$

C_i is the actual exposure time at the noise level L_i, and T_i is the permissible exposure time at the level L_i as determined by a noise standard. For example, let us assume the criterion level L_c to be 90 dB, (the criterion time at that level $T_c = 8$ hr), and the exchange rate is 5 dB per halving of duration. If the sound is at $L_1 = 100$ dB for 3 hr and $L_2 = 95$ dB for 1 hr, the permissible times T_1 and T_2 would be equal to 2 and 4 hr, respectively. Then dose, D, is equal to $100 (3/2 + 1/4) = 175\%$.

Dosimeters can be used in two ways: as an area monitor or as a personal noise dosimeter carried on the person. The same device can be used for both purposes, but usually the area monitor is a larger device, while the personal dosimeter is small, compact and light as shown in Figure 3.11. The personal type can be designed to provide an on-the-spot noise exposure reading, or it can be used in connection with a readout device that can service a number of personal devices. This last one can use electronic exposure accumulation or the electrochemical exposure accumulation.

Generally, the dosimeter worn by a person on the chest gives larger read-outs than an area monitor, but the difference

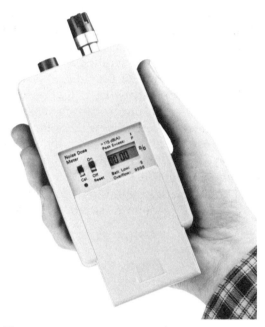

Figure 3.11. A personal noise dosimeter which can be worn in a shirt pocket with the microphone either at the chest or at the shoulder. (Reproduced by courtesy of Brüel and Kjaer Instruments.)

on the average is small. Large differences were observed between noise-dose measurements from stationary area monitors and ear-level dosimeters (3), especially at high frequencies. However, these differences were found to be neither systematic nor recurrent. They vary with occupation, mobility of the test subject, and reverberant field in the work position.

Vibration Meters

Vibration is a fast alternating (to and fro) movement of a body. It is usually understood as the motion of structures, and is termed as solid-borne, or mechanical, vibration. The frequency range of vibrations can be very large. The human body is sensitive to vibrations mainly in the 1 to 2000 Hz region.

The basic quantities related to vibrations are displacement, x (the distance of a point of the body from its equilibrium, reference position); the velocity, v (the time rate of change of displacement); and acceleration, a (the time rate of change of velocity). The reference quantities for vibration levels are 10^{-8} m/s for velocity, and 10^{-5} m/s^2 for acceleration. This latter value is approximately equal to 10^{-6} g (1 μg) g being the gravitational acceleration.

Vibration measurements can be performed with the aid of the so-called vibration pick-ups. They can be used as input devices for vibration meters or some sound level meters. The pick-up is a transducer which, when attached to a surface at the point where vibration is to be investigated, generates voltages proportional to its acceleration. If the pick-up is followed by an electronic integrating network, the velocity, or displacement can be read.

The sensitivity of accelerometers is expressed in terms of open circuit output in millivolts (mV) corresponding to gravitational acceleration g (g = 9.81 m/s^2). The sensitivity varies with the orientation of the pick-up relative to the direction of the vibration. The proper orientation is specified by the manufacturer. A misalignment up to 10° is usually not critical.

Microprocessors allowed the development of the so-called "smart sensors." They consist of transducers coupled to various microelectronic circuits which provide fully processed signals directly from the sensor package.

Recorders

When a permanent record of the result of a measurement is required, a graphic recorder should be used. When a sound is to be preserved for further analysis, magnetic-tape recorders are employed. Graphic recorders can provide a permanent record of various data, like levels, spectra, histograms, and transfer characteristics (frequency responses).

Graphic Level Recorders

Graphic Level Recorders use long strips of paper continuously driven by a motor. Usually, the paper speed is adjustable over a large range—from fractions of millimeter per second to several centimeters per second. A pen mechanism produces a trace corresponding to input levels. The writing speed, or the speed of the pen mechanism, determines how fast the recorder reacts to the changes in input level. Slower speeds can be used if average values are of interest, but higher speeds are required if fast variations of the level are to be studied. A very high writing speed can produce overshoots due to the inertia of the mechanism. Because the pen-drive system acts as a low pass filter, a certain averaging is always present.

Depending on the type of graphic recorder, a direct current (DC) or alternating current (AC) signal input can be used. In a DC mode, the averaged rms level is applied to the input. The AC signal has to be rectified, appropriately filtered, and then the envelope curve of the wave as a function of time can be traced.

Graphic level recorders are often used in place of indicators on sound level meters. It is, therefore, desirable that the dynamic characteristics of the graphic recorder correspond to the dynamic characteristics of the sound level meter.

When graphic recorders are connected to the output of a sound level meter, a time history profile of the monitored sound can be obtained. Statistical distribution analyzers can provide histograms, profiles, and some (like dB-301/652 Metrologger system by Metrosonics) also provide time history profiles, L_{eq}, and other quantities.

A recorder connected to a frequency or wave analyzer can provide results of the narrow band analysis as a form of spectra. The averaging time given by the recording system has to be appreciably shorter than the filter response time if the short-term rms level is to be able to follow the envelope of the filter response curve. For more details about the choice of the writing and paper speeds see Randall (4).

X-Y Plotters

X-Y plotters are now widely used for plotting spectra, results of computations and similar data. The pen position on the chart is determined by electrical signals supplied to the inputs of the plotter. The two signals move the pen in the direction of the x- (horizontal) and y- (vertical) co-ordinate, respectively. There is provision to adjust the starting point and the sensitivity, so that the displacement units can be made to correspond to an appropriate graph paper.

Magnetic-Tape Recorders

Magnetic-tape recorders are employed for storing actual noise signals for future processing or analyzing, or for preserving a reproducible record of progressive changes in sound. In general, each recording introduces some distortions into the signal and, therefore, a direct analysis of the original signal is preferable. However, in various situations, recording of the signal is necessary. Sometimes the time spent on site has to be minimized or the required analyzing equipment for a complex analysis can not be brought to the site. Sometimes different techniques of analysis are to be performed on the same data or, if a short transient has to be analyzed, it needs to be played back repetitively. If the recorded noise is to be translated in frequency by recording at one speed and replaying at another, then very low frequency recordings can be shifted into a frequency range of normal audio frequency analyzers, or very fast transients can be slowed down and observed on a more convenient time scale.

The sound should be recorded as faithfully as possible, and therefore the recorders have to be of high quality. They should also be light, compact and battery driven. If the recorder has several channels, signals from several microphone locations can be stored simultaneously. Some of the recorders have frequency-modulation (FM) channels which allow recording of very low frequency signals, down to direct current. FM recorders can provide very good low frequency phase linearity, amplitude stability and wave-form preservation. They are, therefore, very useful for storing signals from vibration or shock pick-ups, and static or dynamic strain gauges. FM recorders should also be used if the stored data are subjected to correlation analysis, cross-power spectrum analysis and other forms of processing in which time coincidence is to be preserved.

Some tape recorders have companders for preserving good signal-to-noise ratio. The input signal is compressed by an automatic gain control for recording and later expanded for replaying.

Digital magnetic-tape recorders are used for storage of digital data of large quantities. Such recordings last for a lifetime.

Frequency Analyzers

Information about the overall level of the noise is often not sufficient for determination of annoyance, hazard to hearing or other health hazards to the exposed person. For these reasons, the frequency analysis of the noise is often needed. Frequency analysis provides information about the frequency distribution of the sound energy. Analysis of machine vibrations helps determine what remedies should be implemented for reducing such vibrations.

Frequency analysis can be performed using an analog or digital technique or a combination of the two. The fundamental difference between the two techniques is in the continuity of the signal. An analog device continuously responds to the situation at the input of the device. A digital device takes discrete samples of the signal in time, converts them to numbers, on these numbers performs calculations, and delivers a coresponding signal at the output.

Filters used in frequency analyzers are sometimes classified as active or passive. A passive filter is composed only of capacitors, coils or resistors. It does not need any power for its function. An active filter contains capacitors, coils, resistors and amplifiers for which power has to be supplied from batteries or a power line. Analog filters can be passive or active, the digital ones can be only active.

Analog Frequency Analysis

Filtering can be direct or indirect. Direct filtering takes place if filters are operating directly at the desired bands of frequencies. It can be both analog or digital. For indirect filtering, the signal is transposed to another frequency region.

Analog frequency analysis can be based on serial or parallel operation.

Serial Analysis

The serial type of analysis can be performed with a filter whose cut-off frequencies can be sequentially adjusted for passing appropriate bands of frequencies. The filter is followed by a detector. This type of analysis requires time and, therefore, is suitable for analyzing a continuous signal or a signal that is repetitious (as from a magnetic-tape loop).

The same type of analysis can be performed using a bank of filters of appropriate bandwidth and center frequencies. The signal is connected parallel to the inputs of all filters, but outputs of individual filters are switched sequentially to a single detector. The switching can be done manually whenever a reading is made, or automatically in sychrony with the graphic level recorder on which the output of the sequential filters is recorded. This type of analysis is also called discrete stepped filter analysis.

The switching should not occur too rapidly because the filters have their own response time that depends on the filter bandwidth. A too rapid switching would not allow the filters to reach the proper output value.

In addition to the response time of the filter, the averaging time of the detector has to be taken into consideration.

Analog discrete stepped filter analysis is suitable for bands ⅓-octave wide or wider. For narrower bandwidths, the number of filters would be large and the cost of the analyzer too high. Therefore, for narrower bands (narrower than ⅓ octave) a continuous sweeping filter analyses are used.

Sweeping Filter Analysis

The sweeping filter analysis is suitable for narrow frequency bands which can provide greater resolution than ⅓-octave filters. The center frequency of the filter can be tuned continuously and swept over the whole range of frequencies. The bandwidth of the filter can be adjustable.

Some instruments have a constant absolute bandwidth, others have constant relative (percentage) bandwidths. The first type should be used when the signal is stationary and its frequency spectrum has discrete components. When the signal is stationary and random, and has a spectrum with resonance maxima, the constant relative bandwith analysis should be performed.

The bandwidth of the filter should be sufficiently narrow for separation of individual discrete spectral components of a signal. It should be equal to about one-third of the smallest frequency difference between the components. For random signal analysis the relative bandwidth of the filter should be smaller than one-third of the spectral maxima bandwidths, other-wise the maxima would be flattened.

The bandwidth of the filter should not be too wide but neither should it be less than discussed above. Narrowing of the filter prolongs its response time. The sweeping then must be slowed down, and the analysis prolonged.

Parallel Analysis

If the spectra of nonstationary signals or transient events are to be observed, the analysis must be performed rapidly. Parallel analysis has to be used.

The signal is fed to a set of filters each of which has a separate detector. This way the outputs of all channels are continuously available for a display.

Parallel analyzers use more components and are usually larger and more expensive than the corresponding serial types. It would not be economical to use this type of analyzer with narrower than ⅓-octave-wide filters, as the number of components and the cost would be too large. The response of the narrow filters could be too slow for fast-transient analysis.

Band-pass filtering can be done digitally. Analysis with this type of filtering has now generally replaced the analog parallel analyzers.

Heterodyne Analysis

Often it is economical, especially if a wide range of frequencies is to be analyzed, to translate the input signal frequency to the pass-band of a single highly selective filter. This can be done by combining the input signal with the signal of a built-in oscillator in a nonlinear circuit. At the output of the nonlinear circuit, sum and difference frequencies of the two signal frequencies are present, but from these only the difference frequency is allowed to reach the indicator.

The heterodyne principle has been widely used with time-compression systems and in serial analyzers with narrow constant absolute bandwidth. The frequency translation can be performed by both analog and digital processing. The latter one can be used for "zooming" as described later.

Digital Frequency Analysis

Periodic signals can be analyzed by the so-called fourier analysis, while for impulses or bursts the so-called fourier transform has to be used. Rather complicated mathematical calculations required considerable computer time for the fourier transform until the so-called fast fourier transform (FFT) was developed. The FFT is a calculation scheme that replaces the fourier transform itself. The special version of the scheme, the so-called discrete fourier transform (DFT), can be dealt with by digital computers.

To be handled by a digital computer, the signal has to be transformed into a digital time series by "sampling" in an analog-to-digital (A/D) converter. The output of the converter has discrete steps into which the sampled values are rounded (quantized). The size and the total number of steps determines the total range of input values that can be covered. The quantization introduces an error that can reach up to one-half of the quantum step. The resulting equivalent noise has an average rms value of about 0.3 times the step. This value can be decreased by narrowing the filter bandwidth used in the analysis.

After digitization, a number of digits corresponding to the input values in a time segment of the signal is stored in memory and processed as a group (block). The calculation is performed as if this group of samples were periodically repeated. We can consider such a group of samples as that part of the signal which the computer "sees" through a "window." The window may be framed and, therefore, such a group is called a "frame." (Sometimes it is called a "sample" but this term may be confused with a sample corresponding to a single instantaneous value of the input signal.) In real-time FFT analyzers, samples of the signal are stored in one memory while samples in the other memory are analyzed; the duration of performing the analysis must not last longer than the loading time of a frame, if no information is to be lost, and if the analysis be "real-time."

The number of output values from the analysis is equal to the number of samples in the original frame, but it is divided into two pairs of sets: either into real and imaginary values or into the absolute magnitude and phase angle of each individual component. These components are harmonics of the fundamental frequency given by the duration of the frame. Often in acoustics the phase is not interesting and many FFT-analyzers display only the magnitude of the components. The result is the average spectrum of the signal in the frame. If the signal is continuous and deterministic, not random, a transform of a single frame should give adequate information on the spectrum of the signal. If the signal is random, noise-like, several transforms should be combined and averaged to provide statistical stability of the spectrum.

The manufacturers of FFT-analyzers have to decide on the number (N) of points in the frame (framesize). That number determines the relations between the duration of the frame, the frequency resolution and the highest frequency component of the spectrum. The frequency domain resolution, Δf, is the reciprocal of the frame duration T. In FFT-analyzers with frequency range starting at 0 Hz and with frame size of N points, the frequency of the highest component F_{max} is related to Δf or T by the formula:

$$F_{max} = \frac{\Delta f \cdot N}{2} = \frac{N}{2T}.$$

For a fixed N, the frame duration has to be short if the frequency range is to be large, but for a short frame duration the frequency resolution is low. For a given F_{max} the frequency resolution can be increased by increasing the number of points N in the frame, but such an increase would increase the digital processing time and size of the memory.

The frequency range, or F_{max}, cannot be chosen freely. It is related to the sampling rate which can be performed by the analyzer, or more specifically, by the A/D converter. At least two samples have to be taken during the shortest period in the signal. That means, that the highest frequency of the signal at the input of the A/D converter must not be higher than half of the sampling rate. If the signal had frequency components higher than half of the sampling rate (of the so-called "Nyquist frequency"), erroneous frequency information would be given. Components higher than F_{max} would appear below F_{max} and would be "misnamed" or "aliased." To prevent aliasing, components higher than F_{max}, have to be removed from the signal by antialiasing filters. Such filters have become a standard part of FFT analyzers.

The spectrum is displayed in the form of lines. It gives the information on the spectrum through samples of the spectrum. We see the spectrum as if through a picket-fence and, therefore, can miss correct values of narrow peaks in the spectrum. This, the so-called "picket-fence effect" is a source of error which can reach up to 3.9 dB for a rectangular time window or 1.5 dB for the so-called Hanning window (5).

Generally, the signal submitted for analysis is truncated by the time windows. Discontinuities are introduced at the beginning and at the end of the window and harmonics are produced which were not present in the original signal. This effect has been termed "leakage."

The leakage can be large if the shape of the time window is rectangular. It can be considerably reduced by tapering off the edges of the window. The Hanning window is one of the most common windows used for this purpose. It has a form of $cosine^2$ function with the maximum in the center of the window. Such a window has a smaller selectivity (the main spectral lobe of the function is broader than the main lobe of the rectangular window) but its highest sidelobe is −32 dB below the main one. The corresponding value for the rectangular window is −13 dB (4).

Tapering is not desirable when an analyzed signal of transitory character is completely contained within the observation window of the analyzer, or if the placement of such a signal in the middle of the window cannot be secured. Fast transients near the edges of the window would be inappropriately modified by the tapering effect of the window function.

Digital Filtering

Digital filtering is another digital method that has been successfully used for frequency analysis. In a digital filter, the signal is digitally processed in such a way that some of the frequency components present at the input are eliminated from the output. Whereas the FFT analysis processes whole blocks of data at a time, the recursive digital filtering, which is generally used for analysis, processes the input data continuously. For every digitized input value, a digitized output value is obtained. The filtering effect is based on addition of appropriately delayed fractions of the passed values to the present value. The desired properties of the filter are determined by the proportions of the delayed values to the present value and by the number of delays inserted into individual values. By the choice of filter coefficients used in the calculations, virtually any filter shape can be generated. The same hardware is used, the coefficients are easily changed and, therefore, digital filters are very flexible. They also have a larger dynamic range than analog filters.

Analysis with both Analog and Digital Processing

The serial analysis is not suitable for analysis of signals changing in time, unless the signal is first converted into a continuous or repetitive one by using magnetic tape loops containing sections of the signal. Still, the time for analysis may be considerable and the time constants of the filters may be too long for analysis of very short transients.

The process can be considerably speeded up by time compression analysis.

Time Compression Analysis

If the speed of the tape loop in replaying is faster than the original recording speed, all frequencies of the signal and the spacing between them are increased by the speed ratio. Then the corresponding analyzing filters have larger center frequencies and bandwidths, the response time of the filters is shortened by the speed ratio, and the analysis can be performed faster. Principally, tape recording could be used for this purpose, but it is much more practical to use digital memory. The analysis, itself, can be performed by analog heterodyne filtering.

Time compression principle can be employed in real-time as well as nonreal-time high speed analysis. As noted earlier, in real-time analysis, the time required for processing data of a memory must not be longer than the time required to load that memory with data. Then no data is lost. During the analysis, the recorded signal is played back at high speed and is continually updated.

By using a combination of analog and digital processing, the filters carry out the analysis very fast, but are subjected to the general limitations of digital processing. Generally, each individual spectrum represents the average spectrum of a segment. If the averaging time of the detector following the filter is longer than the segment duration, then the display represents the average spectrum of the corresponding number of segments. As the signal changes, the displayed spectrum changes correspondingly. The averaging time is usually equal to at least 3 times the segment duration. An average spectrum over a rather long time interval can be obtained.

Advanced Frequency and Time Domain Analysis

The signal to be analyzed can be translated in frequency by digital processing.

By this method, which is related to heterodyning, an increase of frequency resolution in the spectrum can be secured without increasing the window (transform) size. As it was discussed before, in FFT analysis, better resolution can be achieved if either F_{max} is decreased or the transform size is increased.

By the so-called zooming technique, an increased resolution is achieved by analyzing only a small part of the original frequency range at a time. By this technique high frequency information is not lost.

Two methods of zooming have been used (6): (a) by frequency shifting and low pass filtering, or (b) by recording of signal segment of long duration and transforming it by parts, using a smaller transform.

The second type of zoom has smaller zoom factors (up to 10) than the first one (up to 128) and does not provide for real-time analysis. However, the first type needs to store a new signal segment for zooming in a new frequency range, while the second type can perform the zooming in all bands on the originally stored time function.

Correlation can be used for determination of the degree of similarity of two waveforms. In case that there is a similarity between waves, correlation is a function of the time displacement between them. If the waveform is compared with itself we speak about autocorrelation, and if two different waveforms are compared we speak about cross-correlation. For zero time displacement, the autocorrelation is the mean square value of the wave. The autocorrelation function is symmetrical around the point of zero delay, and periodic, if the waveform is periodic. At zero delay, the function has its maximal value.

The maximum of a cross-correlation function can occur at other than zero delay. That delay can be used for identifying the source of noise disturbance by determining the direction of the source.

Cepstrum (a paraphrase of "spectrum") can be defined as the "amplitude spectrum of the logarithmic spectrum", but also other definitions have been used (7). Ceptrum can be obtained by using a one- or two-channel FFT-analyzer using an appropriate program; for one-channel type, a calculator is needed.

Transfer functions, time delays which vary with frequency, and the similarities between signals as a function of frequency, can be determined by the cross-spectrum. The cross-spectrum is the fourier transform of the cross-correlation, which expresses the similarity of two signals as a function of time.

Transfer Function (also called "frequency response") of a device is the complex ratio of the output to the input as a function of frequency. It is also equal to the ratio of the cross-spectrum of the input and output to the autospectrum of the input. To use the cross-spectrum for determination of the transfer function of the device is very useful in conditions of considerable extraneous noises in which a simple measurement of the transfer function is unreliable. In the cross-spectrum, components that are not common to both input and output are eliminated. The determination of transfer function is useful for handling vibration and noise problems of the devices. When the transfer functions betwen various points of a system are known, the effects of various inputs to the system can be determined.

A function which is related to the transfer function is called the coherence function. This function is defined as the ratio of the square of the magnitude of the cross-spectrum to the product of the input and output autospectrums. Its value (between 0 and 1) depends on how well the input and output values at each frequency are related. The importance of the coherence function lies in the checking of validity of cross-spectra and transfer function measurements, in determination of contributions of a number of independent sources to a given signal, and for the study of systems with partially correlated sources.

Amplitude Distribution Analyzers

Sound level meters give information on the sound level averaged over a very short time; integrating SLMs give the sound level averaged over longer times (up to several tens of hours) and the dosimeters give, so to speak, the average excess of time (in percentage) for which a particular sound level would be acceptable. But, unless a number of readings is collected during the time interval of interest, we do not know how the noise fluctuates.

Such information is provided by amplitude distribution analyzers, also called statistical distribution analyzers. These instruments are essentially combinations of SLMs and digital microprocessors. They indicate various sound levels L_N (or sound pressure levels) which are exceeded during the total measuring period for N percent of time. For instance, L_{10} indicates the level that was exceeded for 10% of the measuring period, L_{50} the level exceeded for 50% of the measuring period, etc. The values L_{10} and L_{90} have been used for determination of the so-called traffic noise index (8) and noise pollution level (9, 10). Levels L_1 and L_{99} have been used for determination of peak and background noise levels, respectively. L_{50} indicates the median value. Printouts of amplitude distribution analyzers in the form of histograms can give a complete picture of the level distribution over a measurement period, and the plots of cumulative distributions provide information on levels that were exceeded for any particular percentage of the measuring period.

Monitoring Systems

For evaluation of a noise problem around noisy establishments, or for evaluation of noise control measures, automatic long-duration measurements of noise are required. Such measurements can be provided by noise-monitoring systems. These systems have to be portable, versatile, and flexible to be suitable for use in various environmental conditions, both indoors and outdoors. Outdoors sound propagation is greatly influenced by weather conditions, like air temperature, temperature gradient, wind, precipitation, and humidity. Therefore, the monitoring system should provide a record of both noise and atmospheric data.

A monitoring system consists typically of a microphone with rain cover and protection against moisture penetration and corrosion, preamplifier (with a heating element), windscreen, mounting rod, A-weighting circuit, amplifier, calibration oscillator, battery, and outputs for attachment of recording and analyzing systems. Units not protected against moisture by weather-proofing have to be housed in a weatherproof enclosure, in an automotive or in an appropriate building. Monitoring systems can be relatively simple, composed of few units, but also very complex, with computers, if a number of sites, like around airports, have to be monitored simultaneously.

Sound Intensity Meters

Development of digital signal processing has made it possible to design an instrument sufficiently precise for direct measurement of sound intensity, I, which is equal to the product of the sound pressure and particle velocity. The input to the digital processing circuitry is provided by a probe of two pressure microphones. These are placed close together and the difference of their outputs is approximately equal to the gradient of the sound pressure. The time integral of this difference is a measure of the particle velocity. The sound pressure at the same point is given by the average output of the two microphones.

The sound intensity measurement has several advantages over the conventional sound pressure level method. There are no special restrictions upon acoustic characteristics of the room; if the sound field is stationary, measurement can be performed in both near and far field; no restrictions are imposed on the shape and size of the measurement surface; and finally, intensity measurements are not influenced by continuous background noise. However, there are limitations imposed on the useful frequency range of the intensity meter due to the distance of the two microphones in the sound intensity probe. The higher the frequency is, the smaller the wavelength is, and the larger the error between the pressure gradient and the pressure difference between the microphones is. This error causes an underestimation of the intensity at high frequencies. The error of 1 dB occurs at 1.25 kHz for 50-mm distance between the microphones, at 5.0 kHz for 12-mm distance, and at 10 kHz for the 6-mm distance between the microphones (11). Another error occurs if the probe is too close to the center of the sound source. This error is generally smaller than 1 dB if the distance of the centers of the probe and of the sound source is 2 to 3 times greater than the microphone spacing (12).

The third error can occur if the two channels for the two microphones are not matched in phase. Digital filtering technique can minimize this problem, especially if the same digital filter is time-shared by the two channels (13).

The axis connecting the two microphones should coincide with the direction of the wave propagation to secure the largest sensitivity. Also, the higher the frequency is, the smaller the microphones should be to prevent an introduction of unwanted pressure differences by shadowing of the microphone membranes.

Calibration

An instrumental set-up for measuring sound and noise has to be calibrated if it is to be useful as a measuring tool. Each individual component, as well as the instruments as a whole, should be calibrated by the manufacturer before delivery. In the field we are interested in the performance and the calibration of the whole set-up, from the microphones to the indicators. Calibrators specially pro-

duced as accessories for acoustic measuring devices serve that purpose.

The calibration of the equipment starts with checking of the battery, if the instrument is battery operated. This can be generally done by switching the instruments in the "battery check" position. The amplifying section can be checked by using an internal or external voltage source. The internal source is often controlled by a crystal for securing a very stable reference. Adjustment to the proper reference mark on the indicator is achieved by adjustable potentiometers.

The calibration of microphones should be done according to ANSI standard "Method for calibration of microphones" (Appendix II-A4). This standard describes absolute calibration based upon the reciprocity principle as well as comparison calibrations of standard laboratory pressure microphones using pressure (coupler), free-field, and random-field methods. Secondary standard microphones which are used for calibration of microphones for consumers, are periodically compared with microphones calibrated at the National Bureau of Standards. Microphones for general use can be calibrated by comparison with secondary standard microphones either by coupler calibration or free-field calibration. Larger laboratories possess their own reciprocity calibration systems, including anechoic chambers for free-field reciprocity calibration.

For microphones rated for uniform random-incidence response, manuals should contain data permitting convergence to perpendicular- or grazing-incidence calibrations. The frequency response of microphones with a flat surface, like the condenser microphones, can be determined by the use of electrostatic actuators. The electrostatic actuator is basically a conducting plate that is placed close to the diaphragm of the microphone. The plate is electrically isolated from the diaphragm and forms with it an electrical capacitor. When voltage is applied on this capacitor, electrostatic force which is independent of frequency, acts on the diaphragm. The exact distance between the actuator plate and the diaphragm of the microphone is, however, difficult to determine and limits the usefulness of this method for absolute calibration.

Sound Level Meter Calibrators

Sound level meter calibrators (pistonphones) are small, battery-driven instruments which produce a specified sound pressure level at the diaphragm of the microphone properly inserted into the measuring cavity of the calibrator. The cavity can usually be adapted for microphones of various dimensions. Simple calibrators allow calibration at one or two frequencies, usually in the range between 200 and 1000 Hz. They produce sound pressure levels of 94 dB (which corresponds to 1 Pa), 114 dB, or 124 dB. At other frequencies the level readings have to be corrected according to a calibration curve. For actual measurements, the directional characteristic of the microphone should be taken into account at frequencies above 1 kHz.

More elaborate calibrators, like the GenRad 1986 Omnical Sound-Level Calibrator, permit comprehensive checking at octave frequencies between 125 and 4000 Hz at sound pressure levels of 74, 84, 94, 104, or 114 dB re 20 μPa. The GenRad 1986 Calibrator also provides 200- and 500-ms tone bursts which can be used for testing the detector-averaging characteristics and the accuracy of the squaring circuit.

Vibration Calibrators

Vibration Calibrators are used for calibration of accelerometers. They consist of an electromechanical oscillator with a mass to which the calibrated accelerometer can be coupled. With additional mass of the accelerometer taken into account, the accelerator can be adjusted to a reference value, like 1 g at 100 Hz, and the excursions noted.

Calibration of Frequency Analyzers

Amplitude spectrum scale can be calibrated in the same dimension as the input signal or can be presented by a logarithmic scale. On such scale a voltage ratio of 10 corresponds to 20 dB. For a reference signal of known value the input potentiometer is adjusted so that the full scale of the recording paper corresponds to a round value of the input. In x-y plotters, the zero points and magnitude of excursions can be adjusted to the grading of the graphic paper. For example, each dB step might correspond to one step on the scale of the paper.

Calibration of Recorders

For determination of correct levels at the time of the recording, a reference signal level must be recorded at both the beginning and end of the graphic level record and the tape recording. Otherwise, the correct level could not be later determined.

Calibration of Personal Dosimeters

Calibration of personal noise dosimeters is described in ANSI S1.25-1978 (Appendix II A 8) standard "Specifications for personal noise dosimeters." It is required that the manufacturer prescribes a method for verification of calibration. The calibration should be acoustical so that the microphone is included in the test, and should permit verification of all circuits including the integrator and display. A single sound level at the top of the operating range is acceptable for the test, but a level near the bottom of the operating range is also recommended.

The absolute sensitivity of the complete instrument should be calibrated at 1000 Hz and the frequency response tested at frequencies between 20 and 10,000 Hz. Directional characteristics should be measured at several frequencies between 31.5 and 8000 Hz. The crest-factor capacity of the amplifier and the accuracy of the square-law and averaging circuits have to be measured with a 1-kHz sine wave with rectangular modulation.

Techniques of Sound Measurement

How to Decide on Instrumentation

The decision on instrumentation depends on the goal of noise measurement. In general, the measurement permits assessment of the noise situation and evaluation of the noise control measures.

Often we want to know if the noise is such that it can lead to permanent hearing damage, if the noise is annoying or disturbing the population around a noisy facility or if noise control measures are needed for the source of noise under investigation.

The initial choice of instrumentation can be sometimes based on the consumer's information. More often though, a site visit is necessary for determination of the characteristics of the noise and of the general situation where the noise is located.

In different situations, one instrument may be more suitable than another. Some, like SLMs and frequency analyzers, have general applicability, others have more specific applicability. Integrating SLMs, statistical distribution analyzers or dosimeters are suitable for determination of the harmful or annoying effects on humans. Others, like dual channel FFT analyzers, vibration pick-ups and sound intensity meters are suitable for the evaluation of noise sources and determination of measures for noise reduction. Of course, all measurement devices should comply with the standards.

For preliminary surveys of noise conditions and identification of problem areas in the field, the S2A sound level meter is recommended. The same type of instrument can often be used for the main sound level measurement, if the noise does not change rapidly, does not have an impulsive character and has only a few spectral components above 3000 Hz. If those conditions are not met, type 0 or 1 instruments should be employed. If the

greatest precision is required for both continuous and impulsive noises, type 0 SLM, the laboratory type, is to be used. When the noise is impulsive, the SLM should have a peak measuring circuit.

If octave or ⅓-octave analysis is to be performed for subsequent calculation of loudness of the noise, evaluation of transmission losses of partitions, effectiveness of barriers, or enclosures, and for the design of noise reduction schemes, the SLM should include a flat characteristic and provide an output for the appropriate analyzing system. Such instruments are usually type 1 if designed for field usage. Type 0 and 1 instruments usually have a set of filters as accessories.

For determination of exposure, the choice of instrumentation depends on the true characteristics of the noise. If the noise level does not change more than 5 dB over a long period, a SLM with A-weighting can be used. If the noise is intermittent, but otherwise approximately constant, the A-weighted level, the exposure time and L_{eq} are determined either by a sound level meter or by an intergrating sound level meter. When the noise is periodically fluctuating, L_{eq} and also the noise dose can be determined using the same instruments as used for the intermittent noise. If the fluctuation is nonperiodic, the noise dose, L_{eq}, and the statistical distribution should be determined using a noise dosimeter, integrating sound level meter and amplitude distribution analyzer, respectively. An impulse sound level meter should be used for noise with single or repeated pulses. For them, peak values, L_{eq}, noise doses and impulse noise levels should be determined. A "maximum hold" feature is useful, for instance, for determination of maximum level of a pass-by vehicle.

Determination of average dosage of an exposed worker in a noisy environment, can be done using area monitoring dosimeters. However, because the noise levels are not uniformly distributed over the working area, workers employed in close proximity to noisy machines can receive considerably higher doses than indicated by the area monitors. Personal dosimeters would help to estimate real doses received by individual workers.

Type 2 instruments are usually designed for one-hand operation. They are simple and very easy to use even by less experienced personnel. For a comparison of type 2 instruments available on the market see Hynes (14). Integrating sound-level meters and dosimeters are usually type S2A instruments.

If daily determination of community noise equivalent levels (CNEL) are required for noisy spots around highways or airports, more or less complex monitoring systems have to be employed. Such systems should contain the same components as a SLM (microphone, A-weighting network, squaring, and averaging circuits) but also circuits performing integration, conversion, timing, and a recording or logging device as a terminal. The terminal can be connected to a computer for calculation of various quantities, like the CNEL, noise exposure level, (NEL), the day-night equivalent level (L_{dn}), etc. The use of a computer permits simultaneous monitoring of several devices covering a large area.

Noise rating of machines whose function is accompanied by noise production requires knowledge of noise power radiated by the device. This knowledge can help to estimate the level of noise which will be found after the machine is installed or used.

For diagnostic purposes, the simplest instrument to use is the sound level meter. At a prescribed distance the sound level (A-weighted) can be measured at several points to see if the manufacturer's specifications are accurate.

Sound power can be determined using sound intensity meters or simple SLMs. Generally, only the sound pressure at several points has to be measured. If the reverberation method is used, the reverbation of the room in which the sound power is measured has also to be determined. In that case, the SLM output is connected to a graphic recorder. Noise is produced, then the source of the noise is suddenly switched off, and the decay of sound in the room is graphically recorded. The slope of the decay determines the reverberation.

Levels at prescribed positions around the noise source can be sequentially measured by holding the SLM by hand. The procedure can be speeded up using more sophisticated instrumentation with various degrees of automation. Several microphones can be located in fixed positions and their outputs connected to multichannel amplifiers scanning the outputs of the microphones. Octave-band analysis can be performed and obtained noise level data displayed on a plotter.

Precision sound level meters have to be used, e.g. for noise-certification tests of aircraft. The noise levels during take-offs and landings must be measured and recorded on magnetic tape at a number of specified points in and around the airport area. A ⅓-octave band spectrum should be obtained twice a second from those noises, fed into the computer memory, calibration corrections applied, and effective perceived noise levels (L_{EPN}) calculated. For this purpose a minicomputer-based system housed in a mobile trailer was developed (15). A multiuser system with microcomputer-controlled digital frequency analyzers performs acoustic and telemetered data acquisition, analysis and data base storage. All data are integrated, properly corrected and, within minutes, acoustic time histories, spectra and L_{EPN} values are printed and displayed on on-line color monitors.

Machinery vibration can be very effectively investigated using various single channel FFT spectrum analyzers. These FFT analyzers should have a frequency range of at least 25 kHz, a dynamic range of 70 dB, and provide a spectrum analysis with 400 or more lines. They should have a digitized time-domain display, provide the capability of measuring differential time, and should be equipped with IEEE 488 or RS 232 interfaces for instant transmission of data to a plotter or computer. For more information see Eshleman (16). By triggering the analyses in the same adjustable phase of rotation of the machine, time domain as well as frequency domain averaging can be performed. Such averaging enhances those components of the input signal which are synchronized with the trigger but eliminates noise and those components which are unrelated to the rotation of the machine.

Vibrations from rotating machines can be studied, and gearbox and ball-bearing problems diagnosed using zoom-transforms. These transforms provide high resolution spectra, in which even large numbers of harmonics, or closely spaced resonances, can be distinguished. For detection of harmonic patterns or for detection and separation of families of sidebands in vibration spectra, cepstra are very useful (7, 17, 18). For detection of echos and of the periodicity buried in noise autocorrelation function can be employed. All these can be performed with single channel FFT analyzers.

For identification of the source of the noise, for mechanical impedance studies, for investigation of systems with partially correlated sources, for transmission path identification, and other, cross-correlation, cross-spectra, transfer function analysis, and coherence are applicable. For these, two channel FFT analyzers should be employed.

What to Measure

For noise evaluation, the measurement of sound pressure level (SPL) and of some quantities derived from it, like sound levels, is fundamental. Practically all other measures and analyses are based on the SPL measurement. For diagnostics of machinery noise the vibration measurement plays a role analogous to the SPL measurement.

When a stationary noise source is evaluated and the effectiveness of a noise control measure determined, only sound levels are measured. However, if the noise sources are not stationary (such as vehicle traffic) information on statistical distribution of levels is more appropriate.

For evaluation of noise levels in shops or offices, average sound levels, and/or dosages, if sound levels are above 85 dB, should be determined. First, average noise levels are surveyed with a portable sound level meter. That measurement is followed by more detailed sound analysis (levels in various frequency bands, or statistical distribution of levels). If noise control is required, the most serious noise source is identified, submitted to an analysis of its noise-producing mechanism (of vibration patterns) and treated with appropriate noise-control measures. Then another series of measurements are performed to see if additional noise sources need to be treated.

The most important derived quantities for noise-pollution measurements are the noise levels L_A and statistical sound levels that are exceeded for a certain percentage of observation intervals, like L_{10}, L_{50}, or L_{90}. Equivalent sound levels L_{eq}s for 1 min, 1 h, or longer times, are very useful for varying noises. For these quantities additional noise-related measures, the so-called noise descriptors can be determined. Most of the noise descriptors are primarily related to annoyance evaluation of aircraft noise, but others, like loudness levels (in phon units), loudness (in sones), or speech interference level (SIL, in dB) have broader applicability.

The perceived noise level (EPNL, L_{EPN}) takes into account duration of a single overflight of an aircraft and any pronounced tonal components in the noise. It is calculated (19) by the formula:

$$L_{EPN} = L_{PN} + C + D.$$

C is the correction factor for tonality, usually between 0 and 3 dB, and D is the duration of noise between the instant of reaching a level 10 dB below maximum and the instant when it drops below that level again.

Noise pollution level (NPL, L_{NP}) takes into account the annoyance effects of the level of noise and its fluctuation (20, 21):

$$L_{NP} = L_{eq} + 2.56\sigma,$$

where L_{eq} is the equivalent sound level, and σ is the standard deviation representing the variability of sound level.

Statistical sound levels allow determination of traffic noise index (TNI) (21, 22):

$$TNI = 4(L_{10} - L_{90}) + L_{90} - 30.$$

Other descriptors useful for planning and evaluation of community noise pollution around airports are composite noise rating (CNR), noise exposure forecast (NEF), noise and number index (NNI), community noise equivalent level (CNEL), and day-night average sound level (DNL, L_{dn}). All these are related to perceived noise levels (L_{PN}) and the flight frequency. Sound exposure level (SEL), also called single event noise exposure level (SENEL), represents the sound energy accumulated over the duration of the noise event as the equivalent level for 1-s duration (23, 24, 25, 26).

Where to Measure

Sites for noise measurements are usually chosen on the basis of site inspection and preliminary measurement with a type 2 SLM. For general community noise investigation, the principles of sound propagation, atmospheric conditions and terrain peculiarities (type of surface, barriers) have to be taken into account (24, 27). With doubling of the distance from a point source, the level tends to decrease by 6 dB and from a line source (like a highway with heavy traffic) by 3 dB. This trend can dramatically change if reflecting objects, like buildings and barriers interfere with sound propagation. Therefore, the sites of the measuring microphones should be free of interfering objects. Grass or heavy snow on the surface increase sound attenuation. The micro-

phones should be mounted about 1.2–1.5 m above the ground (Appendix II C12).

When urban noise is investigated, the measuring equipment is typically placed at a number of places in the streets, including corners of busy intersections. In streets with high buildings, the sound propagation differs from a free-field propagation.

In the case of a noise establishment, points close to it as well as points near the closest residences should be included in the measurement.

The same is true for traffic noise evaluation. If the main concern is the traffic noise itself, the microphone should be close to the highway (around 15 m), if general noise conditions are being determined, the measurement points should be farther away.

If barrier construction is planned, a measurement should be performed before the barrier erection and another measurement taken after the barrier erection is completed. Two microphones should be used. One for the barrier data and the other one for the control data. The data microphone should be placed close to the planned and constructed barrier. There should be no additional fences that could act as barriers and microphones should be at least 3.5 m from any reflecting walls (28). Ideally, the microphones should be surrounded by a flat terrain and be at the same elevations as the highway. The site for the control microphone should have a similar configuration as the data site (except for the barrier) or as is done most often, the control microphone should be located at least 2.5 m above the top of the planned or constructed barrier. For research purposes, microphones should be located along a straight line perpendicular to the highway and at various heights for vertical propagation of the noise (28).

Noise From a Single Machine

The positions of the microphones or vibration transducers (pick-ups) for determination of noise power and vibrations of machinery are prescribed by ANSI standards that were previously mentioned and which are listed in Appendix II.

The conditions for aircraft noise measurement are specified in *Federal Aviation Regulations "Part 36 Noise Standards"* and *"Environmental Protection, Volume 1, Aircraft Noise"* to which the reader is referred (29, 30).

Noise Level from Several Machines

When noise exposure of personnel in noisy areas is to be evaluated, the area is first surveyed with a type 2 SLM. If places are found at which employees are exposed to more than 85-dB sound level (A) for 8 hr, the doses should be measured. Personal dosimeters should be used where a considerable contribution of the daily dose is from direct radiation. Area monitors dosimeters can be used in areas where reverberant sound prevails and the sound field is diffuse. In the case of personal dosimeters, the ideal location of the measuring transducer would be at the ear level of the exposed person (usually attached on the shoulder), nevertheless, a chest-level dosimeter should give a reasonable estimate of the dosage, if the sound source is not very directive. Directivity can play a larger role if high frequency components are present in the noise. The dosage measurement has to be performed for several employees exposed to the highest levels and also at several points in the general reverberant field.

When to Measure

Urban traffic noise is characterized by long-term changes and superimposed short-term changes of average levels. The long-term, daily changes show maximum average noise levels in the midafternoon hours and minimum at early morning hours.

The noise around the center of a community is dominated by urban vehicle traffic; the contribution of aircraft or industrial noise is minimal (31). For daily profiles, a 24-hr monitoring should be provided with calibration rechecking each hour. If the measurements are provided for estimating the insulation of a building from outside noise, the periods of highest traffic noise are the most important. According to Harnapp and Noble (31) the noisiest day is Friday.

At airports, it is the airplane traffic which is the most significant for the overall level. Again, the periods of highest noise have to be identified. The late evening and early morning flights can be the most troublesome. Around the industrial areas of cities, the industrial noise may be the largest contributor to the noise, and for such an environment typical daily noise profiles have to be determined. The overall levels may vary with the seasons of the year. When multiple shifts are present, evening and overnight levels, while possibly lower than daytime levels, may need to be evaluated for annoyance value.

Traffic noise levels depend on pavement condition. On a wet and snow-covered pavement, the tire noise increases. Generally, we are interested in data obtained for dry pavement.

For noise exposure, measurements have to be performed throughout several days so that a realistic representation of daily dose can be obtained. It is important to include a day when the worst noise conditions occur. Daily routines of the workers should be investigated to determine what kind of job is performed during the day. The dose is determined by a dosimeter or calculated from a record of time spent at each work site and of the appropriate levels. If the level varies, L_{eq}s should be determined. If the noise varies regularly, the dose is estimated from the levels at corresponding time segments.

How to Measure

The collected data on noise should be valid and reliable. The validity and reliability of the results are determined by various factors—environmental conditions, locations of instruments (especially microphones), characteristics of the instruments, characteristics of the noise, method employed and, last but not least, by the observer.

Choice of the method, should be determined by the most recent standard covering the task (see Appendix II). Sometimes the recommended method has to be modified to fit the available instrumentation and specific conditions of the task. All cases of noise measurements have not been standardized yet and probably never will be. If modification of the standardized method (code) is desirable, the instrument manuals should be consulted. The manuals of equipment for noise measurements usually contain a discussion of various applications.

The treatment of the problem usually starts with listening, observation, and measuring L_A sound levels with a portable sound level meter. If the levels are too high, then continue: (a) examine the object of measurement and decide which method to use; if possible and appropriate, use the pertinent standard test code; (b) set up the microphones and the devices at the points required by the standard or according to the analysis of the needs for each particular situation; be sure the microphone does not respond to structure-borne vibration; (c) calibrate the whole instrumentation system before beginning the measurement and after you have finished, if the measurement lasts for many hours, recalibrate periodically during the whole measuring period; (d) determine the level of the background noise; (e) make a drawing or plan of the situation including each object which could influence the sound distribution, show the distances, especially of the microphones from the sound source, walls, or other large objects; (f) if outdoor measurement is performed, note the meteorological conditions; (g) note all settings of the instruments (weighting, speed of response) directly on the paper of the graphic level recorder or record them on the magnetic tape if a tape recording is made; (h) briefly describe the task, goal, place, dates and times of the day in a log and note all changes that were introduced during the measurement in the instrument settings, block diagram, makes, models, and serial numbers of the measuring equipment; and (i) note each unusual acoustic event.

It is very important to examine the first few data to see if their values are reasonable and that the equipment is functioning properly. An omission of such examination may be very costly in the loss of time spent by collecting invalid data. Often a simple cause, like a connector improperly plugged-in, can be the cause for malfunction. Such cases can be usually easily corrected on the spot.

When measurements of sound levels are performed, reflections from surrounding objects—including the measuring person—and the background noise have to be taken into consideration.

When the size of an object or obstacle is comparable to the wavelength (usually at relatively high frequencies), reflections occur. For objects smaller than the wavelength (at relatively low frequencies), diffraction can be observed. Therefore, the microphones have to be located so that they will not be in the acoustic shadow of an obstacle or in an appreciable field of reflected waves. To avoid disturbance of the sound field by the person holding the SLM or the microphone, the microphones with preamplifiers can be located on a tripod and connected with the amplifier, recorder or analyzer by a cable. If the observer has to hold the SLM, it should be held to the side of the line connecting the source and the microphone. Precision SLMs have extension rods for microphones so that the observer and meter do not influence the sound level at the microphone. This may be important if the frequency range above 1 kHz is studied.

The absorption of sound by a person increases with frequency and the reflections become more attenuated; also the "cylindrical" or "spherical" shape of the human body causes the sound reflection to be more diffused at high frequencies.

Therefore, the influence of the reflections from a person standing behind the microphone is not greatest at high frequencies but at around 400 Hz. In a diffused, reverberant field, the influence of close objects on measurement is usually not very serious.

Single Machine Noise

When community noise is measured, the microphone should be omnidirectional and, in general, should be pointing vertically. In single machine noise measurement, the microphone orientation depends on the method and microphone calibration. If the microphone is calibrated in a diffused field, and the reading takes place in the free field or close to the source in the reverberant field, there should be an angle between the axis of the microphone and the direction of sound. This angle, specified by the manufacturer, is typically around 70°. If the microphone has a flat frequency response for perpendicular incidence, the microphone should be pointing at the source.

Background noise from several sources can obscure measurements of the noise from the investigated source. If the background noise level (determined when the studied source of noise is shut down) is at least 10 dB less than the noise of the measured source in any frequency band, the background can be ignored. If the total noise is between 3 and 10 dB higher than the background noise itself, a correction should be applied (Fig. 3.12). If the difference is less than 3 dB, at least some of the background noise sources should be shut down for the time of the measurement, or the measured object should be moved to a place with a low noise level.

Internal Noise

The measurement of low level noises can be confounded by internal noise of the equipment. This noise is usually higher for smaller microphones than for the larger ones, and worse for C than for B or A weighting. If the measured and the

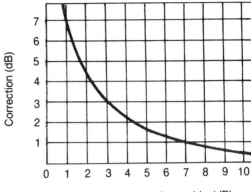

Figure 3.12. Background noise correction for measurement of sound level. L_{SN} stands for the total level of signal with background noise and L_N is the level of the background noise only. The correction has to be subtracted from L_{SN} to obtain the level of the signal (of the measured noise of interest).

internal noise are of the same order, improvement can be usually achieved by performing octave-band analysis.

If hum is picked up (this can be checked by listening through well fitted circumaural earphones or by comparison of C- with A-weighted reading, or by using an analyzer), it can be often eliminated by a reorientation of the instruments. Otherwise, the equipment should be removed from the vicinity of the source of the electromagnetic field. Rechecking the grounding, or simple repluging (reversing) of the power plugs can be effective.

Time Characteristics of Noises

The choice of the proper averaging of the SLM depends on the character of the noise. Noise can be considered to be: steady (Appendix II A5) if its SPL remains essentially constant during the period of observation, i.e. when the fluctuations of the reading with the "slow" characteristic are less than ±3 dB; fluctuating, if its SPL measured with the slow characteristic varies more than 6 dB but does not drop to the ambient environmental level more than once or, when measured with the "fast" characteristic, shows larger than 6-dB changes between some steady state levels; nonsteady, if its SPL shifts, or spectral distribution changes during the period of observation; impulsive, if the SPL is above the ambient level for a brief time (usually less than 1 s); and intermittent, if its SPL drops to the ambient level two or more times during the period of observation, and the periods of greater pressure are on the order of 1 s. or more. Impulsive noise can have a form of isolated impulses, or can consist of a sequence of two or more bursts during observation. If the repetition rate of the impulses is such that it is difficult to distinguish individual bursts by a SLM, the noise is called quasi steady. With a repetition rate of 10 or more/s, the noise is generally quasi steady.

Steady noise level is equal to the average of the maximum and minimum levels measured in the slow mode. If, in such a case, the fast mode readings indicate that the level alternates between two or more well defined levels less than 6 dB apart, and remain at those levels for longer than 1 s, the fast readings should be recorded. If the steady-state portions of the sound are shorter than 1 s, the maximum value of the fast reading is to be recorded. In such a case, the noise can also be treated as impulsive noise. If the repetition rate of impulses is equal to 10 or more/s, the noise is generally quasi steady and can be measured as a steady noise. For a repetition rate between 1 and 10, the noise is either close to being quasi steady or to being isolated bursts. The noise can then be described in terms of estimates of average level and of the magnitude of the SPL fluctuations.

If the meter reading in the slow mode fluctuates between ±3 dB and ±5 dB, "the level corresponding to the rms sound pressure is approximately 3 dB below the maximum level; when successive excursions are observed to have different maximum levels, the level is approximately 3 dB below the mean of the maximum levels for several excursions" (Appendix II A5). If the fluctuations are over ±5 dB

(10 or more) readings are recorded and the average level calculated.

If a single burst lasts longer than about 1 s, the fast mode reading should be used. If the single burst is shorter than 0.5 s, or if the repetition rate is less than 5/s, and the peak values are 15 or more decibels above the A-weighted SPL, the impulse or peak circuitry is employed.

Transients

Transients can be captured on a screen of the storage cathode-ray oscilloscope for observation of the waveform, on the tape recorder for further analysis in the laboratory or in the memory of a digital processor. In the field, short duration acoustic impulses, like sonic booms, gun shots, explosions, etc., often are not repetitive and therefore should be recorded for follow-up analysis. Because such impulses often have very low frequencies, an FM magnetic recording should be employed. Condenser microphones should have the pressure equalization hole sealed for such measurements. For preserving all audible components, the recording speed has to be high. If later a much slower replaying speed is used, the waveform of such an impulse can be graphically charted. Analysis can be performed by sequentially filtering the signal by a tunable, very narrow filter or by a parallel digital analyzer.

Digital spectrum analyzers can usually perform a continuously on-going fourier transformation of the input signal. They have a fixed number of samples, like 1024, on which the transformation is performed. The larger the proportion of these 1024 points that represents the samples of a short-lasting wave, the larger is the amount of transient energy per measurement bandwidth. Therefore, the transient should occupy as much as possible of the time window or, in other words, the time window should be as short as possible. The shorter the time window is, the larger the frequency range is. That means, for very short transient signals, the measurement frequency range should be as large as possible. If a transient is repetitive, a number of the transients can be averaged and the statistical reliability of the results improved.

When sonic booms are measured, the microphone should have the diaphragm facing upwards and be flush with a rigid plane baffle which should be flush with the ground. The location should be essentially without terrain undulations. The baffle should be at least 1.5 m in diameter. Important characteristics of a sonic boom are the positive peak, the initial rise time and the delay time between the incident and the reflected shock waves.

Sound Intensity

For sound intensity measurement a suitable measurement surface has to be selected. Any surface completely enclosing the source can be used. In practice, a hemisphere, a rectangular parallelepiped or a conformal surface which closely follows the actual surface of the source are usually chosen. The intensity probe should be oriented perpendicular to that surface. The accuracy of the measurement will be a function of the chosen microphone distance, of the size of the microphones in the probe, of the phase and amplitude mismatch, and of the time-averaging procedure (32).

Locating The Source

A sound intensity meter, like the sound analyzing system 3360 by Brüel & Kjaer, can be used for finding the location of the source of noise (12). The sound intensity probe is moved along a line in such a way that the axis connecting the membranes of two microphones is identical with the line of motion. When the probe is on one side of the noise source, the output of the microphone closer to the source is ahead in phase with the second one. When the probe reaches a position in which the source is in a plane perpendicular to the connecting line of the microphones, the outputs of the microphones are the same and the difference signal is minimal.

When the probe is moved further along the line, the phase relation between the microphones outputs reverses. The sudden drop of the output at the minimum, or the indication of the phase reversal at the display, gives information on the direction of the source. Repeating the procedure in a direction perpendicular to the first line determines the second direction of the source. The source is then located at the intersection of the two directions.

Noise of Moving Sources

If noise production of a single vehicle is to be determined, the so-called "moving vehicle test" can be used (Appendix II C5). For this test, a flat hard surface (concrete or asphalt) of about 40 m in diameter surrounded by an open space reaching about 30 m beyond the hard surface circle can be used. The vehicle should be in second gear (if it has four gears) and the speed should be the lower of three-quarter of the maximum engine speed or 50 km/hr vehicle speed. The throttle should be fully opened when the front of the vehicle reaches 10 m from the microphones and closed when the rear of the vehicle is 10 m behind the microphones. The microphones (1.2 m above the ground) are 7.5 m distant at each side of the path of the vehicle.

Aircraft noise can be measured and analyzed at a large number of points around the airport area. Because the data should be collected during several days, weeks or even months, this procedure is time consuming. However, noise contours for individual types of aircraft can be estimated from ground measurements at several points and these estimates can serve for a relatively reliable evaluation of noise distribution around the airport. The surface at the points of measurements should be flat and hard, the microphones should be 1.2 m above the ground, and a type 1 SLM with a flat frequency response with quality FM magnetic tape recording should be used. The data are later analyzed in the laboratory, preferably using parallel filtering and digital processing. As mentioned before, data of all ⅓-octave filters at 0.5 sec-intervals are analyzed and converted to the effective perceived noise level (L_{EPN}).

Vibration Measurement

When vibrations are to be measured, several considerations have to be taken into account.

The fastening of the pick-up to a vibrating surface should be as direct and as rigid as possible. Simple fastening by a double-sided adhesive tape, magnet or petroleum jelly (on a horizontal surface) can be applied if the fastening is temporary, the acceleration is smaller than the gravity, and if the vibration has only low frequency components. When high accelerations are present the pick-up must be fastened by a bolt or stud. For permanent attachment, a thin layer of cement can be used.

If the vibrating device is massive, one can make a quick check of the vibration magnitude by holding the pick-up by hand against the vibrating surface; however, the vibrations are usually considerably modified by such a procedure and the results are not accurate. A noncontacting modal probe has been recently developed by which a small microphone senses acoustic pressure near the surface of the vibrating test specimen (33).

Tremor of the hand has to be taken into account at low frequencies and small vibrations. The hand-produced vibration has components mainly below 20 Hz, peak-to-peak magnitude of acceleration about 12.5 cm/s^2 and of velocity 0.5 cm/s when the pick-up is held against a stationary surface (24).

Computers and microprocessors permitted the development of new tests. For instance, the so-called "system mapping" can depict on one plot the entire history of machine behavior for a sweep of a variable over a prescribed range; or the "modal analysis" is used for determination of modal parameters (effective mass,

stiffness, damping, resonance frequency, and mode shape) of the structures (34).

Calibration

Calibration should be checked at least before and after the measurement. Older equipment stabilized its performance over a period of time, during which the equipment performance drifted. In such case, calibration checks had to be done more often (in about 15-min intervals) until the performance stabilized. With modern instruments, this is generally not necessary. However for long-lasting measurements it is recommended that one checks the calibration at about hourly intervals.

Reporting of Survey Measurements

A report of the survey measurement should contain information on the object and purpose of the measurement, on the acoustic environment of the object, on the method and instrumentation used in testing, results of measurement (testing), conclusions, and recommendations. If applicable, the following information should be included in the main text of the report or, if more appropriate, in the appendix:

1. The dates of the report preparation and of the measurement; daily times of the measurements
2. Description of the object and the purpose of the survey
3. Description of the noise sources and their operating conditions and installation (mounting)
4. Description of the area and spaces of testing and location of sound sources; of reflecting or otherwise interfering objects; placement and the number of persons exposed to noise; dimensional sketches, possible photographs; for indoor measurements, the acoustical treatment of walls, ceiling and floor; for outdoor measurements, description of buildings, trees, and other reflecting objects; physical and topographic description of the ground surface; location of closest residences; in reports on vehicle testing, the loading of vehicle during the test and the horse power rating; in reports on aircraft noise measurements

aircraft type, model, engine, weight, flap, landing gear positions, speed, flight path, altitude, take-off power, etc.

5. Method, instrumentation, results and conclusions from a preliminary survey, including the identification of the principle sources of noise and of the critical points of exposure in the area
6. Method of main measurements, including the standard test codes
7. List of microphones, vibration pick-ups and all other instruments including identification of individual devices of the instrumental set-up by make, model and serial numbers
8. Block diagram and arrangement of the measuring equipment
9. Specifications of bandwidth of frequency analyzer, of frequency response of the measuring system, including weighting used, of the time response (slow, or fast, impulse or peak)
10. Method of calibration and its results, including applied corrections
11. Locations and orientations of microphones, placement of vibration pick-ups
12. Positions of observers
13. Test of standing wave pattern and decreasing of the sound level with distance
14. Air temperatures in degrees Celsius, relative humidity in percentages, and barometric pressure in pascals (1 atm = 101.34 kPa) for indoor and outdoor measurements and additional data on wind direction and speed and precipitation for outdoor measurements
15. Data on background noise
16. Collected data and applied corrections of over-all and band-level measurements; estimation of the extent of level fluctuations; data on audiometric examination of personnel exposed to noises over $L_A = 90$ dB, or even 85 dB
17. Time pattern of exposure
18. Comparison of data with other measured values or with prescribed values
19. Summary of data and conclusions
20. Recommendations for improvement, if any
21. Any changes in equipment settings and unusual events occurring during the testing
22. Names and qualifications of observers

A well documented report is important for future reference, in cases of litigation and for drawing conclusion on possible improvement of the method when surveying similar situations. High quality of the report is very important for the success of recommended improvements in each particular situation (47, 48, 49).

CONTROL OF NOISE

Measurement of noise can serve as the basis for implementation of noise reduction. In this section a brief outline of general procedures of noise control is presented.

Two approaches can be distinguished: (a) noise prevention, primarily connected with planning of new facilities, and (b) noise reduction in existing facilities.

Prevention can be achieved by, (a) properly planning the site of the noisy and quiet facilities; (b) by choosing the quieter option of various operational procedures and methods of manufacturing; (c) purchasing machines with respect to their noise ratings; (d) by designing proper mountings to prevent machine vibration transfer to the supporting structure; (e) by planning enclosures for noisy machines to prevent the spread of air-borne noise; and (f) designing the building with proper noise control and with proper relative placement of noisy and quiet operations in the building.

The task of noise reduction in existing locations requires (a) locating the sources of noise; (b) identifying the noise-producing mechanism; (c) determining the time and frequency characteristics of the noise; (d) deciding: if noise reduction can be achieved by alteration of the noise production mechanism, if the noise can be confined to the area around the source and if the noise protection should be introduced at the receiver site; (e) designing and introducing noise reduction measures; and (f) checking the effectiveness of those measures.

Before discussing the above listed steps in more detail, general principles of sound and vibration production and propagation are reviewed.

Rule 1: Vibrating surfaces are sources of sound waves

Rule 2: Large surfaces radiate the sound

more efficiently than the small ones

Rule 3: Prolongation of vibration increases the energy of sound in space

Rule 4: Reduction of vibration is the most desirable method of noise treatment

Rule 5: Large, fast changes of motion of a mass produce more noise than small, slow changes

Rule 6: Heavier objects tend to vibrate more slowly than lighter ones

Rule 7: Objects with small mass and small stiffness can be set into vibration easier than those with large mass and large stiffness

Rule 8: Large deformations by large masses are connected with low frequencies and small deformations by small masses are connected with high frequencies

Rule 9: Sound-absorbing and damping materials attenuate resonances and shorten the natural vibrations of the surface

Rule 10: Turbulence in air is a source of noise; this noise increases with the volume of space occupied by the turbulence

Rule 11: Spreading of the noise into the structure should be prevented

Rule 12: Energy transfer from one point in space to another is small if the sound passes through impedance mismatches

Rule 13: Vibration transfer from one part to another is easy when the connection between the parts is rigid; it is difficult when the connection is soft and flexible

Rule 14: A material with large compliance isolates the vibration of a mass from the supporting structure effectively if the resonance frequency of that compliance and mass is lower than the frequency of forced vibration of the mass

Rule 15: Reaching of the receiver by noise through the air should be prevented

Rule 16: The noise level decreases with distance from the source

Rule 17: In absorptive materials, the sound energy is dissipated into heat. In air and other absorbing materials, the high frequency energy is absorbed more than the low frequency energy

Rule 18: Low frequencies bend around obstacles and pass easily through holes and openings; high frequencies do not

Rule 19: Obstacles large with respect to the wavelength reflect more sound than small ones

Rule 20: Obstacles large with respect to the wavelength create a larger area of acoustic shadow than the small ones

Rule 21: Two waves of equal amplitude but of opposite phase cancel each other

Rule 22: High frequencies are more annoying than low frequencies

Noise Prevention in New Facilities

When planning a new facility many measures can be implemented relatively simply and economically. Later, implementation of such measures could be difficult, much more expensive, and probably also less effective.

Planning of the Site

First, the effect of distance (Rule 16) and terrain pecularities (Rule 20) on noise levels should be exploited. The larger the distance and obstacles (hills, large existing buildings) between the noise source and the receivers, the smaller the noise level at the receiver.

Choice of Quieter Procedures (Rule 5)

For instance, bolting or welding is preferable to riveting; squeezing to hammering; continuous cutting to chopping; low speed processing to high speed processing; using plastics to metals; and application of continuous steady force to an impact of heavy mass.

Quieter Machines

Purchasing of quieter machines according to specifications, or for which an additional noise control can be easily introduced later. For instance, a belt drive is generally less noisy than a gear drive, a plastic gear less noisy than a metal gear, electrically powered carts less noisy than vehicles with combustion engine.

If a device, like a fan, radiates sound directly into an occupied room, the lower noise frequencies are preferable to the higher ones (Rule 22). On the other hand, industrial fans radiating noise into the atmosphere should have higher noise frequencies (more blades) because then the noise travels only a short distance (Rule 17) and, being more directional, can be directed, e.g., toward the sky (Rule 18).

Machine Mountings

Mountings of machines generating vibrations should be soft or elastic to prevent spreading of vibration into the supporting structure (Rule 13). Large machines with large vibrations should have their own foundations that are separated from the building foundation.

Machine Enclosures

Machines producing air-borne sound should be located in separate chambers with walls thick enough to provide large transmission loss to adjacent rooms (Rules 12, 17) and lined inside by absorptive material for reducing the noise level in the chamber.

Building Design

Other noise control measures include (a) construction of ceilings, windows, door, etc. with sufficient sound insulation to prevent noise transmission from outside into the building and from one room of the building to the other; (b) lining of the heating and ventilation ducts with sound-absorptive materials to prevent spreading of noise from one room to another through ducts (Rule 17); (c) using absorption on the ceiling of offices (and possibly on the walls) to reduce sound reflection and reverberation in the rooms (Rules 3 and 17); (d) using floating floors, or at least carpets, to prevent transmission of impact noise through the ceilings (Rules 12 and 13); and (e) providing partial partitions in open-space type of spaces (Rule 20).

Noise Prevention in Existing Facilities

If existing conditions have to be improved, any of the four main approaches have to be considered: (a) reduction of sound production by the source (Rules 1 and 14); (b) reduction of vibration transfer from the source into the structure (Rule 11); (c) reduction of sound transfer from the source into the air (Rule 15); and (d) reduction of the amount of sound energy of sound reaching the receiver from the air (Rule 15).

Reduction of Sound Production at the Source

In reduction of sound production, the noise source has to be located first. Often, this is a very easy task. For example, a steel mill can be a rather obvious noise source. Often the machine, or its part, that produces substantial noise in a factory hall can be easily identified by listening or using a type 2 SLM. It helps, if individual machines can be measured with all other machines shut-down. If all machines have to operate continuously, identification of major noise sources may be more complicated. In the later case, a careful measurement of noise and vibration at various points in the hall may be required. If the machine identified as the source of noise has large dimensions, it may be difficult to pinpoint the noisiest part of it. An intensity meter with an indicator of phase of vibration can be helpful.

Clues for source identification frequently can be obtained if the operating conditions of the machine can be changed (for example run in segments), while simultaneously measuring the changes in noise level.

Identify Noise-Producing Mechanism

After the source of noise has been pinpointed, the noise production mechanism has to be identified. Often a simple inspection discovers a loose or damaged part, but sometimes a careful analysis of noise and vibration is required. In a motor, the noise can be generated by various means, like the air-flow, magnetic field, bearings and gear drives, and unbalanced rotors, to name just a few. A frequency analysis using spectra, zooming or cepstra can usually distinguish among noises resulting from variety of mechanisms. For proper conclusions an understanding of mechanical operation of the machine and its relation to data displays are needed. It is beyond the scope of this chapter to discuss all these relations in detail. A brief overview is shown in Table 3.1.

Engineering Modifications of Machines

After the noise production mechanism of the source has been identified, engineering type of modifications of the machines have to be undertaken for the reduction of noise. General concepts are given here. For details of solving the practical problems, the reader should refer to publications on noise control, like *Handbook of Noise Control* (35), *Handbook of Noise Measurement* (24) the AIHA *Industrial Noise Manual* (36), the American Foundrymen's Society *Control of Noise* (37), or *NIOSH Compendium of Materials for Noise Control* (38), and journals like *Sound and Vibration*, or *Noise Control Engineering*.

Vibrations

Noise is always produced by vibrations. If the vibration is eliminated, the noise is eliminated, therefore, the best solution is to eliminate the cause of vibrations (Rule 4). If that cannot be done, the size of the vibrating body has to be reduced to the minimum (Rule 2), and the vibration has to be damped as much as possible. A small surface radiates noise less effectively then a large one and the shortening of the duration of vibration decreases the energy (power × time) of the radiated sound. Damping materials shorten and also reduce the magnitude of vibration, especially at resonance. The sources of vibra-

tion are impacts, friction, alternating forces, and turbulences.

Impacts occur if two bodies come in a sudden contact because of differences in their speed, if explosions or implosions take place, or if sound waves are made to coincide in time, like in a sonic boom. Impacts have a continuous spectrum, which is spread over a wider or narrower frequency range. Pronounced vibrations can occur if resonance frequencies of the mechanical system (the so-called natural, or eigenfrequencies) are in the frequency range of the impact spectrum. If the impacts are repeated with a frequency corresponding to the resonance, amplitude of the vibration can become large and dangerous. Impacts of large masses have low frequency content, while impacts of small masses have more high frequency content (Rule 8). The former are more difficult to attenuate than are the latter (Rule 17).

Explosions are inherent in combustion engines. Their control is in the hands of the designers. Implosions in hydraulic systems accompany the so-called cavitation. If the cross-section area of a pipe changes suddenly (like at the valves), the pressure and velocity changes in the flow of the liquid are quick and large, and vapor bubbles are formed. These bubbles collapse nearly immediately and produce noise and erosion of the material. Cavitation can be reduced if the changes of the cross-sections of the pipes are gradual.

Friction prevents a smooth motion of one part on the other. Small jerks take place which have a wide, continuous spectrum. Friction causes faster and larger wear off of the parts like ball bearings, sliding bearings, gear teeth, cams, etc. These parts become loose, friction increases, small impacts between them take place. Those frequency components of the continuous spectra of jerks and impacts which are equal to the resonance frequencies of the system (or subsystems), are amplified and the systems (or subsystems), are set into vibrations. Various parts of the machines have various natu-

Table 3.1
Relation between components of noise or vibration spectra of machines and possible causes.[a]

Component Frequency / Shaft speed[b]	Usual cause	Other possibilities
<½	Oil whirl	Defective drive belt (if pulley speed) Vibration from other machines or slower speed components Gear train modulation Friction whip (if speed > critical)
Between ½ and 1	Defective drive belt	Friction whip (if speed > critical) Vibration from other sources Gear train modulation
1	Unbalance (radial motion) Misalignment (axial motion also)	Bent shaft Defective drive belt (if belt speed) Unbalanced magnetic force
2 or 3	Misalignment Unbalance	Mechanical looseness Bent shaft Defective drive belt
>3	Bad gears Cam impulses Fan vibration Reciprocating actions Hydraulic forces	Parts colliding Broken pieces
Noninteger	Bad gears	Gears on other shafts Modulation of gear vibration Toothed belts with modulation by belt speed Aerodynamically driven galloping
High noninteger	Bad bearings	Friction-induced vibration Chatter Rubbing Induction motor vibration Slipping clutches
Broadband	Aerodynamic Fluid flow Air leaks Hydraulic leaks	

Component frequency / A-C line frequency	Usual cause	Other possibilities
1× 2 or higher	Defective motor rotor Magnetostriction Defective electrical components Distorted electrical wave	Unbalanced phases (electrical) Loose laminations

[a] Reproduced with permission from Peterson APG: *Handbook of Noise Measurement*. Concord, Mass, GenRad, 1980 (24).
[b] Shaft speed is a ratio of component frequency in H_2 and shaft speed in rotations per second and is therefore a dimensionless number.

ral frequencies which depend on their sizes, masses and stiffnesses. In general, small components have high resonance frequencies, large components have low resonance frequencies.

The fundamental frequency of vibrations from the gears is equal to the product of the number of gear teeth and the number of revolutions per second. The vibration from the gear has various harmonics, especially when the profiles of the teeth are worn out. Resonances of shafts, gear cases, etc., coinciding with any of these components can increase vibrations significantly.

Alternating force sets various parts of matter into motion that is eventually transferred to air. Such forces in machines result from various causes: unbalanced rotating masses; misalignment of the shafts with adjacent structures; piston-like motion, as in combustion engines or hydraulic equipment, or magnetic forces in electrical motors, transformers or fluorescent lamp ballasts.

For unbalanced rotors the vibration frequency is characteristically equal to rotations per second; for misalignment and bent shafts it is usually twice as high; for transformer noise the vibration frequencies are the multiples of the power line frequency (of 60 Hz in the USA and 50 Hz in Europe). Proper balancing, alignment, isolation from the supporting structures, tightening the laminations of the iron core of the transformer, and proper design of rotor slots and of the number of poles of the motor are some of the means for vibration reduction.

Turbulences—erratic variations of the magnitude and direction of the fluid flow—can occur if the flow of the fluid is obstructed or if the velocity of the fluid in a pipe is so large that the so-called Reynold's number (39) is larger than 2000. Reynold's number increases with the fluid density and velocity, and the diameter of the pipe, but decreases with the viscosity of the fluid. If it is less than 2000, the fluid flow is laminar, above 2000 it is becoming turbulent.

Turbulence is accompanied by irregular pressure variances which are the source of noise. Such noise can be reduced if changes in diameter of the pipes or in the direction of the fluid are gradual, and if the cross-area of the ducts (or pipes) is subdivided into several sections. The space occupied by the turbulent flow should be maximally reduced. That can be achieved if, for instance, the intake air of a fan is undisturbed and free of turbulences, or the outlet of a pipe is divided into several smaller ones.

Reduction of Vibration Transfer from the Source into the Structure

When vibration transfer from the source of vibration into the supporting structure is eliminated, the size of radiating surface (Rule 2) and the transfer of structure-borne sound to distant places are reduced.

Fundamentally, all vibration sources can be very effectively isolated from the supporting structure by resilient, flexible mounts (Rules 12 and 13). These can be in the form of springs, when heavy machines, or whole rooms, are to be isolated. For mounting of relatively light machines, pads of resilient material, rubber, cork, polystyrene can be used. Mounts are on the market containing resilient materials between a screw which is fastened to the machine and a plate which is fastened to the support.

The isolating mounts should have high internal damping (Rule 9). Such damping significantly reduces the vibration at resonance frequency while retaining the isolation effectiveness at other vibration frequencies. This is important for cases when the machine running speed remains relatively long around the resonance frequency during run-ups or run-downs.

As mentioned before, heavy machines with large vibrations should have foundations separate from the foundation of the rest of the building. Such machines should also be separated from the foundation by a spring support. Smaller machines should use a spring support; their foundations should be heavy (Rule 7), but not necessarily separated from the building.

The mass of the machine and the compliance of the support represent a resonant system. It is necessary that the resonance frequency of this system be lower than the vibration frequencies of the machine and under the resonances of the floor (Rule 14). Sometimes the floor has to be stiffened by reinforcement.

If the mass of the object to be isolated is small, it may be necessary to increase its mass by an "inertia block" inserted between the machine and the vibration isolators.

If the center of gravity of the machine is high, above rather tall and flexible mountings, a rocking motion can occur. To prevent this, the static displacement of each mount should be the same. The best results are obtained, if the center of gravity of the machine is at the same elevation as the isolators.

To secure an effective isolation of vibrating objects, the connecting pipes, supply ducts, electrical connections, etc., have also to be isolated from the supporting walls, floors or ceilings, or from the machine itself. Such isolation can be achieved by layers of soft materials (Rule 13), like foam-rubber washers mounted between the piping and the walls, by hanging the "plumbing" on rubber or spring hangers, by inserting flexible hose segments between the machine and outgoing piping, by inserting flexible collars into the ducts, and by using flexible electrical cables.

Reduction of Sound Transfer from the Source into the Air

The sound transfer from the source to the air may be the result of spreading of the noise through the inlets and outlets of the machine, of the gas flow out or around the machine, or it can be the result of the vibration of the surface of the machine, if the engineering measures discussed before have not been completely satisfactory.

Ducts

The prevention of spreading of noise through ducts can be achieved by lining the inside walls of the ducts with sound absorptive materials. For low frequencies the lining should be thicker than for the high frequencies (Rule 17).

Ducts with smaller diameter provide larger attenuation of sound than the wider ducts. If the velocity of gas through the ducts or pipes is not so high that turbulence becomes a significant source of noise (less than about 500 m/min), large changes in cross-sectional area or bendings of the duct can be used as efficient means of sound emission attenuation. Large cross-sectional changes mean large mismatch of acoustic impedance (recall that the acoustic impedance, z_a, is indirectly proportional to the cross-sectional area) and that means large reflection of acoustic energy (Rule 12). An enlargement in a duct forms an expansion chamber which can be used as an effective low-frequency attenuator.

Branching is another way of reducing tones or narrow bands of noise present in the sound. If the branch is in a form of the Helmholtz resonator, the energy at the resonance frequency of the resonator can be absorbed in the resonator. A branch can also return to the duct at such a distance that the tones from the two branches meet in opposite phase and cancel out (Rule 21).

Combustion engines, either stationary or mobile, have to be provided with mufflers (silencers) for attenuation of sound radiated from the exhaust pipe (40). Two kinds of mufflers can be used: reactive and absorptive.

Reactive mufflers are represented by a series of expansion chambers, branch ducts, and openings between concentric ducts, which form an acoustical filter. Chambers, openings and friction represent compliances, masses and resistances of the filter elements. The attenuation of sound in the desired frequency range can be achieved by mechanical arrangement of those elements.

Reactive mufflers usually do not contain absorptive lining. High flow velocities or high temperature of the gas or air could erode such linings.

Absorptive mufflers (silencers) use sound-absorptive linings on the walls or on the baffles inside the silencer. Sound energy is absorbed in the linings. Thick linings are effective absorbents at low frequencies and thin linings with narrow passages are effective absorbents at high frequencies. For attenuation in the widest frequency ranges, baffles covered with thick absorptive layers and only with narrow passages between them are the best.

The sound attenuation of mufflers can be expressed in terms of its insertion loss. Insertion loss is the difference in the sound pressure level at a certain point measured before and after the muffler has been inserted between that point and the noise source.

Surface Damping

If the engineering measures for vibration reduction discussed above are not fully effective, additional measures for vibration reduction should be undertaken. The first step could be the painting or spraying of the vibrating surfaces by paints or other materials having high internal damping properties. Gluing of damping materials or simply covering the vibrating surface with laminates with damping layers can be also very effective.

Damping layers on the surface might not be applicable if they prevent adequate cooling of the machine. In such cases, the machine should be placed in a sound-insulating enclosure. If low frequencies are predominant, and the machine should be mobile, such enclosure should encapsule the entire machine; it should be well sealed to prevent any noise leaks. The enclosure can be single- or double-walled and lined from the inside with sound-absorbing material. Air for cooling purposes should be carried through ducts having acoustic louvers for inlet and outlet. If high frequencies are predominant, complete sealing is not necessary (41, 42).

Perforating

Sometimes the source of noise can have the form of a large vibrating panel. If its vibration can not be eliminated, the radiation of sound can be reduced by providing a "short circuit" for waves in front and behind the panel by perforating the panel. The waves on two sides of the panel have opposite phases and cancel out if added together (Rule 21). Further cancellation takes place around the edges of the panels if passage for the waves around them is provided.

Noisy, heavy and stationary machines should be placed in sound-insulated rooms with walls with high transmission losses (see below) and a sound attenuating door. Inside, the ceiling and walls should be covered with sound-absorptive material. The absorption on the walls reduces the overall level of the noise in the enclosure by reducing the intensity of the reflected waves.

Reduction of Sound Reaching the Receiver from the Air

Insulation of machines by enclosure should confine the noise to their immediate vicinity and protect the environment from noise pollution. Unfortunately, this cannot be always achieved. For instance, noise from highways and airports spreads into a large space. Then it is the receiver that has to be protected from the environmental noise. The pathways of the sound from the source to the receiver have to be interrupted by an obstacle in the form of a barrier; alternatively, the receiver (instead of the noise source) is placed in an enclosure, such as a building.

Partitions

Noise can enter the building through the walls and roof as an air-borne sound, or through vibrations via foundations as a structure-borne sound. The first way—by the air-borne sound—is the most common one. The ground can be usually considered to be an excellent insulator of sound.

Air-borne sound can pass through a partition in several ways. If the partition is rigid and nonporous, the fraction of incident sound which penetrates it, propagates through the material and radiates into the space on the other side. Because of the impedance mismatch between the air and wall material, this type of energy transmission is generally negligible. If the material is porous, the sound penetrates it easily. Part of it changes into heat by friction, but most of it passes through the pores to the space behind the partition. Porous materials are poor sound insulators; their transmission loss is small. If the partition is flexible, the incident sound can set it into vibration and acoustic waves are generated by it in the space behind. Sound can pass through a partition by flanking paths like ventilation ducts, joints in panels, etc.

Various terms are used to define the insulating properties of partitions. The most widely used are transmission loss (TL), noise reduction (NR), and sound transmission class (STC).

The transmission loss (TL) is the difference between the power level of the sound incident on one side of the partition and the power level of the sound transmitted to the space on the other side of it. It is assumed that the size of the partition is very large, and the space behind it is a free field. In practice, the partition has limited size and the space on the receiver side can be completely or partially closed.

The noise reduction (NR) does not depend only on the TL of the partition itself, but also on the acoustic properties of the receiver room. The NR is equal to the difference between the average sound-pressure level in the room containing the sound source and the average sound-pressure level in the receiving room. It can be determined as:

$$NR = TL + \log(a/S) \text{ dB,}$$

where a is the total absorption in the receiving room and S is the area of the wall transmitting sound in m^2. (Absorption is discussed later.)

The TL is frequency dependent and that makes its use complicated. A single average value of TL over the frequency could be given, but such a value would not generally correspond to subjective impressions resulting from sound insulation. The sound transmission class (STC) attempts to represent insulation effectiveness in a single number. Weighted transmission losses at different frequencies according to subjective importance are built into it.

Standard STC contours have been determined (ASTM 1973, Appendix II D1) to which the transmission loss curve corresponding to the partition is to be matched. The sum of deviations of the partition curve down from the standard STC contour at 16 test frequencies should not be more than 32 dB and none of the deviations must exceed 8 dB. When that is achieved, the STC value is read as the TL value corresponding to the intersection of the STC contour and the 500-Hz frequency line.

Transmission losses for some types of partitions are shown in Table 3.2 (41).

Partitions separating various rooms and spaces can be of the single-leaf or two-leaf (multiple-layered) type. A single-leaf partition has both exposed faces rigidly connected and moves essentially as a unit. Such are homogeneous panels, brick and concrete block walls, solid or hollow-core concrete partitions, or glass or plaster panels. Sandwich type of construction, if the connection between the two faces is rigid, also belongs to this category. The two-leaf partitions consist of two single leafs a few centimeters apart and with the minimum structural connection between them. Multiple layered partitions have several such layers.

The sound transmission loss of a single-leaf partition increases as the mass increases, according to the so-called "mass law" (Rule 7). As was shown before, the mass reactance increases proportionally with the mass and frequency. However, the mass law holds only between about the lowest natural resonance frequency of the panel and the frequency at which the "coincidence effect," or "coincidence

Table 3.2.
Transmission loss in decibels for common building constructions.[a]

No.	Material	Total thickness (inch)	(cm)	125	250	500	1K	2K	4K	STC rating	IIC rating
						Frequency (Hz)					
Walls[b,c]											
1.	Solid concrete	3	8	35	40	44	52	59	64	47	—[d]
2.	Concrete (6, 15), layers of plaster	7	18	39	42	50	58	64	66	53	—
3.	Concrete wall (6, 15), wood-wool + plaster on furring	10	25	31	40	52	58	60	60	52	—
4.	Solid concrete blocks, layers of plaster	16	41	50	54	59	65	71	68	63	—
5.	Brick (4.5, 11), layers of plaster	5.5	14	34	34	41	50	56	58	42	—
6.	Brick (9, 23), layers of plaster	10	25	41	43	49	55	57	59	52	—
7.	Brick (12, 30) without plaster	12	31	45	44	52	58	60	61	56	—
8.	Stone (24, 61), layers of plaster	25	64	50	53	52	58	61	68	56	—
9.	Hollow concrete block wall	12	34	47	43	45	52	54	56	48	—
10.	Hollow concrete block	6	15	32	33	40	48	51	48	43	—
11.	Cinder block (4, 10), layer of plaster	5.25	13	36	37	44	51	55	62	46	—
12.	Cement block painted at both sides	3.75	10	40	40	40	48	55	56	44	—
13.	Hollow gypsum block (3, 8), layers of plaster	4	10	39	34	38	43	48	46	40	—
14.	Hollow gypsum block (3, 8), resilient one side, plaster	5	13	38	37	44	51	56	59	46	—
15.	Hollow gypsum block (4, 10), gypsum lath + resilient clips	6	15	25	37	46	53	56	63	47	—
16.	Hollow concrete (9.25, 23), layers of fiberboard	10.25	27	41	42	47	51	52	39	43	—
17.	Double brick (4.5, 11) wall, cavity (2, 5), layer of plaster	12	31	37	41	48	60	60	61	49	—
18.	Double brick (4.5, 11) wall, cavity (6, 15), layer of plaster	18	46	48	54	58	64	69	75	62	—
19.	Wooden studs (4, 10), gypsum wallboards	5	13	22	30	35	40	41	40	39	—
20.	Wooden studs (4, 10), gypsum laths + plaster layers	5.75	15	32	36	42	48	48	62	46	—
21.	Steel truss studs (3.75, 8), metal lath, plaster	5.25	13	30	28	35	40	43	53	39	—
22.	Steel truss studs (3.75, 8), double layers gypsum boards	4.75	12	35	38	44	50	50	51	48	—
23.	Metal channel studs (1.625, 4), gypsum wallboards	2.625	7	20	30	38	47	48	45	39	—
24.	Solid sanded gypsum plaster	2	5	36	28	35	39	48	52	36	—

Table 3.2.—(Continued)

No.	Material	Total thickness (inch)	(cm)	Frequency (Hz) 125	250	500	1K	2K	4K	STC rating	IIC rating
25.	Solid sanded gypsum plaster with metal channels	2	5	35	25	32	38	47	54	36	—
26.	Solid gypsum core movable partition	2.25	6	34	34	37	38	39	45	36	—
Floors-Ceilings											
1.	Reinforced concrete slab	4	10	48	42	45	55	57	66	44	25
2.	Reinforced concrete as above + carpeting and pad	4.5	11	48	42	45	55	57	66	44	80
3.	Reinforced concrete slab (6, 15), layer of plaster	7.5	19	42	39	44	49	54	60	47	31
4.	Concrete (4.5, 11), wood flooring, layer of plaster	7	18	35	37	42	49	58	62	46	47
5.	Concrete (4.375, 11), screed, suspended plaster ceiling	10	25	38	41	45	52	57	59	48	47
6.	Concrete (6, 15), wood, battens floating on glass wool, layer of plaster	9.5	24	38	44	52	55	60	65	55	57
7.	Concrete (6, 15) with hollow blocks, wood on screed, plaster	8.165	21	40	42	46	52	58	60	50	48
8.	Concrete (5.5, 14), floating floor, suspended ceiling	15.25	38	40	46	54	59	62	68	55	53
9.	Hollow tile beam (5, 13), screed + linoleum, plaster	6.75	17	36	40	43	49	55	60	47	40
10.	Hollow concrete slab (6, 15), cement mortar + cement finish, plaster	7.5	19	39	38	43	49	54	57	46	30
11.	Concrete channel slab, sand cement finish	6.25	16	34	34	38	46	55	61	42	32
12.	Ribbed concrete (7.25, 18) screed, wooden lath + plaster	9.50	24	33	37	42	52	58	62	46	42
13.	Hollow concrete beam (6, 15), screed + floor, plaster	7.50	19	32	41	43	44	54	64	45	31
14.	Wooden joists (8, 20), floor, gypsum wallboard	9.50	24	19	24	31	35	45	42	34	32
15.	Wooden joists (7, 18), wood + linoleum, reeds + plaster	9.50	24	24	27	35	44	52	58	39	40
16.	Wooden joists (10, 25), paperboard + pad + carpet, wallboard	12.5	32	27	32	38	44	49	60	38	57

Table 3.2.—(Continued)

No.	Material	Total thickness (inch)	(cm)	Frequency (Hz) 125	250	500	1K	2K	4K	STC rating	IIC rating
Windows											
1.	Sliding, aluminum frame	0.09375[e]	0.2	10	14	17	18	18	20	—	—
2.	Projected (awning), aluminum frame, exceptionally good weather strip	0.09375[e]	0.2	16	22	25	28	32	28	—	—
3.	Double window 0.09375,[e] 0.2), air-space (0.1875, 0.5)	0.375	1.0	18	21	19	24	27	18	—	—
4.	As (3) with a storm window, air-space (2, 5)	2.375	6.0	16	24	27	33	37	29	—	—
Doors											
1.	Hollow-core flush, 30 lb (6.7 kg)	1.75	4	11	16	16	16	21	23	—	—
2.	Solid-core flush, 95 lb (21.1 kg)	1.75	4	20	25	23	25	25	28	—	—

[a] Reproduced with permission from Nábělek AK, Nábělek IV: Noise control by acoustical treatment. In Lipscomb DM, Taylor AC Jr., Noise Control: Handbook of Principles and Practices, (eds): New York, Van Nostrand Reinhold, 1978 (41).
[b] Numbers in parentheses indicate thickness of layer, in inches and centimeters, respectively.
[c] Data for walls and floors-ceilings from Berendt et al., 1967. Data for windows and doors from Bishop and Hirtle, 1968.
[d] Not applicable.
[e] Conventionally described as 3/32 inch.

Table 3.3
Sound absorption coefficients for common materials.[a]

No.	Material	Frequency (Hz)						NCR rating
		125	250	500	1K	2K	4K	
Walls								
1	Brick	0.03	0.03	0.03	0.04	0.05	0.07	0.05
2	Concrete painted	0.10	0.05	0.06	0.07	0.09	0.08	0.05
3	Window glass	0.35	0.25	0.18	0.12	0.07	0.04	0.15
4	Marble	0.01	0.01	0.01	0.01	0.02	0.02	0.00
5	Plaster on concrete	0.12	0.09	0.07	0.05	0.05	0.04	0.05
6	Plywood	0.28	0.22	0.17	0.09	0.10	0.11	0.15
7	Concrete block, coarse	0.36	0.44	0.31	0.29	0.39	0.25	0.35
8	Heavyweight drapery	0.14	0.35	0.55	0.72	0.70	0.65	0.60
9	Fiberglass wall treatment, 1 in (2.5 cm)	0.08	0.32	0.99	0.76	0.34	0.12	0.60
10	Fiberglass wall treatment, 7 in (17.8 cm)	0.86	0.99	0.99	0.99	0.99	0.99	0.95
11	Wood paneling on glass fiber blanket	0.40	0.90	0.80	0.50	0.40	0.30	0.65
Floors								
1	Wood parquet on concrete	0.04	0.04	0.07	0.06	0.06	0.07	0.05
2	Linoleum	0.02	0.03	0.03	0.03	0.03	0.02	0.05
3	Carpet on concrete	0.02	0.06	0.14	0.37	0.60	0.65	0.30
4	Carpet on foam rubber padding	0.08	0.24	0.57	0.69	0.71	0.73	0.55
Ceilings								
1	Plaster, gypsum, or lime on lath	0.14	0.10	0.06	0.05	0.04	0.03	0.05
2	Acoustic tiles 0.625 in (1.6 cm), suspended 16 in (40.6 cm) from ceiling	0.25	0.28	0.46	0.71	0.86	0.93	0.60
3	Acoustic tiles 0.5 in (1.2 cm), suspended 16 in (40.6 cm) from ceiling	0.52	0.37	0.50	0.69	0.79	0.78	0.60
4	The same as (3), but cemented directly to ceiling	0.10	0.22	0.61	0.66	0.74	0.72	0.55
5	Highly absorptive panels, 1 in (2.5 cm), suspended 16 in (40.6 cm)	0.58	0.88	0.75	0.99	1.00	0.96	0.90
Others								
1	Upholstered seats	0.19	0.37	0.56	0.67	0.61	0.59	0.55
2	Audience in upholstered seats	0.39	0.57	0.80	0.94	0.92	0.87	0.80
3	Grass	0.11	0.26	0.60	0.69	0.92	0.99	0.61
4	Soil	0.15	0.25	0.40	0.55	0.60	0.60	0.45
5	Water surface	0.01	0.01	0.01	0.02	0.02	0.03	0.00

[a] Reproduced from data from American Board Products Association, 1975 (43).

dip" appears. The natural resonance frequency of the partition is given by its mass and stiffness. The coincidence dip occurs around the frequency at which the wavelength of free bending waves in the partition coincides with the wavelength of sound in air. The width of the dip depends on the homogeneity of the material and its internal damping.

Ideally, the coincidence dip should be either above or below the frequency range in which good sound insulation is required. Thick, dense, concrete or brick walls have such dips below that range, lightweight masonry partitions may have the dips in the midfrequency range.

Masonry walls are often porous. Therefore, they should be plastered or sealed with block sealers.

High sound insulation by a single-leaf partition would require a very massive construction. For each doubling of the mass of the partition, only 4–5 dB increase in insulation could be obtained. Two leafs completely separated should provide a doubling of insulation achieved by one-leaf partition. Such an increase of insulation cannot be achieved, because some coupling between the two leaves with reasonable spacing always exists. Even if no structural coupling is present, the air space between the leaves provides an elastic connection between them. In general, the increase of TL with respect to one-leaf partition is substantial. The sound insulation of a two-leaf partition is determined by the properties of each leaf and by the coupling between them.

Absorption material between the leaves contribute somewhat to sound insulation. The density of such material is not important as much as its thickness. A blanket of fiberglass, mineral wool, or similar porous material, may improve the rating by about 5 dB. However, even this contribution to insulation may be reduced if the framing is rigid and provides a secondary transmission path between the two leaves.

Composite partitions have components with various values of TL. It should be emphasized that the overall attenuation of sound by a structure is determined by its weakest component. If one component is a poor insulator, then the other components do not need to be excellent insulators either (43, 45).

Noises passing into a room through a partition and the noises created in the room, itself, are reflected from the walls, ceiling and floor. Therefore, the sound power in the room is increased. By absorbing incident sound energy at the walls, etc., the sound pressure level in the room can be reduced (Rule 17).

Absorption of Sound

The absorption of sound is a phenomenon in which the sound energy is dissipated into heat by friction between the particles of the media and absorptive material. The absorptive unit is sabine; it is the absorption of an open window of 1 m² area. The sound absorption coefficient is defined as the ratio of energy which is not reflected back by the surface and the incident energy. It depends on frequency. The noise reduction coefficient (NRC)—do not confuse with "noise reduction" defined above—is the arithmetic average of absorption coefficients for 0.25, 0.5, 1.0, and 2.0 kHz.

Absorption coefficients of some materials are shown in Table 3.3.

In general, high frequencies are absorbed more than low frequencies. Sometimes, proper balance of wide range absorption requires special provision for low frequency absorption. This can be achieved by using wooden panels mounted a certain distance from the wall and with absorptive material in the space so created. Such panels represent damped resonators. Their resonance frequency is determined by the thickness (mass) of the panel, and by the compliance of the panel and of the air space behind the panel (that means, by the distance from the wall).

Carpets on the floor primarily reduce the surface-generated noise of footsteps. They are good absorbers for high frequency air-borne sound, but poor ones for low frequency sounds.

The noise reduction by absorption (NR_A) inside the enclosure can reach up to 15 dB.

The ceiling and the upper parts of the walls are usually the most appropriate places for location of absorbers. The mounting of absorbers influences absorption efficiency. Direct application to the surface by adhesives results in poor absorption at low frequencies. In the form of suspended ceilings they provide absorption balanced over a large frequency range (45, 46).

Barriers

Complete enclosure of the noise source or of the receiver is often not possible. In such a case barriers are introduced between the source and the receiver. Barriers can protect whole residential areas against highway traffic noise, protect the operator from the machinery noise, or separate (acoustically and visually) groups of people in open-space type of offices and schools.

The effectiveness of the barrier depends on its dimensions, its location relative to the source and receiver, on the surrounding terrain, and on the frequencies of the sound. As mentioned before, when the size of the barrier is smaller than the wavelength of the sound, diffraction occurs and the barrier is not effective. The effectiveness of the barrier increases when it is placed close to the sound source, especially when the side facing the noise source is sound absorptive, and when the tip of the barrier is high above the line of sight between source and receiver.

The barriers for open-plan offices should be at least 1.5 m high and 2.5 m wide if they are to be effective for separation of sitting persons. The barriers should extend to the floor and be tied to the walls or other dividers to reduce vertical leaks. The ceiling above the barriers should be sound absorptive to reduce the sound connection between the two places by reflections.

The attenuation of 5 dB by a solid barrier is rather common. A good design can provide around 10-dB attenuation. It is unlikely that 15 dB noise reduction could be exceeded.

SUMMARY

At the beginning of the chapter, a short outline of physical characteristics of noise and of acoustic events related to sound propagation in air are discussed, and concepts of sound pressure levels and of frequency spectra of sound are introduced. In the section on measurement of sound, sound level meters, noise dosimeters, vibration meters, various types of recorders (graphic and magnetic tape), frequency analyzers, time-domain analyzers, amplitude distribution analyzers and sound intensity meters are described. This description is followed by the section on calibration of the measuring equipment,

and by the section on techniques of sound measurement. Criteria are introduced which should be applied to the choice of instrumentation, what to measure (various noise descriptors are defined here), where to measure, when to measure, and how to report the results of noise survey measurements.

In the section on noise control, prevention and noise reduction are discussed. Considerations for new facilities as well as old facilities are listed and methods to reduce noise are suggested. Means are described which are effective in reduction of vibration transfer from the source into the structure, and of the sound into the air. The chapter ends with the role of partitions and barriers in noise control.

References

1. Kryter ID Concepts of perceived noisiness, their implementation and application. *J Acoust Soc Am* 43:344–361, 1968
2. Stevens SS: Perceived level of noise by Mark VII and decibels (E). *J Acoust Soc Am* 51:575–601, 1972.
3. Erlandsson B, Hakanson H, Ivarsson A, Nilsson P: Noise dose measurements with stationary and ear-borne microphones. In Ivarsson A, Nilsson P (eds): *Advances in Measurement of Noise and Hearing.* Malmo, Sweden, Litos Reprotryck, 1980.
4. Randall RB: *Application of B & K Equipment To Frequency Analysis.* Naerum, Denmark. Brüel & Kjaer. 1977.
5. Thrane N: The discrete fourier transform and FFT analyzers. *B K Technol Rev* No. 1. 1979.
6. Thrane, N: Zoom-FFT. *B K Technol Rev* No. 2. 1980.
7. Randall, RB, Hee, J: Cepstrum analysis. *B K Technol Rev* No. 3, 1981.
8. Griffiths, ID, Langdon FJ: Subjective response to road traffic noise. *Sound Vibration* 8, No 1: 16–32, 1968.
9. Robinson DW: An outline guide to criteria for the limitation of urban noise. *National Physical Laboratory Aero Report AC.* Tebbington, England, National Physical Laboratory, Aerodynamics Division, 1969.
10. Jensen P: Community noise. In Lipscomb DM (ed): *Noise and Audiology,* Baltimore, University Park Press, 1978, p 245.
11. Gade S: Sound intensity. *B K Technol Rev* No. 3. 1982.
12. Upton R: Sound intensity—a powerful new measurement tool. *Sound Vibration* 16, No 10:10–18, 1982.
13. Roth O: *A Sound Intensity Real Time Analyzer.* Senlis Congress on Sound Intensity. Naerum, Denmark, Brüel & Kjaer, 1981.

14. Hynes GM: How to select a low-priced sound level meter. *Sound Vibration* 17:20–22, 1983.

15. Boston DW, Cashar EE, Cope DA, Glover BM Jr: A computer system for aircraft flyover acoustic data acquisition and analysis, D6-51888. Seattle, Boeing Co., 1983.

16. Eshleman RL: Machinery diagnostics and your FFT. *Sound Vibration* 17, No 4:12–18, 1983.

17. Sapy G: Une application du traitement numerique des signaux au diagnostic vibratoire de panne: la detection des ruptures d'aubes mobiles de turbines. *Automatisme* 20:392–399, 1975.

18. Syed AA, Brown JD, Oliver MJ, Hills SA: The Cepstrum: available method for the removal of ground reflections. *J. Sound Vib* 71:299–313, 1980.

19. Young RW: Measurement of noise level and exposure. In Chalupnik JD (ed): *Transportation noises; A Symposium on Acceptability Criteria.* Seattle, University of Washington Press, 1970, 45–58.

20. Robinson DW: Towards a unified system of noise assessment. *Sound Vibration* 14:279–298, 1971.

21. Pearsons KS, Bennett RL: *Handbook of Noise Ratings.* Washington, D.C., National Aeronautics and Space Administration Report NASA CR-2376, 1974.

22. Schultz TJ: Noise assessment guidelines: technical background. Washington, D.C., Department of Housing and Urban Development Report TE/NA 172, 1971.

23. Goldstein J: Fundamental concepts in sound measurement. In Lipscomb DM (ed): *Noise and Audiology.* Baltimore, University Park Press, 1978, p 3.

24. Peterson APG: *Handbook of Noise Measurement.* Concord, Mass, GenRad, 1980.

25. Sperry WC: Aircraft and airport noise. In Lipscomb DM, Taylor AC (eds): *Noise Control Handbook of Principles and Practices.* New York, Van Nostrand Reinhold, 1978.

26. Williams K: An introduction to the assessment and measurement of sound. In Lipscomb DM, Taylor AC (eds): *Noise Control Handbook of Principles and Practices.* New York, Van Nostrand Reinhold, 1978.

27. Kurze U, Beranek LL: Sound propagation outdoors. In Beranek LL (ed): *Noise and Vibration Control.* New York, McGraw-Hill, 1971.

28. Desormeaux J: Field assessment of highway noise barriers. *Sound Vibration* 16, No 12:23–25, 1982

29. Federal Aviation Administration. *Federal Aviation Regulations, Part 36-Noise Standards: Aircraft type certification,* Washington, D.C. FAA, Department of Transportation, 1978.

30. International Civil Aviation Organization: *Environmental Protection, Vol. 1, Aircraft Noise.* International Standards and Recommended Practices, Annex 16 to the Convention on International Civil Aviation. Montreal, Canada, ICAO, 1981.

31. Harnapp VR, Noble AG: Time variations in urban traffic noise—a case study in Akron, Ohio. *Sound Vibration* 16, No 12:20–22, 1982.

32. Pleeck D, Petersen EC: *Real Time Sound Intensity Measurements Performed with an Analog and Portable Instrument.* Senlis Congress on Sound Intensity. Naerum, Denmark, Brüel & Kjaer, 1981.

33. Lang GF: Using sound to measure vibration. *Sound Vibration* 16, No 11:8–10, 1982.

34. Smiley RG: Vibration and performance testing with small digital test systems. *Sound Vibration* 16, No 4:8–15, 1982.

35. Harris CM (ed): *Handbook of Noise Control.* New York, McGraw-Hill, 1979.

36. American Industrial Hygiene Association: *Industrial Noise Manual.* Akron, Ohio, AIHA, 1975.

37. American Foundrymen's Society: *Control of Noise.* Des Plaines, Ill, AFS, 1980.

38. National Institute for Occupational Safety and Health: *Compendium of Materials for Noise Control.* Superintendent of Documents, U.S. Government Printing Office, Washington, D.C., 1975.

39. Gray DE: *American Institute of Physics Handbook,* ed 3. New York, McGraw Hill, 1972, p 2.

40. Eriksson LJ, Thawani PT, Hoops RH: Acoustical design and evaluation of silencers. *Sound Vibration* 17, No 7:20–27, 1983.

41. Nábělek AK, Nábělek IV: Noise control by acoustical treatment. In Lipscomb DM, Taylor AC (eds): *Noise Control Handbook of Principles and Practices.* New York, Van Nostrand Reinhold, 1978.

42. Nashif AD: Control of noise and vibration with damping materials. *Sound and Vibration* 17:28–36, 1983.

43. American Board Products Association, *Performance Data Acoustical Materials.* Park Ridge, Ill, ABPA, 1975.

44. Kopec JW; Variations in sound transmission on steel studded, gypsum walls. *Sound Vibration* 16. No 6:10–15. 1982.

45. Berendt RD, Winzer GE, Burroughs CBA: *Guide to Airborne, Impact, and Structure Borne Noise-Control in Multifamily Dwellings.* Washington, D.C., U.S. Dept. of Housing and Urban Development, 1967.

46. Bishop, DE, Hirtle PW: Notes on the sound-transmission loss of residential-type windows and doors. *J Acoust Soc Am* 43:880–882, 1968.

47. Council on Environmental Quality: *Preparation of Environmental Impact Statements: Guidelines.* 38 *Federal Register,* 20550, August 1, 1973.

48. U.S. Department of Agriculture: *Environmental Impact Statements: Proposed Guidelines.* 38 *Federal Register,* 31904, November 19, 1973.

49. U.S. Department of the Army, *Handbook For Environmental Impact Analysis.* Champaign, Ill., Construction Engineering Research Laboratory, April 1974.

CHAPTER 4

Federal Regulations Dealing with Occupational Noise

ALAN S. FELDMAN

BACKGROUND

The safety and health of American workers have been the focus of increasing concern in this country. At both state and federal levels, legislation has evolved which is directed toward such protection. When no minimum standards are established, such as is the case with Workers Compensation (see Chapter 11), rules pertaining to safety and health in the workplace are haphazardly developed from state-to-state. This can even result in the complete absence of statute for worker health and safety protection.

Federal statutes serve to set the pattern for occupational safety and health of workers. Under existing law, individual states may elect to develop safety and health standards as long as they are at least as effective in providing worker protection against safety and health hazards as do standards promulgated under federal auspices. Furthermore, the states may elect not to participate in the enforcement program. In this latter instance, enforcement would be solely the responsibility of the U.S. Department of Labor (DOL). This chapter will not consider those regulations that may be established by particular states which deal with occupational noise and which may exceed federal regulations. The reader should be aware that more stringent rules and regulations may exist in some states.

The problem of hazardous noise in the workplace and resultant occupational hearing loss has only recently been the object of serious federal regulation. Until 1969, although permissive legislation existed, and the damaging effects of noise on hearing were well documented, no specific regulation had been developed which would serve either to limit personal exposure or to monitor the development of noise induced hearing loss.

The longest standing legislation dealing with the protection of the health and safety of the worker is the 1936 Walsh-Healey Public Contracts Act (1). As with other federal statutes addressing the welfare of the worker, development of regulations and their enforcement is under the aegis of the DOL. Within the DOL, responsibility for implementation of the safety and health aspects under the Walsh-Healey Act was assigned to the Bureau of Labor Standards. The first attempt to evolve rules dealing with occupational noise occurred in 1964. At that time, regulations were promulgated which required "reasonable control" of occupational noise exposure in order to minimize fatigue as well as the probability of accidents. From this starting point the long process of evolution of a final standard was initiated. As is the fact today, it was not easy to establish consensus for a regulation, either on the basis of documented scientific evidence or prevailing practice. It was not until 1969 that the Bureau of Labor Standards adopted guidelines for a noise regulation that, in many ways, was the forerunner of todays rule (2).

The Walsh-Healey regulations first specified (a) measurement based on dBA sound level meter readings; (b) a 90 dBA,

8-hr damage risk criterion; (c) the summing of exposures over time; (d) the specification of need for engineering and administrative controls to reduce worker exposure to 90 dBA for an 8-hr period; (e) a halving of exposure-time/intensity trade-off relationship of 5 dB; and (f) the use of personal hearing protective devices when engineering and/or administration controls are not feasible. All of these features continue to exist as components of current regulation.

In 1970, Congress passed a new statute which provided the authority for protection of what amounted to the workforce in general, rather than to the small number of workers covered under the Walsh-Healey legislation. This was the Williams-Steiger Occupational Safety and Health Act (OSHAct) (3). Two rather dramatic differences exist between this legislation and its predecessors. Compliance with established regulations under this statute not only became mandatory, but it applied to the breadth of industries engaged in any facet of interstate commerce. Whereas the old legislation only affected a small number of businesses (industries having government contracts in excess of $10,000), the new legislation impacts on millions of small and large commercial and industrial settings. In fact, there would be very few settings outside of governmental agencies that would not be covered by the regulations promulgated under the aegis of the OSHAct which took effect in April, 1971. Specifically exempted were employees engaged in construction, oil and gas well drilling and servicing operations.

Another important feature of this legislation was the establishment of the National Institute of Occupational Safety and Health (NIOSH). The Institute was provided for within the Department of Health, Education and Welfare (now the Department of Health and Human Services). It is charged with the task of ongoing research in the area of occupational safety and health and for the development of recommendations for new or revised standards pertinent to occupational safety and health. For example, in 1972 NIOSH produced a publication identified as the NIOSH Criteria Document on Occupational Exposure to Noise (4), that provided the background, terminology and theoretical foundations and recommendations for a noise standard. Much of this, in one or another form, served as a basis for what eventually developed as regulation.

During the period of transition following the 1970 enactment of the OSHAct, many of the existing rules originally generated under the Bureau of Labor Standards were carried over under the authority of the newly developed Occupational Safety and Health Administration (OSHA) within the DOL. Enhancement of Public Law 91-596 (OSHAct of 1970) specifically subsumed other safety and health standards previously promulgated through earlier legislation and specified that regulations promulgated under this new act would supercede all previous regulations. The Secretary of the DOL was charged to insure coordination between the OSHAct and other federal laws. Temporary and standing rules and regulations are constantly reviewed and modified or eliminated by OSHA.

REGULATION PROCESS

The process by which regulations are developed in conformity with the OSHAct is detailed in the statute (3) as follows:

Sec. 6. (b) The Secretary may by rule promulgate, modify, or revoke any occupational safety or health standard in the following manner:

(1) Whenever the Secretary, upon the basis of information submitted to him in writing by an interested person, a representative of any organization of employers or employees, a nationally recognized standards-producing organization, the Secretary of Health, Education, and Welfare, the National Institute for Occupational Safety and Health, or a State or political subdivision, or on the basis of information developed by the Secretary or otherwise available to him, determines that a rule should be promulgated in order to serve the

objectives of this Act, the Secretary may request the recommendations of an advisory committee appointed under section 7 of this Act. The Secretary shall provide such an advisory committee with any proposals of his own or of the Secretary of Health, Education, and Welfare, together with all pertinent factual information developed by the Secretary or the Secretary of Health, Education, and Welfare, or otherwise available, including the results of research, demonstrations, and experiments. An advisory committee shall submit to the Secretary its recommendations regarding the rule to be promulgated within ninety days from the date of its appointment or within such longer or shorter period as may be prescribed by the Secretary, but in no event for a period which is longer than two hundred and seventy days.

(2) The Secretary shall publish a proposed rule promulgating, modifying, or revoking an occupational safety or health standard in the *Federal Register* and shall afford interested persons a period of thirty days after publication to submit written data or comments. Where an advisory committee is appointed and the Secretary determines that a rule should be issued, he shall publish the proposed rule within sixty days after the submission of the advisory committee's recommendations or the expiration of the period prescribed by the Secretary for such submission.

(3) On or before the last day of the period provided for the submission of written data or comments under paragraph (2), any interested person may file with the Secretary written objections to the proposed rule, stating the grounds therefor and requesting a public hearing on such objections. Within thirty days after the last day for filing such objections, the Secretary shall publish in the *Federal Register* a notice specifying the occupational safety or health standard to which objections have been filed and a hearing requested, and specifying a time and place for such hearing.

(4) Within sixty days after the expiration of the period provided for the submission of written data or comments under paragraph (2) or within sixty days after the completion of any hearing held under paragraph (3), the Secretary shall issue a rule promulgating, modifying, or revoking an occupational safety or health standard or make a determination that a rule should not be issued. Such a rule may contain a provision delaying its effective date for such period (not in excess of ninety days) as the Secretary determines may be necessary to insure that affected employers and employees will be informed of the existence of the standard and of its terms and that employers affected are given an opportunity to familiarize themselves and their employees with the existence of the requirements of the standard.

(5) The Secretary, in promulgating standards dealing with toxic materials or harmful physical agents under this subsection, shall set the standard which most adequately assures, to the extent feasible, on the basis of the best available evidence, that no employee will suffer material impairment of health or functional capacity even if such employee has regular exposure to the hazard dealt with by such standard for the period of his working life. Development of standards under the subsection shall be based upon research, demonstrations, experiments, and such other information as may be appropriate. In addition to the attainment of the highest degree of health and safety protection for the employee, other considerations shall be the latest available scientific data in the field, the feasibility of the standards, and experience gained under this and other health and safety laws. Whenever practicable, the standard promulgated shall be expressed in terms of objective criteria and of the performance desired.

DEVELOPMENT OF THE OCCUPATIONAL NOISE EXPOSURE RULE

With its inception, OSHA adopted the preexisting rules regarding occupational noise exposure until such time as a comprehensive final rule could be developed (5). The process of finalizing the occupational noise rule took approximately 12 yr, from April 1971 to March 1983. As noted above, a major thrust was generated in 1972 with the NIOSH Criteria Document. This was followed by recommendations from a DOL Standards Advisory Committee on Noise. This committee deliberated for over 1 yr and submitted its recommendations to the OSHA. Pursuant to the requirements for rule promulgation, in October 1974 a proposed rule was published in the *Federal Register* (6). This was followed by a prolonged period of comment. Public testimony was offered by a variety of interested parties including industry, labor, the scientific community, and the public in general. Over the years the public record on this topic became so large as to be almost meaningless. The record contains in excess of 40,000 pages of public comment.

During this period a rule was always in place (29 CFR 1910.95). However, it was essentially the 1969 Walsh-Healey rule, which was basically a vague performance standard without objective criteria and left questions about many facets of compliance—such as how often, by whom, how, or even if at all, hearing testing must be performed. It stated the need for a hearing conservation program (HCP) but did not establish criteria for one. Specifically, 29 CFR 1910.95 has always stated:

(a) Protection against the effects of noise exposure shall be provided when the sound levels exceed that shown in Table G-16 (see Table 4.1) when measured on the A scale of a standard sound level meter at slow response

(b) [1] When employees are subjected to sound exceeding those listed in Table G-16 (see Table 4.1), feasible administrative or engineering controls shall be utilized. If such levels fail to reduce sound within the levels of Table G-16 (see Table 4.1), personal protective equipment shall be provided and used to reduce sound levels within the levels of the table

[2] If the variations in noise level involve maximum at intervals of 1 second or less, it is to be considered continuous

[3] In all cases where the sound levels exceed the values shown herein, a continuing effective hearing conservation program shall be administered

Table 4.1.
Permissible exposure time by intensity in dB sound pressure level (SPL)

Exposure in hours	SPL
8	90
6	92
4	95
3	97
2	100
1.50	102
1	105
0.50	110
0.25 or less	115

The debate over the details of the ultimate rule continued for another 6 yr. In January 1981 there was published in the *Federal Register* what was supposed to have been the final rule specifying in detail the specific features in of a HCP for noise exposed employees (7). Other components of the rule were left intact. The timing coincided with a change in presidential administrations, and the rule was stayed pending another review, this time by the incoming Reagan administration. This was followed by an opportunity for additional comment which further engorged the public record.

In August of 1981, parts of the regulation were put in place (8), but others were stayed, and further study still was deemed necessary before the stayed elements of the rule could be dealt with. Finally, on March 9, 1983, the revised Occupational Noise Exposure; Hearing Conservation Amendment, Final Rule was published in the *Federal Register* (9). It reflected the new administration's goal of reducing some of its specificity and placing greater emphasis on a performance standard which allows for achieving compliance in a more discretionary manner. Goals are specified but the routes by which the goals may be reached are, in many instances, discretionary. The newly published section is an amendment to the previously (October 1974) published 29 CFR 1910.95, and it became effective on April 7, 1983. The entire rule 29 CFR 1910.95 is detailed in Appendix I.

FEATURES OF THE OCCUPATIONAL NOISE EXPOSURE RULE

The high degree of interest that surrounded the developments leading to promulgation of the Hearing Conservation Amendment sometimes obscured the fact that the already existing standard (parts a and b) had continued to be in effect, and that a permissible noise exposure level and requirements for engineering controls, or personal hearing protection when engineering control was not feasible, had already been established and put in place. It is important for the professional, as well as for industry, to bear in mind that the final rule still requires the employer to reduce employee exposure to below 90 dBA by the use of feasible engineering controls or administrative controls. While the OSHA is presently reviewing this aspect of the standard, it is in effect, and a full industrial occupational noise program must demonstrate that it has paid attention, not only to measurement of employee exposure, but also to the possibility of adopting feasible engineering or administrative controls to reduce exposure.

In 1983, OSHA did issue instructions to its field compliance officers that seemed to imply citations would not be issued when engineering or administrative control costs were in excess of the costs of an effective HCP and when hearing protectors may reliably reduce the noise level at the ear to below 90 dBA. The use of hearing protection was not deemed reliable when noise levels border on 100 dBA (10).

A major impact of the amendment was to insure inclusion of employees whose noise exposure equaled or exceeded a time-weighted average exposure of 85 dBA within the HCP. This had been included in the 1974 proposal but had not been finalized. The old rule had set 90 dBA as the action level for inclusion. The overall effect of the amendment was not to remove the previous elements of the standard regarding the engineering and administrative controls or the necessity for a HCP but, rather, it augmented the existing standard and detailed a number of specific goals and requirements that needed to be included in HCPs.

Many of the elements of an occupational noise exposure program were previously among the debatable issues. They fundamentally deal with (a) monitoring of employee noise exposure, (b) the responsibility for the professional supervision of the HCP as a whole, (c) the audiometric testing programs, (d) the identification and qualifications of personnel involved in the program, (e) the selection and use of personal hearing potective devices (HPDs) as a means of minimizing exposure, (f) employee education and training programs and (g) the maintenance of records detailing the features of the HCP.

The flow chart depicted in Figure 4.1 exemplifies the steps that any program must follow in order to be in compliance with existing regulations. It should be noted that, while the damage risk criteria in the occupational noise rule remains at 90 dBA, the action level is 85 dBA. This represents a 50% dose and is intended to serve as an added measure of protection. It means that employees exposed to a time-weighted average (TWA) of 85 dB measured on the A scale of a sound level meter for an 8-hr work period shall be included in the program. The rule continues to assume a 5 dB exchange rate for doubling or halving of exposure.

MONITORING OF NOISE LEVELS

The monitoring of existing noise levels and employee exposure to the noise levels is considered in some detail in the regulation. The existence of work place noise is only a matter of importance when there is exposure to the noise. Monitoring of the noise exposure is to be done in a manner which will accurately identify those employees exposed at or above an 85 dBA, 8-hr TWA. Included in the measurement of exposure must be all noise generated between 80 to 130 dBA. The choice of monitoring technique is left to the employer depending upon the uniqueness of the particular situation. In all instances, employees or their representatives are entitled to observe monitoring and, regardless of whether or not monitoring is observed, employees must be advised of the results of the exposure monitoring whenever exposure exceeds the action level (85 dBA). The method of notification is unspecified and the posting of warning signs is optional.

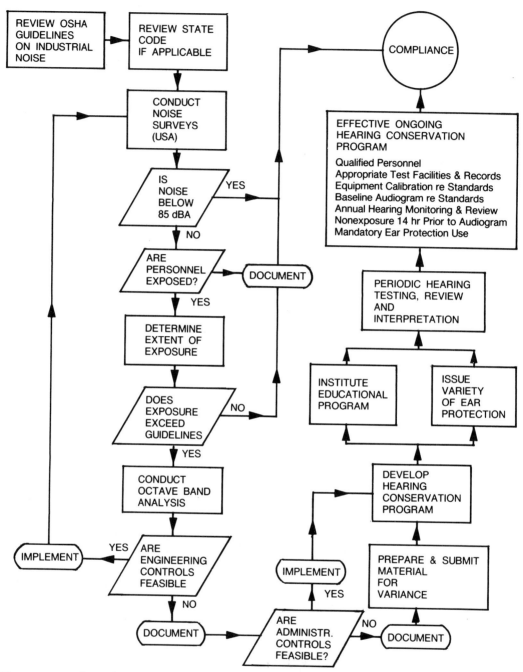

Figure 4.1. Flow chart to be followed to determine compliance with occupational noise exposure regulations and determining the need for a hearing conservation program. (Reproduced by courtesy of Environmental Hearing and Vision Consultants, Ltd., E. Syracuse, NY).

The relationship between dose and TWA is displayed in Table 4.2.

To establish the dose in percent the following formula is applied:

$$\text{Dose } (D) = 100(C1/T1 + C2/T2 +, \ldots, Cn/Tn)$$

where Cn is the actual duration of exposure at a specific level and Tn is the permissible exposure time at that level.

The conversion from Dose (D) to TWA is given by:

$$\text{TWA} = 16.61 \log 10\ (D/100) + 90.$$

Table 4.2.
Sample of conversion between dose (%) and TWA (dB) expressed in the nearest dB.[a]

Dose	TWA
(%)	(dB)
10	73
25	80
50	85
75	88
100	90
115	91
130	92
150	93
175	94
200	95
400	100

[a] See Appendix I, Table A.1 for a more detailed conversion.

Employee monitoring is a good example of the manner in which the modification of the rule resulted in a more broadly based performance standard rather than a very specific detailed "how to" standard. Employers are entitled to use a variety of techniques and have the choice of applying "worst case" measures to all employees or may, by individual employee monitoring through dosimetery, include only those employees within the program who are identified as having a dose of 50% or greater. Repeated occasions of monitoring are not required if levels of exposure are not considered to have changed.

Monitoring of the noise levels in the work place provides the data which (a) identifies those employees who shall be included in the HCP as a consequence of exposure to 85 dBA or greater for an 8-hr period, (b) identifies employees for whom the use of HPDs is required (exposure to 90 dBA or greater for an 8-hr period), (c) establishes how much attenuation HPDs must provide, and (d) acts as a means of acquainting both employers and employees with the degree of noise hazard.

TYPES OF MONITORING

There are two fundamental types of noise monitoring approaches: (a) personal sampling and (b) area sampling. The former may be achieved through dosimetry or sound level meter readings, although dosimetry is far more accurate in establishing the actual individual exposure. Because employees are not immobile during the work day, they may be subject to wide fluctuations in exposure that may not be accurately reflected when monitored with a nonintegrating device such as a sound level meter. If selective inclusion in the HCP is to be based on individual monitoring, then dosimetry would appear to be the procedure of choice.

Selective inclusion within a program presents numerous monitoring obstacles and management problems. For example, it is difficult to monitor employee compliance when some employees are required to wear HPDs while others are not. It also results in lower worker morale when seemingly different rules are applied to some workers. Furthermore, changes in exposure due to worker mobility, changing job responsibilities (bumping), work load changes, and similar variables make it advisable that broader criteria for inclusion within the program be adopted.

As a result, area monitoring with a sound level meter is often selected by management as the procedure by which to identify those groups of workers to be included in the HCP. This procedure allows for a mapping of noise zones which can be flagged as hazard areas and employees within them are automatically included within the HCP. The extreme of this approach would be to use a worst case approach whereby the highest exposure measures are applied to all potentially exposed employees. In fact, this procedure is frequently used because it is the easiest to administer. There is no question that area monitoring is less costly than individual dosimetry. Application of the worst case approach with either individual monitoring or area monitoring can result in a more expensive program because it will be overly protective and include employees whose exposure does not exceed the criterion level of 85 dBA. However, it may actually be administratively easier and result in better employer compliance. Depending on workforce size, fluctuation in noise levels across different locations and other factors, management may opt for more protective programs than the minimum specified by the OSHA standard. It is important to weigh enforcement and compliance considerations along with cost considerations before deciding on the specificity of the monitoring approach management may select.

PROFESSIONAL SUPERVISION

Earlier proposals included hearing testing and other HCP features under the rubric of medical surveilance. This was to distinguish it from the engineering and administrative controls component. The final document, which includes both a lengthy preamble and rule, established the HCP as the umbrella for the program which includes professional supervision of the hearing testing. The preamble provides insight into OSHA's intent and expands and clarifies the concise phraseology of the regulation. It is clear from this document that the technician in the HCP is to be responsible to qualified professionals. These professionals are defined as audiologists, otolaryngologists or other physicians. Presumably the latter would be physicians well versed in hearing and hearing conservation. Supervisory responsibility of the professionals extends well beyond the supervision of persons performing the audiometric test. It includes judgements about test validity, work relatedness, existence of standard threshold shift (STS), stability of the STS, establishing referral criteria and numerous other professional judgements and decisions about the HCP. It could include all phases of the program, with the possible exception of engineering, noise control and reduction, and noise measurement and monitoring. Depending upon qualifications and interests, some of these latter may also be under the auspices of the above specified professionals.

AUDIOMETRIC TESTING PROGRAMS

Annual audiometric testing at the employer's expense is a required component of HCPs. The rule specifies that baseline audiograms be offered to all employees exposed to a TWA of 85 dBA or above. The *baseline* audiogram serves as the reference threshold with which subsequent *annual* monitoring audiograms are compared. In theory, protected employees will demonstrate no progressive hearing loss as a consequence of exposure to hazardous workplace noise.

The *original* audiogram is that audiogram obtained either at the onset of the HCP or, in the case of new or previously unexposed employees, prior to or within 6 months of placement in an area with noise identified as being at or above the action level (85 dBA). While at the outset they will be identical, it is likely that over time the original and baseline audiograms will cease to be the same. The professional who reviews the audiograms may update the baseline audiogram when changes in threshold are deemed to be persistent. In such an instance, a more current annual audiogram may be substituted for the earlier baseline audiogram. The new baseline may reflect thresholds that are better or worse, whatever the case may be, for individual employees.

The rule does allow new employees to not be tested for a 6-month period for in-house programs and 12 months when annual testing is performed by mobile vans. The latter is only permissible when hearing protection is worn by noise-exposed employees, at least for the period after the first 6 months. The prudent employer will recognize that other considerations may enter into the decision to defer testing for a full year. Workers compensation rules (see Chapter 11) sometimes make it appropriate to notify a prior employer of a pre-existing hearing loss found in a new employee. Notification to the prior employer of such a preexisting condition must usually occur within 90 days of exposure in order to establish liability. Thus, delaying the first hearing test for as long as 6 months, let alone 12 months, would hardly be advisable, even though it is permissible under OSHA regulations.

EQUIPMENT AND ENVIRONMENT FOR AUDIOMETRIC TESTING

The rule does specify standards for equipment performance and calibration background noise and personnel as well as for follow-up. The requirement that hearing baseline testing be performed following a 14-hr period of nonexposure to noise (both occupational and nonoccupational) may be satisfied through the use of HPDs. Although it is not professionally advocated, according to the regulation, the annual audiograms need not be preceded by a noise-free period. Presumably the nonprotective condition would exaggerate the effect of exposure.

Audiometers must meet ANSI standards (American National Standard Specifications for Audiometers, S3.6-1969) and a functional calibration must be performed prior to use each day. Deviation in listening checks or changes in thresholds of 10 dB or greater would require an acoustic calibration. In any event, an acoustic calibration is an annual requirement, and an exhaustive calibration must be performed at least every 2 years. The details of these requirements are specified in Appendix E of the Hearing Conservation Amendment (9) which is included in Appendix I of this text.

The background noise permitted for audiometric testing must not exceed the limits as noted in Table 4.3.

PERSONNEL QUALIFICATIONS FOR AUDIOMETRIC TESTING

To the professional, one of the major deficiencies in the rule is the lack of spec-

Table 4.3.
Permissible background noise levels specified by 29 CFR 1910.95

	Octave band center frequency				
Hz	500	1000	2000	4000	8000
db SPL	40	40	47	57	62

ification of credentials for those persons performing the hearing testing. Although supervision of the program and responsibility for review of audiograms is properly vested in either an audiologist, otolaryngologist or other physician, the qualification specifications of the technician leave something to be desired. Even the minimal training exemplified by the requirements established by the Council for Accreditation in Occupational Hearing Conservation (CAOHC) as set forth in Chapter 7 are diluted in the current rule which implies all that is needed is the approval of the supervising professional. It is likely, however, that in view of professional liability constraints (Chapter 12), the astute professional will set higher standards for the technicians than does OSHA.

AUDIOMETRIC SPECIFICATIONS AND REVIEW

The audiogram specifications include the requirement that threshold testing for each ear include at least the frequencies 500, 1000, 2000, 3000, 4000, and 6000 Hz. Many programs will choose to also test at 8000 Hz. However, the rule only requires analysis of a change at 2000, 3000 and 4000 Hz. An average change of 10 dB or more at those frequencies is defined as a STS. The average of the threshold shift may be reduced by anticipated hearing loss due to presbycusis. Appendix I includes the presbycusis adjustment table.

The audiometric review and determination of the appropriate course of action is the responsibility of the supervising professional (audiologist, otolaryngologist or other physician). There are no criteria in regulations for hearing loss detected in baseline audiograms. The rule only deals with changes. Most professionals will report losses detected on baseline hearing tests.

While the criteria for determination of an STS are established in the rule along with the specification of some necessary follow-up procedures, as in the case with the credentials of technicians, the responsible professional will, again, be likely to impose additional criteria relating to changes in hearing that may be revealed in an annual audiogram. The qualified and astute professional is well aware of the implied professional liability that would be the consequence of failure to identify and report a potentially debilitating or treatable condition first revealed by a developing hearing loss.

Changes in audiometric threshold frequently act to suggest problems other than noise exposure and such changes should certainly be identified and reported. For this reason, it would be an abrogation of professional responsibility for the professional in charge to permit review by the technician even though regulation is permissive in that regard. The rule only requires "problem" audiograms be reviewed by the professional. The question of whether to seek additional professional consultation following an identified change in the annual audiogram must also be weighed against the likelihood that such consultation would provide additional information. Unproductive follow-up consultations are costly because medical expenses incurred as a consequence of work-related changes in hearing are the responsibility of the employer. The rule does allow for the professional reviewer to interpret the test and provide recommendations without necessitating additional follow-up evaluation. At the same time, the professional might consider additional follow-up to be warranted in some instances. Such recommendations would be based upon professional judgement following a review of the current, baseline and prior hearing tests as well as the history.

EMPLOYEE NOTIFICATION AND RECOMMENDED COURSE OF ACTION

Whatever the criteria established for review by the responsible professional, the employee must be notified in writing within 21 days of the receipt of the report of the professional review. This would include notification about the results of the hearing test and the recommended course of action. Once again, although the rule specifies that only those employees exhibiting a standard threshold shift must be informed in writing of such findings, good management principles dictate that all employees be notified of the test outcome. This is especially true in light of the rule's annual training requirement. The reporting of results can be developed as a component of the training program.

For those employees whose change in hearing is deemed to be a consequence of noise exposure, the rule specifies that they shall be fit (or refit) and instructed (or reinstructed) in the use of hearing protectors. When hearing thresholds are not permanently shifted, as revealed by a lack of persistence of STS on subsequent tests, then use of hearing protection may be discontinued for those employees not exposed in excess of an 8-hr TWA of 90 dBA.

When other than noise-related hearing loss is suspected, the rule provides for referral for additional professional evaluation. This could apply not only when medical conditions may be suspect, but also when other forms of aural rehabilitation (such as a hearing aid) may be considered.

HEARING PROTECTIVE DEVICES

All employees exposed to a TWA of 90 dBA or greater must be included in a mandatory hearing protection usage program. For employees exposed to a TWA of between 85 and 90 dBA, the use of hearing protection is optional but is still at the expense of the employer. The selection of hearing protection shall be such that a variety (muff, plug, disposable, reusable) of suitable protectors is made available.

All employees using HPDs must be properly fit and instructed in their use and care. Reinstruction and refitting is required when an STS is observed on an annual audiogram. Employers are entitled to require payment for the HPDs if employees are negligent in their care. The selected HPDs must provide attenuation that is sufficient to reduce exposure below 90 dB for employees who have not exhibited an STS and 85 dB for those who have.

As with other features of these programs, the monitoring of HPD compliance is a requirement of the employer. Many companies institute an 85 dBA action level for hearing protection usage for all employees in order to facilitate compliance monitoring.

TRAINING PROGRAMS

Perhaps the most crucial feature of the occupational noise regulation is the requirement of an annual training program for all exposed employees. The premise of such a program is that knowledge about the hazard of noise exposure will enhance participation in a program geared toward the prevention of hearing loss.

The annual program must include the following:

(a) The effects of noise on hearing
(b) The purpose of hearing protectors; the advantages and disadvantages and attenuation of various types, and instructions on their selection, fitting, use, and care
(c) The purpose of audiometric testing as well as an explanation of test procedures

The method by which the educational program is offered to the employee is left to the discretion of the employer. Segments may be provided at different times or at a single time each year. It can be via print material, audio visual presentation or lecture/discussion or any combination of these. OSHA recognizes training programs as being a critical step in promoting safety and health programs in the workplace. More than 100 current OSHA standards contain training requirements. In the August 30, 1983 *Federal Register*, OSHA elicited comment on proposed guidelines for training that are designed to educate employees about safety and health in order to reduce risk and enhance safety and health in the workplace (11).

RECORD KEEPING

The record-keeping requirements in the regulation are not extensive. The employer is required to maintain an accurate record of all required employee exposure measurements for a period of 2 yr. Audiometric test records must be retained. Included with the test record must be the employee name and job classification, the date of audiogram, the examiner's name, the audiometer's most recent calibration date (acoustic or exhaustive), the employee's most recent noise exposure assessment, and verification of ambient noise levels during audiometric testing. The employee audiometric test data must be retained for the duration of employment and records shall be accessible to employees or their designee. Most employers will maintain audiometric records longer than the duration of employment. These records may have value in future workers' compensation claims.

PENALTIES

Failure on the part of employers to comply with health and safety rules under the OSHAct does carry penalties that can be quite costly, particularly when violations are uncorrected. In most instances, in establishing the extent of a fine, OSHA will consider whether the employer has exhibited good faith in attempting to comply.

The willful or repeated violation of a standard or order promulgated under the statute may result in a civil penalty of up to $10,000. Citation for a serious or nonserious violation may result in a penalty of up to $1000 for each citation.

Any employer who fails within due time to correct a violation for which a citation has been issued may be assessed a civil penalty of not more than $1000 for each day during which such failure to comply or the violation continues. Employers have recourse to challenge citations and fines through the courts.

MINE SAFETY AND HEALTH ACT

Federal regulations dealing with safety and health, in general, and occupational noise exposure, specifically, are not totally encompassed by the OSHAct. Separate safety and health standards exist for miners. While also under the umbrella of the DOL, they are established and monitored by the Mine Safety and Health Administration (MSHA).

Within MSHA, the administrative structure is such that there are discrete rules established for coal mining on the one hand and all remaining metal and nonmetal mining on the other. The rules pertaining to noise exposure in both instances are quite similar and, while they parallel the general industry noise standard set by OSHA in the area of damage risk criteria (90 dBA), they are presently more performance standard oriented and do not include anything comparable to the OSHA hearing conservation amendment. The specifics of the health standard for coal miners are set forth in CFR 30 parts 70.500–70.511 for underground miners and part 71.800–71.805 for surface miners.

Essential differences are that hearing testing is provided for, but not mandated, although HPDs are mandated when engineering and administrative controls are not feasible. It is anticipated that MSHA regulations will ultimately be more specific in the areas covered by OSHA.

ADDENDUM

As noted in the Preface, the entire Hearing Conservation Amendment Final Rule (8) has been vacated by court order effective November 7, 1984. OSHA petitioned for a review en banc on December 27, 1984. Pending a reversal or a rewriting of the amendment, the components of the HCPs are advised but not mandated.

References

1. Walsh Healy *Public Contracts Acts* Title 41 CFR Chapt. 50, Washington, D.C., 1936.
2. U.S. Department of Labor: Safety and health standards. *Federal Register* 34:96, May 20, 1969 P 7948, Superintendent of Documents, Washington, D.C.
3. Williams-Steiger: *Occupational Safety and Health Act*. Public Law 91-596 Title 29 CFR Chapt. 17, Washington, D.C., 1970.
4. National Institute for Occupational Safety and Health: Criteria for a Recommended Standard for Occupational Exposure to Noise, HSM 73-11001, Department of Health, Education and Welfare, Cincinnati, 1972.
5. U.S. Department of Labor: *Guidelines to the Department of Labor's Occupational Noise Standards for Federal Supply Contracts* (Bulletin 334), Superintendent of Documents, Washington, D.C.
6. Occupational Safety and Health Administration: Proposed requirements for occupational noise exposure. *Federal Register* 39:207, October 24, 1974, p 37773, Superintendent of Documents, Washington, D.C.
7. Occupational Safety and Health Administration: Occupational noise exposure; hearing conservation amendment. *Federal Register* 46:11, January 16, 1981, 4161, Superintendent of Documents, Washington, D.C.
8. Occupational Safety and Health Administration: Occupational noise exposure; hearing conservation amendment; rule and proposed rule. *Federal Register* 46: 162, August 21, 1981, 42632, Superintendent of Documents, Washington, D.C.
9. Occupational Safety and Health Administration: Occupational noise exposure; hearing conservation amendment; final rules. *Federal Register*, 48:46, March 8, 1983, 9776, Superintendent of Documents, Washington, D.C.
10. OSHA Office of Compliance: Assistance Instruction CPL 2-2.35, November, 1983.
11. Occupational Safety and Health Administration: Training guidelines; request for comments and information. *Federal Register*, 48:169, August 30, 1982, p 39317, Superintendent of Documents, Washington, D.C.

CHAPTER 5

Types of Hearing Conservation Programs

ALAN S. FELDMAN

GENERAL FEATURES OF HEARING CONSERVATION PROGRAMS

The OSHA regulations now define the features of a complete occupational noise exposure and hearing conservation program (HCP) (1). The components of HCPs have been well known for many years. (2–4) These have been reviewed at one level in Chapter 4 and are specified in Appendix I. Whenever noise in the workplace cannot be eliminated and has been defined as hazardous, it becomes necessary to:

1. Identify exposed workers
2. Establish the extent of exposure
3. Institute an audiometric testing program for exposed workers
4. Provide for professional review of audiograms and recommendations for the appropriate course of action
5. Provide appropriate personal hearing protection
6. Provide annual educational programs for exposed employees
7. Insure that appropriately qualified personnel are engaged in all facets of the program
8. Establish and maintain an effective record keeping system encompassing all phases of the program

APPROACHES USED TO ACHIEVE COMPLIANCE

A wide range of approaches may be utilized to achieve compliance with the variety of explicit and implicit requirements that stem from these components of a comprehensive HCP. One approach is not necessarily better than another. Individual corporate considerations will dictate the best route for any particular company. It is important that, regardless of the approach selected, due consideration be given to all aspects of the program. This begins with full management support (2) and must be characterized by communication between those charged with responsibility for various phases of the program (5).

The route any particular company may follow ranges from complete internal management and execution of the program to total use of consultative services. In the present chapter we will review the features of programs and the various procedural options available to management. We will also consider some implications of each approach. The selection of a particular approach will, in the end, depend on company size, personnel, operating practices, resources, both internal and external and, to some extent, how the options may have been marketed. The options consist of:

1. In-house programs
2. On-site consultative and mobile services
3. Off-site consultative programs
4. Combinations of the above

MANAGEMENT RESPONSIBILITY

In some instances, no one person within a particular company has the responsibility for the program. This is sometimes accompanied by a lack of understanding about the totality of the program or by poor coordination between the people involved with various phases of the program. Often this may result in some components falling by the wayside or, perhaps, only superficial attention being afforded parts of the program (5). For example, it is common to assume that as long as hearing is tested and hearing protection is made available, the company will be in compliance. Of course such superficiality is not acceptable, and proper attention must be paid to all features of the program both to demonstrate good faith compliance and to achieve program effectiveness.

Regardless of whether or not consultation services are sought to develop and operate an HCP, a decision must be made by someone with administrative authority to initiate the program. Following that point, ongoing management authority may be delegated to yet another individual or individuals. For example, top level management, once convinced that there must be a program, may delegate the entire responsibility to the personnel manager. Or, the responsibility could be split between the medical director or occupational nurse and the industrial hygiene officer. It is not unusual to see the responsibility for HCPs delegated to personnel, safety, hygiene, medicine, or some other similar administrative entity. Within larger corporations having multiple geographic settings, the responsibility could be different at different plant settings. Furthermore, the extent of corporate control could range from complete to nonexistent. In the former instance, all policy decisions are made at the corporate level, while in the latter they are locally developed.

IN-HOUSE PROGRAMS

The larger corporations with fully staffed medical, safety and industrial hygiene departments will frequently choose in-house programs, if not in their entirety, at least for the noise measurement, hearing protection, hearing testing, and educational components. The presence of an industrial physician or audiologist might result in even the professional review of audiograms being accomplished internally. Some corporations (e.g. Eastman

Kodak, 3M) employ audiologists to administer the programs. Certainly, when computer capability exists, the larger corporations may develop on-line capabilities which permit hearing tests at multiple sites to be directly stored. The data may then be reviewed through a sophisticated review and record keeping system by professionals employed within the corporation or by consultants to the corporation.

ON-SITE CONSULTATIVE PROGRAMS

When companies elect to have consultants provide on-site consultative services these would usually consist of: sound surveys and the identification of exposed workers to be included in the hearing conservation program; hearing testing programs, including the professional review of audiograms; consultation about the hearing protection device (HPD) program; employee annual educational programs; and assistance in record keeping systems. Engineering consultation services may also be utilized in attempts to reduce the noise levels at the source or in the work environment. Most audiologists engaged in large scale industrial consultation practices would provide many of these services to industry within the framework of on-site consultative and mobile hearing testing services. Some may work with, or provide, engineering consultants to complement their own background in that area.

OFF-SITE CONSULTATIVE PROGRAMS

The nature of the problem is such that only about three features of the components of effective programs may be engaged in off-site. One of these would be hearing testing that is accomplished by having the industrial employee go to the site of the professional. For example, employees could be periodically tested at the audiologist's private office. A second, and perhaps most common, off-site service is the computerized review and record keeping system. In this facet, audiograms performed by corporate personnel are sent to consultants who provide the required professional review and recommendations for the appropriate course of action as well as contributing an efficient record keeping system. The third feature, training courses for occupational hearing conversationists, is also commonly provided by professionals off-site.

NOISE SURVEYS AND IDENTIFICATION OF EXPOSED WORKERS

Whether noise surveys are provided by in-house personnel or by consultants, the goals are the same. Fundamentally, they are two-fold. First, there is the need to establish (a) the fact that hazardous noise exists and (b) the necessity to develop plans for the reduction of noise levels. Engineering and administrative controls for the reduction of exposure to hazardous noise continue to be a requirement of OSHA 1910.95 (6). Second, there is the need to identify workers who are exposed beyond the time-weighted average (TWA) of 85 dBA and who, as a consequence, must be included in the hearing conservation program.

Regardless of who performs this task, the minimum requirements are quite explicit. The consultant must be aware that management will rarely be overly enthusiastic about exceeding minimum standards. Consequently, there may be a desire on the part of the employer not to include those employees whose TWA is less than, but close to, 85 dB. Reliance on sound survey data must be tempered with the reality of the work situation. For example, in industry it is not uncommon for workers to change job locations with some regularity. This "bumping" will often result in workers moving from below borderline to above action-level zones. Unless baseline audiograms have been established for these workers, obtaining preplacement audiometric testing could be chaotic. As a consequence, employers should be encouraged to use a liberal designation for initial worker inclusion within the program.

AUDIOMETRIC TESTING PROGRAM FOR EXPOSED WORKERS

The decision to test hearing in-house should be arrived at after an in-depth review of such factors as equipment and space, the continuing availability of qualified personnel, and the advantages and disadvantages of spreading testing over a long period of time. It is not always cost-effective for even large companies to perform their own hearing testing. At the same time, there are some unique advantages to in-house testing. Among these are: (a) it provides a timely opportunity to simultaneously offer at least a substantial portion of the annual educational program; (b) it is an excellent time to review the results of the employees' own understanding of the prior year's results and recommended course of action as well as to review the results of any follow-up that may have taken place; (c) it lends some element of consistency of personnel and an identifiable person to whom the employee can relate. For example, when the program is under the auspices of the medical department there is an ongoing familiarity with the variety of health personnel that is usually not found when using consultant services; and (d) the in-house testing staff may also be trained in, and charged with, review of the manner in which the employee inserts or uses any HPDs, thus allowing for timely review of this important feature of the program.

While many of these activities may also be accomplished when testing is performed by mobile services or at off-site locations, they usually are not. For one thing, they add significant time to the process and would, consequently, substantially increase the cost.

Among the disadvantages of in-house hearing testing are the overhead costs of space, equipment and personnel. The space requirements are such that the testing must be performed in a fairly quiet area in which a properly treated test booth may be located. The space should have convenient access for employees and be contiguous to the usual work area of the personnel assigned to the testing. Frequently this is in the medical department. Equipment must be purchased and regularly calibrated and cared for. Time must be available by qualified personnel on a regular schedule, often on multiple shifts.

When the hearing testing is carried out using on-site mobile consultative services, certain advantages accrue to the company. On-site testing may be promoted by the company as a fringe health benefit for which it obtains consultative services thereby fostering improved employee moral and acceptance of the program. When the program is carried out within a brief and defined period of time it also gains visibility and acts to promote the concept of employee hearing conservation. Even very large companies, especially those working multiple shifts in several different buildings, may find mobile testing services to be cost effective. Certainly, companies that do not have full-time personnel and space that can be devoted to this task will have to use either mobile or off-site services. Smaller companies have little choice beyond the use of consultative testing services, either on-site or off-site.

The primary advantage of a mobile testing service is the ability it offers to test large numbers of employees in short periods of time. Depending on the size and number of vehicles and type of audiometers, from 45 to 500 or more people may be tested in a work shift, although the latter number is not usually advisable. Testing should be coordinated in a manner which minimizes interference with production schedules. Scheduling as many as 400–500 people in a work shift would usually prove to be disruptive. Mobile testing services can be scheduled over

a 24-hr period when a plant has multiple shifts.

Another form of mobile on-site service is one in which the consultant brings a test room that is set up on the employer's site. A modification of this would include testing by the consultant using the employer's booth. Some services have been offered in which the consultant does not use a specific test booth but, instead, carries a sound level meter and audiometer and attempts to test in a "quiet" office. Such an approach is likely to fall well short of both OSHA and prevailing professional standards and would be frowned upon in professional circles.

Problems exist with on-site mobile services, as with any option. The hazards of mobile programs tend to rest more with the provider than the recipient of the service. Moving large trailers or vans from site to site can be a scheduling nightmare, particularly in periods of inclement weather. Vehicle breakdown, accidents and other variables can result in an inability to arrive at test locations on schedule and may result in the inability to test employees as contracted for. Also, each test location must be appraised of electric power and access requirements as well as background noise constraints. Even the best of trailers equipped with standard sound booths must be situated in quieter areas around a plant. Maintaining adequate background noise levels within a vehicle can be a problem when moving large numbers of employees through the program.

Some employers, particularly smaller businesses, will contract for hearing testing services for the employee at fixed off-site facilities, such as at the office of the audiologist or otolaryngologist, or in a hospital or university clinical service program. Such an option may be all that would be available to small companies because the minimum cost of on-site services could make the per-employee test costs prohibitive. Also, geographic consideration may further influence the selection of such an option. The major disadvantage of off-site testing is the cost incurred as a consequence of time off the job and travel expenses. These would usually result in the real costs of off-site testing being quite excessive when more than just a few employees are involved.

In every instance, the decision about which testing approach to take will be based on the consideration of size, cost, facility, availability of other services, personnel, and corporate philosophy. Some large companies may elect to do only preemployment and preplacement testing in-house, but do the annual monitoring with mobile consultative testing services. There is no hard and fast rule that determines which way a company should proceed.

TRAINING OF PERSONNEL INVOLVED IN THE HCP

As has been noted earlier, a variety of disciplines, (e.g. safety, health, industrial hygiene, personnel) may all be involved in various facets of the HCP. It is important that appropriate training be provided to those assigned responsibility for any phase of the program. While the training is frequently informal, it may take the form of structured seminars and workshops specific to one's discipline.

The training of persons to perform hearing testing is most commonly externally provided, even in otherwise totally in-house programs. A few companies with the proper professionals can and do train their own occupational hearing conservationists, but this tends to be the exception rather than the rule.

Despite a statement to the contrary in the regulation that negates the need for training if one is using a microprocessor audiometer, some training must be provided to those persons doing the hearing testing. Responsible professionals, both in-house and consultative, will demand at least the level of training comparable to that set forth for occupational hearing conservationists as detailed in Chapter 7.

While everyone will acknowledge that extensive training is not required to operate a microprocessor audiometer, the task of an occupational hearing conservationist involves more than pressing a switch to initiate the operation of a piece of equipment. The realities of professional liability should insure at least a minimum competence level.

PROFESSIONAL REVIEW OF AUDIOGRAMS

The professional review of industrial audiograms is commonly a consultative service, even in predominantly in-house programs. When properly done, this can be a very time consuming task for the in-house professional. Too often, when done in-house, the review is delegated with only loose criteria being established by the professional. The review of the audiogram, the comparison with baseline, the decision about appropriate course of action, and the employee notification of the outcome together constitute an integral feature of an effective HCP. While it lends itself to computerization, professional review still requires the direct and active involvement of a qualified professional. The professional liability implications of over-delegation of this responsibility to unqualified personnel are immense. Referral criteria and interpretation of industrial audiograms is not without its problem areas (7, 8).

HEARING PROTECTION

The fitting and training in the use of HPDs is frequently a split responsibility with safety, industrial hygiene and medical personnel all being involved. In any event, this aspect of the program is generally performed in-house. Commonly, one of the program features that is poorly handled is education in the use of HPDs. It is important that the responsibility for this task be well identified and strictly adhered to. While consultants can advise about the appropriateness or inappropriateness of certain HPDs and compliance matters, the major ongoing responsibility for the HPD program must reside in-house in order for it to be successful.

Compliance with the HPD program must be mandated and enforced (5). It must begin with a good example being set by foremen and supervisors. No one should be allowed in areas designated as requiring hearing protector use without visible compliance. For this reason, earmuffs are preferable when the exposure is to visitors or others just passing through the noisy area. While the use of reward is a good technique to increase employee motivation and compliance with hearing protector use, and is always advocated, it is essential, at the same time, that the ultimate corporate authority for penalty for noncompliance be negotiated in contracts. As with other mandated safety equipment, HPD use must be a contingency of employment.

ANNUAL EMPLOYEE EDUCATIONAL PROGRAM

The requirement for an annual educational program for exposed employees is explicit. It is also probably one of the poorest handled components of the program. While the regulation does not specify the duration of the program, it does specify its components. The person responsible for the entire hearing conservation program within any company must identify how the annual educational program will be handled. The use of consultants to develop and/or present educational materials and programs is not uncommon. Some consultant services include audio-visual educational programs in conjunction with on-site mobile hearing testing.

In any educational program there needs to be a clear and open statement from management about what the company is doing about the noise in the workplace and the company policy about all phases of the HCP. Union support for that program is essential. Naturally, openness and honesty is an important component for any educational program.

Employee resistance to come off the production line is probably greatest when earnings are related to productivity. Piecework employees will resent time off the production line and this factor must be a consideration in scheduling educational programs. The inclusion of this material as a package in periodic safety meetings is one approach that is often utilized. Regardless of how the program has been presented, it is important to document what was covered and who attended educational programs.

RECORDS

Because responsibility for the HCP program is often divided, record keeping can be fragmented as well. The records of monitoring, testing, review, hearing protection, and related matters should always be integrated and coordinated. The normally responsible individual within any plant should have the overall record keeping responsibilities. Consultant services may be utilized to develop a record keeping format and the report of the review of audiometric testing by consultants contributes to an orderly record, but it is not the entire record. This information must be integrated with internal records of sound surveys, HPD compliance programs, technician certification and the pertinent information about the program.

A comprehensive outline of the occupational noise and hearing conservation program is a record form that serves as an excellent management tool which can provide a number of advantages. First, it affords an overview of the entire program that compliance officers would find impressive and view as evidence of good faith. Secondly, it serves as a document that can acquaint the variety of people involved in the program within any organization about each others' roles, thereby lending a cohesiveness to the program. Thirdly, it is particularly helpful to

Table 5.1.
Superior Metal Working Industries, Inc.
Hearing conservation program policy

I PURPOSE OF PROGRAM

The hearing conservation program is designed to protect the hearing of all employees and identify hearing problems of any type before they become serious. The program is intended to comply with OSHA 1910.95. It also serves as a tool by which compensation cost control may be monitored

A. Survey of Noise Levels

Any area in which workers are likely to be exposed to hazardous (>85 dBA) noise shall be surveyed. Exposed workers shall be identified and spot dosimetry shall be used to verify area measurements. Company policy is to include all workers with any chance of exposure to 83 dB or more within the hearing conservation program

B. Engineering Control

The engineering plan for noise control shall consider all of the following. The detailed plan shall be kept on file in the office of the plant manager. When feasible noise level shall be reduced to <90 dB

1. Maintenance of equipment shall be adhered to in order to reduce noise levels
2. Substitution of machines
3. Substitution of process
4. Vibration dampening
5. Reduction of sound transmission through solids
6. Reduction of sound produced by fluid flow
7. Include noise level specifications when buying new equipment
8. Isolate noise source
9. Isolate operator

C. Administrative Control

Administrative control: when feasible, manipulation of exposure time may be reduced through:

1. Arrange production schedule to distribute heavy noise over time
2. Divide work time at excessive noise levels among several people
3. Shorten run time on noisy machines
4. Perform noisy jobs when fewer people are in the area

D. Hearing Protective Devices (HPDs).

1. Earplugs with poor attenuation are unacceptable
2. Disposable and semidisposable plugs such as Swedish wool (Bilsom) and foam (EAR, Purafoam) are acceptable
3. Issuing of HPDs shall be the responsibility of the Safety Office. The condition of reusable HPDs shall be checked at least monthly by the Safety Office. Plugs or muffs must be fit or dispensed with instructions by someone who has been appropriately trained and supervised
4. The choice of HPDs is restricted to those providing sufficient attenuation so as to reduce the noise level at the ear to below 85 dBA. As a guide, one-half the NRR may be subtracted from the employee TWA exposure to establish effectiveness
5. All employees exposed to more than 85 dB shall be provided with HPDs and required to wear them
6. The use of HPDs shall be a condition of employment for exposed employees

E. Audiometric Testing

1. All new employees shall have preemployment audiograms
2. All employees exposed to a TWA of 85 dB shall have a baseline audiogram and annual hearing tests thereafter
3. Annual audiograms shall be professionally reviewed by Environmental Hearing & Vision

Table 5.1—*(Continued)*

Consultants to establish the existence of a standard threshold shift (STS) of an average 10 dB or more at 2000, 3000 and 4000 Hz, or with shifts of potential medical or other significance as determined by the reviewing professional

4. All employees shall be advised in writing of the outcome of the hearing test and of the recommended course of action as deemed appropriate by the professional reviewer. Advice to the employees shall be transmitted within 21 days of receipt of the report from the reviewing professional

5. S.M.I. Corporation will cover the costs of additional professional evaluation and treatment when the problem is deemed work related by the examining professional

F. Training

1. Environmental Hearing & Vision's tape slide presentation *Noise and Your Hearing* will be shown initially to all employees included in the HCP

2. Training about audiometric testing, the audiogram and hearing protective devices will occur prior to the annual audiometric test. Employees will also be referred to the safety department and instructed in the use of HPDs

3. Employees exhibiting an STS will be refitted and/or reinstructed in the use of HPDs.

G. General

1. Audiometers will be checked biologically prior to daily use. This includes a listening check of cords, switches and earphone wires

2. Audiometers will be calibrated electroacoustically on an annual basis and exhaustively calibrated every other year unless a problem is detected earlier

3. Audiometric sound room will be recertified biannually or more often if a change is suspected

H. Records

1. Plant noise survey records are maintained in the safety office. These records are updated whenever new noise measurements are performed in any area

2. Noise exposure records are regularly updated and maintained with the administrative listing of annual audiometric tests in the medical department

3. Documentation of audiometer calibration (daily biological, annual electroacoustic, biannual exhaustive), sound room calibration, audiometric technician certification verification, sample letters of notification of outcome of hearing test and recommended course of action are all maintained in the medical department

4. Corporate policy and enforcement program for hearing protective devices is detailed and maintained in the safety office

5. Records shall be maintained to document employee participation in the annual educational program. These records are on file in the safety office

6. A copy of OSHA 1910.95 shall be maintained in both the medical and safety offices.

II   RESPONSIBILITY FOR HEARING CONSERVATION PROGRAM COMPONENTS

Function	Department
A. Arrange for 25% of employees to have their hearing tested each quarter. Send test results to Environmental Hearing Vision Consultants for review	Medical
B. Each quarter, when analysis of tests taken during previous quarter are received	
1. Insure that letters of notification of test and recommended course of action are distributed to employees as soon as professional review is completed	Medical
2. Arrange for all employees in category 5 (unreliable test results) to be retested	Medical
3. Meet with all employees in category 7A and 7B (significant shift) to review the history of their hearing loss and the results of their test	Medical

Table 5.1—(*Continued*)

4. Arrange for those employees in category 7B to be referred to an otolaryngologist or audiologist	Medical
5. Determine if employee can continue working in the same environment	Medical & Safety
6. If loss of hearing (or STS) is occupationally induced (as determined by a professional):	
(a) Recheck the level of noise to which exposed	Safety
(b) Determine the effect of the noise level on co-workers in that work area	Medical & Safety
(c) Determine if employee is wearing hearing protection. Check fit and reinstruct and enforce use	Safety & Line Supervision
7. Follow up on each employee's problem to determine:	
(a) Improvement	Medical & Safety
(b) Action required	
8. Provide annual educational program	Medical & Safety
9. Record on OSHA form 200 when hearing loss is professionally established to be work related	Medical

III WORKERS COMPENSATION FILE

   A. Maintain estimate of number of potential claims and cost in the Medical Department. This information is derived from annual hearing tests

   B. Obtain records of evaluation of preexisting hearing loss at time of employment. Notify prior employer of preexisting condition

   C. Maintain roster of audiologists and otolaryngologists who will act as consultants on hearing loss claims

   D. Establish protocol for investigation of hearing loss claims

personnel newly assigned to various phases of the program. Turnover of personnel is not uncommon, and the program outline can function to provide a basis of continuity. It also is a means of enlightening upper level managment about the totality of the program. Table 5.1 serves as an example of a program outline for a large industrial firm.

SUMMARY

In this chapter we have identified the components of hearing conservation programs and explored the approaches that may be followed to achieve compliance with the requirements. The fundamental responsibility for the program resides in-house but a number of consultative services may be utilized to lend support to satisfy the needs of individual companies. Innovative approaches appear all the time. One thing that is clear is that no single approach is the best approach in every instance. Table 5.2 offers an example of how one company offering industrial hearing conservation services assists its potential and current clients in the determination of how well they are achieving compliance.

Table 5.2
Hearing conservation program analysis by proView®[a]

I. **NOISE LEVELS AND NOISE EXPOSURE**

  A. **When were noise levels measured**
    1. Date

  B. **What type of measurements were taken**
    1. Sound level meter
      a. Area monitoring
      b. Individual monitoring
    2. Dosimetry

  C. **Has any change occurred since measurements were taken that would effect sound levels**

  D. **What criteria were used to include employees in the program**
    1. 8-hr TWA of 85 db
    2. 8-hr TWA of _____ dB
    3. Individual monitoring
    4. Area monitoring
    5. Worst case criterion
    6. Other

  E. **Have employees been notified of results of monitoring**
    1. All employees
    2. Only exposed employees
    3. How were employees notified

  F. **Has a copy of the OHSA noise standard (1910.95) been posted in the workplace**

II. **ENGINEERING AND ADMINISTRATIVE CONSIDERATIONS**

  A. **Has a plan been developed for reducing employee exposure to hazardous noise**
    1. Is engineering noise-out technically feasible
    2. Is engineering noise-out economically feasible
    3. Are administrative controls feasible
    4. Are engineering and/or administrative controls less costly than an effective hearing conservative program

III. **ANNUAL AUDIOMETRIC TESTING PROGRAM**

  A. **Have baseline audiograms been obtained for exposed employees**
    1. Either preemployment or preplacement in noisy areas
    2. Were baselines obtained following 14 h of nonexposure to noise (HPD can be used to achieve nonexposure)
    3. Are annual tests obtained following nonexposure

  B. **Does equipment and environment meet standards**
    1. Are tests done
      a. In house
      b. By mobile services
      c. Other
    2. Are tests conducted in test booth
      a. Is sound level in test booth certified
    3. Are audiometers calibrated
      a. Daily biological & listening check
      b. Annual electroacoustic
      c. Biannual exhaustive
    4. Type of audiometer(s)
      a. Manual

Table 5.2— *(Continued)*

      b. Self-recording
      c. Microprocessor

C. What are the qualifications of audiometric technicians
   1. CAOHC[b] certified
      a. Original date
      b. Recertification date
   2. Completed CAOHC course but not CAOHC certified
      a. Original date
      b. Refresher course date(s)
   3. Completed a technical course not registered with CAOHC
   4. Noncertified & did not complete a 20-h technician course

D. Is the audiometric program supervised by a qualified professional
   1. Audiologist
   2. Otolaryngologist
   3. Other physician

E. How are audiograms reviewed
   1. Have original and baseline audiograms been reviewed for validity and maintained in the record
   2. All audiograms are individually reviewed
      a. By technician
      b. By supervising professionals
   3. All audiometric data is entered into computerized data base
      a. Are all hearing tests categorized
      b. Who established criteria for categorization
      c. Does categorization differentiate between amount and type of hearing loss
   4. What audiograms are personally reviewed by supervising professional (audiologist or physician)
      a. All
      b. Only those with standard threshold shift (STS)
      c. Those with STS and other significant hearing losses
      d. How are possible medical problems identified
   5. Who established criteria for baseline audiogram revision
      a. Technician
      b. Supervising professional
      c. Baselines not revised

F. What is the process of employee notification of results of hearing tests
   1. Are employees advised of the hearing test results
      a. Verbally
      b. By letter
   2. Are only certain employees advised of the hearing test results
      a. Those with STS
      b. Those with STS and other hearing loss
      c. Those with STS and possible medical problems
      d. Other:

G. What are employees told about the hearing test results
   1. Test outcome indicates need for referral for professional evaluation
      a. All STS
      b. Certain STS
      c. Other hearing losses
      d. Possible medical problems
      e. If referred with hearing losses other than STS what are the criteria
      f. Are employees with STS instructed or reinstructed in use of hearing protective devices

Table 5.2— (*Continued*)

IV. HEARING PROTECTIVE DEVICE (HPD) PROGRAM

A. HPD use is mandatory for
1. All employees exposed to TWA (8 hr)
2. TWA 90 dB or greater
3. TWA 85 dB or greater
4. TWA 85 dB–90 dB only if demonstrating STS
5. Other

B. What types of HPDs are provided
1. Choice
2. Muff
3. Band
4. Reusable plug
5. Disposable plug
6. Custom earplug

C. What is the procedure for instruction in selection, fitting and use of HPD
1. Individual instruction
2. Group instruction
3. Other

D. Is there a HPD monitoring and enforcement policy
1. HPD use is a contingency of employment
2. Penalties are specified for employee noncompliance (e.g. warning, suspension, termination)
3. Proper and regular HPD use is monitored by
   a. Sporadic inspections
   b. Regular inspections
   c. Other

V. ANNUAL EMPLOYEE HEARING CONSERVATION TRAINING PROGRAM

A. All employees included in the HCP receive annual training through
1. Group safety meetings
2. Individualized instruction via
   a. Lectures
   b. Films
   c. Print material, e.g. brochures
3. No annual program is offered

B. Annual training program includes information about
1. The effects of noise on hearing
2. The appropriate and effective use of HPDs
3. The purpose of hearing testing and it's procedure
4. Other (specify)

C. What procedures and policies are in effect to insure employee participation in annual training programs

VI. A COORDINATED RECORD KEEPING SYSTEM

A. Are records of noise measurement and control programs current and maintained for a least 2 years

B. Are all calibration logs maintained
1. Sound level measurement equipment

Table 5.2— *(Continued)*

    2. Audiometer calibrations
        a. Maintained in the log
        b. Recorded on individual audiograms
    3. Test environment measurements

C. Are audiometric tests properly maintained
    1. At least for the duration of employment
    2. Do audiometric tests include name and job classifications, date of last calibration, employees most recent noise exposure assessment
    3. Is there an individual audiometric report for each employee's record
    4. Is there an administrative listing of all annual audiometric tests

D. Are records made available to employees or their designee upon proper request

E. Is there a centralized record of the occupational noise and hearing conservation program
    1. Is company policy pertaining to program as a whole in the record
    2. Are noise levels and noise exposures maintained centrally
    3. Is there an administrative listing of annual hearing tests
    4. Do policies dealing with components of the program include
        a. Noise measurement
        b. Audiometric testing and review
        c. HPD
        d. Training
        e. Records
    5. Is there a designee responsible for integration of the entire program

VII. PROCEDURE TO MONITOR THE EFFECTIVENESS OF THE HCP

A. Are annual audiograms analyzed to identify the level of effectiveness
    1. Across plant locations
    2. Using what criteria

B. Is the HPD compliance program monitored
    1. Log maintained for employee violations
    2. Standard policy for monitoring

VIII. WORKER'S COMPENSATION CONTROL ANALYSIS

A. Are the results of annual audiometric testing used to protect potential cost of hearing disability claims

B. Are employees advised of possible compensation for hearing loss

C. Is the hearing of all new employees tested within 90 days of initial placement in areas with noise levels in excess of 85 dB

D. Is there notification to prior employers of preexisting hearing loss

[a] Reproduced with permission of Environmental Hearing and Vision Consultants, Ltd.
[b] CAOHC, Council of Accreditation in Occupational Hearing Conservation.

References

1. Code of Federal Regulations, Title 29, Chapter XVII, Part 1910 Subpart G, 36 FR 10466, May 29, 1971; Amended by 46 FR 4161, January 16, 1981 and March 8, 1983, Superintendent of Documents, Washington, D.C.
2. Mass R: Industrial noise and hearing conservation. In Katz J (ed): *Handbook of Clinical Audiology*, ed 1. Baltimore, Williams & Wilkins, 1972.
3. Glorig A: Industrial hearing conservation, In *Noise-Con 73*. Washington, D.C., National Conference on Noise Control Engineering, 1973.
4. Feldman A: Industrial hearing conservation programs. In Henderson D, Hamernik R, Dosanjh D, Mills J (eds): *Effects of Noise on Hearing*. New York, Raven Press, 1976.
5. Royster, LH, Royster JD, Berger EH: Guidelines for developing an effective hearing conservation program. *Am Ind Hyg Associ* 41:48, 1982.

6. OSHA Instruction CPL 2-2.35, Office of Health Compliance Assistance, Nov. 9, 1983, Washington, D.C.

7. Feldman AS, Grimes CT: Review and referral of industrial audiograms: a professional dilemma. ASHA, 19:4, 1977.

8. Feldman AS: Industrial audiogram review: the professional's dilemma, *Hear Aid J* 35:18–20, 1982.

CHAPTER 6

Hearing Protection Devices

LARRY H. ROYSTER and JULIA DOSWELL ROYSTER

INTRODUCTION

Hearing protection devices (HPDs) can be approached either from a perspective emphasizing the practical concerns faced by users in industry or from a perspective focusing on the idealistic HPD performance potentials which can be attained in the laboratory. Since the goal of protecting employees' hearing is achieved only in industrial environments, the authors have elected to stress factors affecting the performance of HPDs in the real world and information which will assist the hearing conservationist in obtaining the maximum utilization of HPDs by wearers.

The Need

The need for HPDs can easily be justified by the sheer number of employees who are exposed to potentially hazardous noise environments. However, individual people tell the real story. During a series of one-on-one interviews with employees who had incurred significant, but not compensable, high-frequency noise-induced permanent threshold shift (NIPTS) at a large industrial facility in North Carolina, a 29-year-old male brought home the personal meaning of noise-induced hearing loss when he commented to one of the authors:

"My young daughters no longer speak clearly anymore."

It is quite unfortunate that this person was not provided with potentially effective HPDs in his initial years on the job, trained in their proper use and maintenance, and required to wear them as a condition of employment. Our primary goal in writing this chapter is to provide the reader with the basic information necessary to minimize on-the-job NIPTS through the use of HPDs.

HPDs in an Effective Hearing Conservation Program

We have studied the audiometric data bases of over 40 industries to assess the degree of protection provided to the noise exposed populations (1). The hearing conservation programs (HCPs) for well protected populations were examined to identify the characteristics shared by successful programs. The basic common element is the absolute *enforcement of HPD utilization* (2). Without exception, at industrial facilities with effective HCPs, management strictly enforced the use of HPDs by all employees, including top managers, when they entered a noise-hazard area for even a brief period of time. Each successful HCP was guided by a *key individual* who made the program work through his/her sincere commitment to the employee's well-being, plus the ability to get the job done. The key individual was extremely familiar with the employees and their working environments. The successful HCPs also exhibited *active communications* among all personnel involved in the program, from production workers right up the administrative line to the boss. All these firms offered a choice of *potentially effective HPDs*. That is, each wearer could find at least one HPD which was practically usable and protective in the work environment.

The hearing protection phase is only one of five phases of effective HCPs (2). All five phases (education, sound surveys, engineering and administrative controls, hearing protection, and audiometric evaluations) are tightly interconnected in achieving employee protection. For example, the moment when the employee steps out of the audiometric test booth is one of the most opportune times to reeducate the worker about hearing loss, check the condition of his/her HPDs, and motivate the individual to wear HPDs faithfully. All of the effective HCPs studied to date have provided the employee with feedback at this contact point. Since supervisors and managers were also audiometrically tested in effective HCPs, the annual retest situation gave the key individual the opportunity to reinforce the needed support of each manager for the hearing protection phase of the HCP. In contrast, in HCPs implemented primarily to achieve regulatory compliance, the program phases were perceived as unrelated requirements rather than as interdependent means of preserving hearing.

Typical Breakdowns in the Hearing Protection Phase

We have been conducting an ongoing series of interviews in industries throughout the USA to collect information about HPD utilization from individuals who are responsible for issuing HPDs to employees (3). Nurses issued HPDs in 54% of sites, but personnel with widely varying backgrounds were responsible for issuing in other industries. These included foremen, safety directors, personnel directors, plant managers, clerks of supply rooms or tool cribs, and others. Unfortunately, many of these individuals lacked the training or experience needed to understand or handle the problems encountered by wearers. In fact, many had never worn the HPDs that they dispensed and were relatively unfamiliar with the environments where HPDs were worn. Consequently, they could not help the employee select the most appropriate HPD or suggest how to use it most effectively within the context of job demands and environmental factors.

Often the issuers did not even attempt to assist the employee in selecting a HPD; they simply displayed the styles available and told the worker to choose! The choice of HPDs available was often inadequate; 40% of sites offered less than the minimum acceptable selection of at least two plugs and one muff. Only 45% of issuers actually checked HPDs for proper fit, and only 37% maintained records of the style and size issued. Employees could obtain replacement HPDs without having size records checked in 76% of sites, so they were free to switch to a smaller size or another style which was more comfortable, but which probably did not seal the ear canal. Some personnel who failed to check HPDs for fit believed they were issuing a universal HPD for which one size fits all. In spite of advertising claims, there is no HPD which can fit all wearers or satisfy the requirements of all industrial environments.

For employees to obtain the maximum benefit from the HPDs made available, the issuer must know the expected real-world attenuation of HPDs in industrial (as opposed to laboratory) settings, the limitations of HPDs in the particular environments where employees will wear them, the types of problems employees may encounter, the proper procedures for fitting, use, and care of HPDs, and methods for monitoring whether HPDs are worn correctly and replaced as needed.

Overview of HPD Utilization Problems in the Real World

During the interviews with industrial personnel responsible for issuing HPDs, the issuers were asked to name any problems wearers encounter in using HPDs and to estimate the frequency of problem occurrence (3). Presented as Figure 6.1 are the percentages of sites where the most common problems were named. These data indicate that some problems are widespread in terms of the number of sites where they occur. However, the percentages of employees affected are gen-

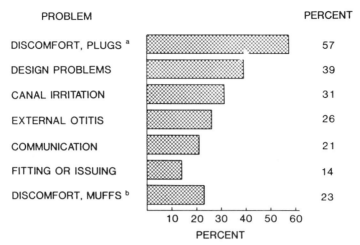

Figure 6.1. The most common problems associated with HPD utilization named by industrial HPD issuers, and the percentage of survey sites where each problem was reported, disregarding frequency of occurrence. ([a] Percent of 72 sites using plugs. [b] Percent of 42 sites using muffs.) (From Royster JD, Royster LH: *Hearing Protection Devices as Used in Real World Environments.* Final report submitted to OSHA. Submission number 501-2 to docket OSH-011. Washington, DC, U.S. Department of Labor, 1982, (3).)

erally small, as shown by the low estimated frequencies of occurrence in Figure 6.2. The estimated rate of 2% for external otitis is no higher than would be expected in the general United States population (4). During these interviews we have not encountered any significant medical or health problems resulting from normal HPD utilization. A few unusual problems were observed when HPDs were used carelessly in conjunction with environmental irritants or toxins.

In light of the inadequate procedures for issuing HPDs and monitoring their use which were reported in many industries, one would anticipate that employees would have reason to complain about difficulties in HPD utilization. However, most of these problems can be prevented or solved if the HPD fitter obtains sufficient training and establishes careful policies for implementing the hearing protection phase of the HCP.

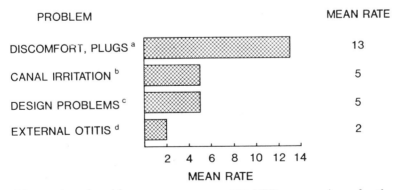

Figure 6.2. Mean rates of problem occurrence per 100 HPD wearers/year for those problems for which at least 10 interviewees estimated the frequency rate. ([a] Mean estimate from 23 of 52 sites. [b] Mean estimate from 10 of 29 sites. [c] Mean estimate from 18 of 22 sites. [d] Mean estimate from 13 of 18 sites.) (From Royster JD, Royster LH: *Hearing Protection Devices as Used in Real World Environments.* Final report submitted to OSHA. Submission number 501-2 to docket OSH-011. Washington, DC, U.S. Department of Labor, 1982, (3).)

Recommended Restrictions on HPD Selection for TWA Ranges

One question managers often ask concerns recommendations for the HPD selection options which should be allowed for employees working in environments with different TWAs. The TWA is the time-weighted average sound level which, if constant over an 8-hr exposure, would result in the same noise dose as actually measured. The OSHA Hearing Conservation Amendment (5) requires mandatory use of HPDs by all employees whose TWAs are 90 dB or above, based on A-weighted sound pressure levels (6). Therefore, managers must decide whether to implement a policy for mandatory HPD use by workers in areas where the TWAs are 85–89 dB. The trend seems to be toward a blanket requirement for the use of HPDs in all environments where the TWA is 85 dB or above. This approach does prevent administrative problems which arise when supervisors in areas with TWAs of 85–89 dB must enforce HPD utilization for those employees who have shown standard threshold shifts, but not for other workers.

Individuals differ in the amount of annoyance, stress and fatigue experienced during noise exposure. Industrial personnel indicate that they encounter greater employee resistance to wearing HPDs in environments with TWAs below 90 dB than in higher exposure areas (3). However, other employees request HPDs for use in environments with noise levels below 85 dB, such as computer rooms and word processing areas with a high density of equipment.

Presented as Table 6.1 are recommended policy guidelines for requiring HPD utilization in varying TWA ranges. Restrictions are needed to control the styles of HPDs which are allowed for use in areas with higher TWAs because HPDs differ much more widely in their real-world effectiveness (their typical attenuation as used by employees) than indicated by manufacturers' published atten-

Table 6.1.

Recommended guidelines for enforcement of HPD utilization in different TWA ranges, and accompanying restrictions on the selection of HPDs with adequate real-world attenuation

TWA, dB	HPD utilization	Selection options
89 or below	Optional[a]	No restrictions
90–94	Required	No restrictions
95–99	Required	Limited choice
100 or above	Required	Very limited choice

[a] See text discussion.

uation data, which are based on laboratory measurements (7).

The recommendation for optional use of HPDs in areas with TWAs below 90 dB is qualified by the assumption that the following conditions are met. First, the company performs annual audiometric evaluations, as required by OSHA, for all employees in the area and requires HPD use for any employees who show a standard threshold shift. Second, the company also requires HPD use for any employees who show a persistent shift of 20 dB or more at any test frequency. Third, the company conducts an annual analysis of the audiometric data base to ensure that the hearing trends for departments with optional HPD utilization do not show hearing loss beyond normal age effects (1, 8).

The degree of hazard from noise exposure in the range of 85–89 dB can be estimated using the predictive model for hearing damage proposed in ISO/DIS 1999 (9). This model predicts that the NIPTS incurred after 40 yr of exposure for the 0.1 fractile (sensitive ears which would show more loss than 90% of all ears) would be a loss at 4 kHz of approximately 9 dB for a TWA of 85 dB, or 18 dB for a TWA of 89 dB. For ears with normal sensitivity to noise (the 0.5 fractile or median), predicted NIPTS at 4 kHz after 40 yr exposure would be approximately 6 dB for a TWA of 85 dB and 13 dB for a TWA of 89 dB. These predicted threshold shifts are approximations because the ISO/DIS 1999 model is based on the equal energy principle, or a doubling rate of 3 dB, whereas the OSHA TWA is based on a doubling rate of 5 dB.

The risk of hearing loss after 40 yr from TWAs below 90 dB is small enough to allow HPD utilization to be a personal choice *if* all employees in these areas are encouraged to wear HPDs and educated regarding the effects of noise, the benefits of hearing protection and the wear and care of HPDs. If the employees who show a shift of 20 dB at any test frequency are required to wear HPDs, then no workers should incur a significant hearing impairment. If individuals who have already developed substantial NIPTS from past noise exposures are required to wear HPDs in low noise levels, they will experience communication difficulties, as discussed later.

When the potential for hearing damage is weighed against the employee resistance and the functional communication problems for some workers, it appears that voluntary HPD utilization is adequate for areas with TWAs in the range below 90 dB, if the HCP fulfills the conditions described above.

For TWAs of 90 dB and above, HPD utilization is required. Most commonly used HPDs are capable of providing sufficient protection to prevent NIPTS from exposures in the range of 90–94 dB. At these noise levels the most important parameter affecting the degree of attenuation attained is the user's attention to correct HPD placement rather than HPD design. Consequently, it is more important to focus on the enforcement of proper HPD usage than on the selection of HPDs to be offered.

When workers' TWAs exceed 94 dB, emphasis must be placed on choosing HPDs which are potentially effective at these higher noise levels. Studies of attenuation attained by industrial employees in the field strongly indicate that some types of HPDs, as typically used by employees, provide inadequate attenuation to protect workers effectively at these noise levels (7).

For TWAs of 100 dB or greater, it is recommended that the HPD choices made available to employees be strictly limited to those designs which maximize the possibility that the user will attain a good fit providing an acoustic seal. The HPDs which appear to be most user-proof, based on field studies, are the foam earplugs and earmuffs. Because less than 3% of American workers have TWAs of 100 dB or higher (10), this recommendation for severely limited HPD choices should not present an implementation problem for the hearing conservationist in fitting the affected individuals with these two types of HPDs.

These recommendations for HPD utilization are based on typical industrial environments. However, there are situations in which HPD selection will be dictated by constraints of the job task and work environment. Management must always be willing to modify existing HPD use policies in order to yield the maximum protection for the employees. The suitability of any HPD use policy for a work environment can best be judged by an analysis of the audiometric data base. In general, the most effective HPD will be the one the employee will wear properly and constantly while on the job.

TYPES OF HPDs
Earplugs

Plugs, or insert HPDs, are designed to be worn in the outer portion of the ear canal, where they should fit tightly against the cartilaginous walls to create an acoustic seal. Earplugs may be divided into premolded, formable, and custommolded types, which differ in their requirements for fitting, issuing and maintenance, as well as their approach to sealing the ear canal.

Premolded

Numerous styles of plugs are manufactured in assorted shapes from flexible materials such as vinyl and silicone rubber. To varying degrees, these plugs bend to follow the curvature of the particular ear canal into which they are inserted; however, their basic shape is determined during the manufacturing process. A few styles have an internal air bubble. Some plugs come in only one size, while others offer a range of sizes, typically two to five. Careful fitting is necessary to ensure that the proper size is selected, and that the shape of the plug is compatible with the shape of the individual canal. Premolded plugs are usually reusable for several months, and most types are sold in small plastic carrying cases. Figure 6.3 illustrates various premolded plugs, including models which seal against the canal with flexible flanges, the body of the plug, or both.

cotton, and the various down plugs must be forced against the walls of the ear canal to conform to its contours tightly enough to create an attenuating seal. In contrast, foam earplugs are rolled down before insertion into the canal, where they expand to adjust to the canal shape and form a seal against its walls. The encased silicone plugs are rolled into a long tapered cone for insertion, then regain their original diameter. Glass down and waxed cotton HPDs are intended to be discarded after one use. Foam plugs may be washed and reused as long as they retain their capacity to expand to their original dimensions after compression. Encased silicone plugs are washable and reusable for several months.

Formable

In contrast to premolded styles, formable plugs are shaped by the wearer to fit each ear, minimizing the need to stock multiple sizes. They are manufactured from materials including acoustic foams, fiberglass down, silicone encased in a bladder, wax-impregnated cotton, and elastomers. Glass down HPDs are available either with or without a thin plastic covering intended to prevent fibers from separating from the plug and lodging in the canal. These varieties of HPDs are shown in Figure 6.4. Elastomers, waxed

Custom Molded

These plugs are made specifically for the individual wearer by making an impression of each ear, similar to a hearing aid mold, which fills the concha and extends into the canal. For some brands, the original impressions of catalytically cured silicone set to become the employee's HPDs; in other cases, temporary impressions are mailed to a manufacturer's laboratory, which returns a finished pair of HPDs. Custom-molded plugs generally may be worn for 2 or more years. The quality of the seal obtained

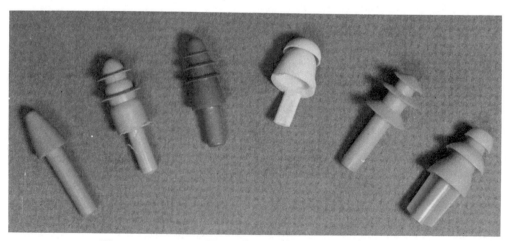

Figure 6.3. Several commonly used premolded earplugs.

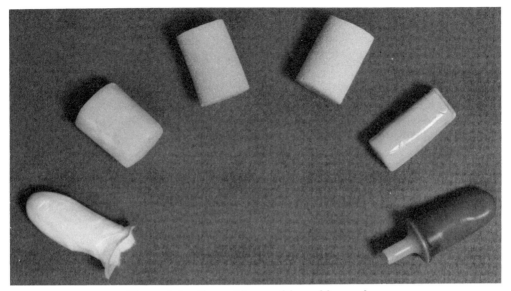

Figure 6.4. Several types of formable earplugs.

depends on the tightness of the impression, the depth of the canal extension, and the resistance of the material to shrinkage and surface wear. Several custom molded HPDs are shown as Figure 6.5.

Earmuffs

Earmuffs, or circumaural HPDs, consist of cups which fit over the pinna and are attached to a tension headband. The interior of the cup is lined with a material such as acoustic foam, and the perimeter of the cup is fitted with a cushioned seal which rests against the head. The cushion may be made of either foam or liquid inside a vinyl skin. The clamping force of the headband presses the cushions against the head to form a seal. Because people differ in head size and pinna placement,

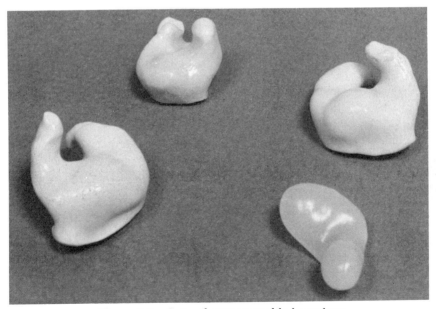

Figure 6.5. Several custom molded earplugs.

muffs should be adjustable for band length and cup orientation. Muffs usually provide greater attenuation when the band is worn over the head rather than under the chin or behind the neck. Figure 6.6 shows sample earmuffs with large-volume cups and small-volume cups. Dielectric muffs without metal parts are available for use around electric hazards.

Semiaurals

Semiaurals, also called canal caps or semi-inserts, consist of flexible caps attached to a tension band. The band is usually worn below the chin or behind the neck, but over-the-head models are available. The caps or pods block the entrance to the ear canal, but they do not insert into the canal. These HPDs are easily carried around the neck, so they are convenient for persons who must occasionally enter noise areas for brief periods or those who need HPDs intermittently. Figure 6.7 illustrates two samples of semiaural devices.

Special HPDs

Nonlinear earplugs have been developed to minimize communication interference by providing amplitude-sensitive and frequency-sensitive attenuation (11). Such HPDs are marketed to sportsmen and provided in military applications for protection against gunfire characterized by infrequent impulses at very high sound levels. A small opening through the plug provides rising attenuation of frequencies above about 1 kHz, while lower frequency sounds pass with little or no attenuation. The opening may contain a valve mechanism or damping material. At levels above about 110 dB SPL, turbulence or valve function increases the attenuation. These designs are *not* appropriate for use in industrial environments, where the noise spectra require more attenuation than these devices provide across the entire frequency range.

Active noise reduction devices depend on an electronic system to attenuate selected noise components without eliminating the wearer's auditory communication ability (12). Flying helmets with active noise reduction systems have been developed for military aircraft personnel. Active attenuation systems are also available in commercial earmuffs with a microphone on the outside of each cup and a speaker inside. The amplifier allows noises below about 85 dB to pass but at-

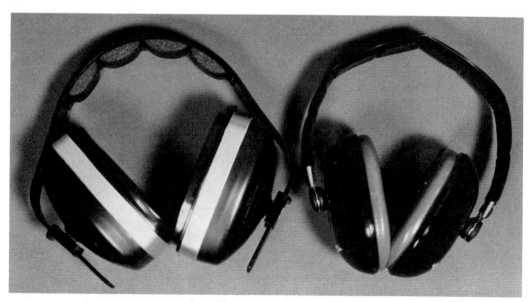

Figure 6.6.   Examples of large-volume and small-volume earmuffs.

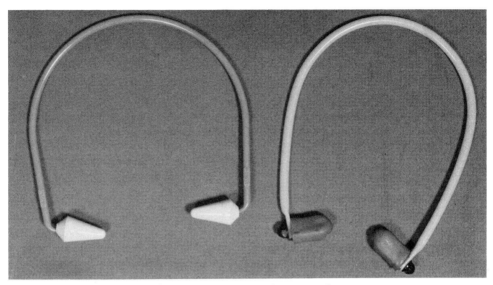

Figure 6.7.   Two types of semiaural HPDs.

tenuates sound above that level. This type HPD might be desirable for use in intermittent noise.

Communication earmuff headsets containing two-way radios are available for isolated machinery operators, such as drivers of heavy equipment.

Combinations of HPDs with Other Equipment

Many industrial workers must wear other items of personal protective equipment such as safety glasses, hard hats, goggles, respirators, welding hoods, or gloves. Earplugs do not interfere with headgear, but earmuffs are incompatible with some headgear, or too heavy in combination with it. Gloves may make the insertion, reseating, and removal of earplugs very difficult. Muffs attached to hard hats are difficult to adjust and typically provide less attenuation than muffs on a headband. The temple bars of glasses usually create a leak in the seal of muff cushions against the head, reducing attenuation by at least 5 dB, even with adaptor pads (13).

Personal radios within non-HPD muffs have been substituted by employees for their HPDs to provide entertainment. These popular radios lack significant attenuation ability (14) and are unsuitable for use in noise areas. Not only do the radio muffs fail to attenuate machinery noise, but the employee adds to his exposure by increasing the radio volume to hear it above the background levels. Other employees have worn miniature earphone speakers within their HPD muffs. Although the attenuation of background noise is possible in this arrangement, the worker still may increase the radio volume to an unacceptable level, and the music can mask external warning sounds. Some industrial facilities have provided audio entertainment by purchasing HPD earmuffs fitted with radio pick-ups which receive local broadcasts from an induction loop system. These systems could include volume governors, and safety warnings could be transmitted, but music might distract employees' attention from safety awareness and production demands.

Cost of Hearing Protection

The annual cost of the hearing protection phase of the HCP includes administrative expenses as well as the purchase price of the HPDs issued to employees.

More personnel time will be required to fit and reissue reusable, sized HPDs than unsized HPDs which are disposable or used for only a few weeks. Purchase prices per item are cheaper for disposable HPDs, but they may be more expensive on an annual basis considering replacement frequency. Purchase prices for the same HPDs vary substantially between distributors as well as depending on the quantities ordered. Additional administrative costs include the time involved in maintaining fitting records for reissuing purposes and monitoring the utilization of HPDs in the workplace. For many industries, the administrative costs exceed the purchase costs.

HPD replacement policies also influence costs. Some industries provide replacement HPDs free of charge regardless of whether they were lost or damaged rather than worn out. Other industries require the wearer to purchase replacements if loss or damage is habitual, especially for expensive muffs, semiaurals, and custom-molded plugs. Management must decide whether to make the employee responsible for maintaining his/her HPDs by limiting the number of HPD replacements per year, or to provide free replacements on demand.

ESTIMATING THE EFFECTIVENESS OF HPDs

An Overview

The protection provided by HPDs in real-world environments can be judged directly only by analyzing the audiometric data base. The estimates of the protection predicted, based on laboratory attenuation data, in-the-field attenuation data for selected employees or other similar measurements provide only indirect evidence of the effectiveness of HPDs as worn by workers everyday. Our experiences in interviewing industrial personnel have identified so many variations in work environments and constraints on HPD users that we doubt it is possible to establish a single number indicator or a multiple factor rating procedure that could realistically estimate the effectiveness of a HPD across all situations.

The air and bone conduction paths by which airborne sound reaches the inner ear are illustrated in Figure 6.8. Usually the air conduction pathway is the dominant route. If a perfect HPD could be developed to completely eliminate sound transmission by air conduction, the wearer's hearing thresholds would be reduced 40–55 dB depending upon the test frequency of interest (15). Practically, with respect to real-world HPD attenuation, the sound transmitted via bone conduction can be neglected. However, in measuring idealistic HPD attenuation in laboratories, bone-conducted sound partially limits the measurable attenuation at 2–8 kHz (16).

The paths by which sound reaches the inner ear of a person wearing plugs or muffs are illustrated in Figure 6.9. These are: (1) sound leakage around the HPD, (2) vibration of the HPD itself, (3) transmission through the materials of the HPD, and (4) transmission by bone conduction. Real-world users obtain less attenuation than predicted from laboratory estimates because they are unable to minimize sound transmission by path 1 and, to a lesser extent, path 2.

The effective protection provided by a HPD is also significantly reduced if the wearer removes the protector for a portion of the exposure time (17). Presented as Figure 6.10 are estimates of the reduction in the NRR (noise reduction rating, or nominal attenuation) for a HPD if it is removed for different percentages of the total exposure time. For example, if an employee wearing a HPD with a NRR of 25 dB removed the HPD for only 4% of the daily exposure time, then the effective NRR would be reduced to 21 dB.

Predictive Procedures

American National Standard

The American National Standard, ANSI S3.19-1974 (18), defines an absolute

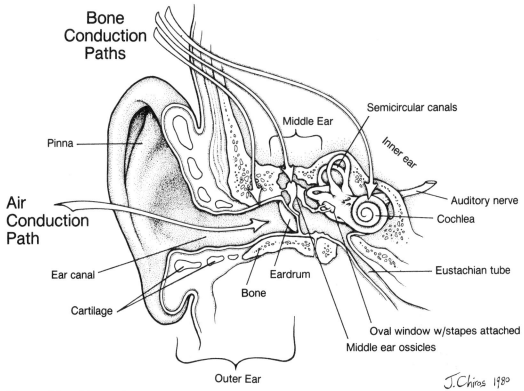

Figure 6.8. Air conduction and bone conduction pathways to the inner ear (courtesy of E. Berger, from EARlog 5).

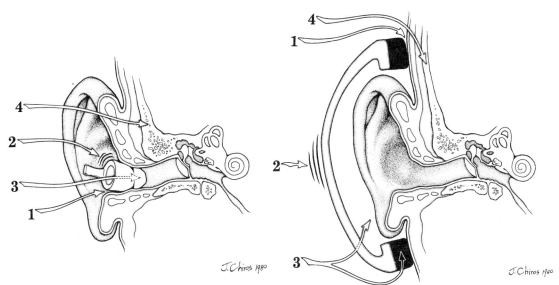

Figure 6.9. Air conduction and bone conduction pathways to the inner ear for an earplug wearer (*left*) and an earmuff wearer (*right*). (Courtesy of E. Berger, from EARlog 5.)

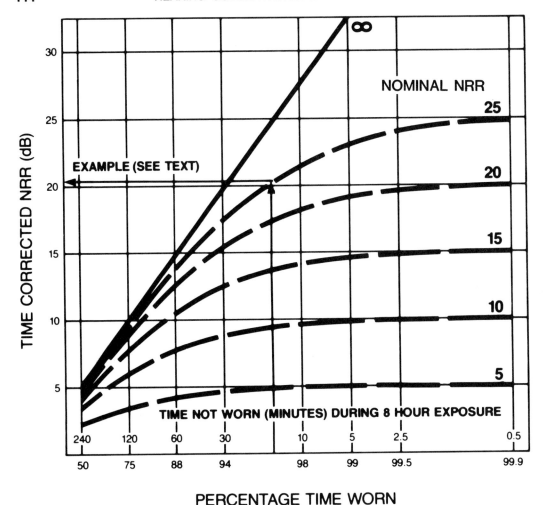

Figure 6.10.   Effective NRR resulting from removal of the HPD for a percentage of the exposure time, based on OSHA's 5-dB trading relationship (courtesy of E. Berger, from EARlog 5).

threshold shift technique for testing HPDs. The standard requires that 10 subjects be tested three times each at nine frequencies, using ⅓-octave bands of noise as stimuli for threshold responses in a diffuse sound field. In this real-ear at threshold method, attenuation is measured as the difference between protected and unprotected thresholds. The resulting data are a set of means and standard deviations for attenuation at each frequency. Sample data obtained according to this standard are presented as Table 6.2 for three earplugs, two muffs and two semiaural devices. The manufacturer's published NRR for each device is also presented.

The data obtained following ANSI S3.19-1974 are measured using trained subjects who wear a particular HPD for only three brief test sessions. The tester places the HPDs to attain the maximum possible attenuation rather than having the subjects place the devices themselves. There is no attempt to simulate the environmental or physical constraints experienced by real-world users. Therefore, results from such idealistic tests should not be expected to produce HPD attenuation data that would be attainable in real-world utilization. The estimates of HPD attenuation based on this test procedure should be viewed as a source of

Table 6.2.
Mean attenuation data with associated standard deviations (ANSI S3.19-1974) for seven hearing protection devices and the corresponding NRR values reported by the manufacturers, dB

Device	Type[a]	Test frequency, kHz									NRR[b]
		0.125	0.25	0.5	1	2	3.2	4	6.3	8	
E-A-R, Decidamp	EP	29.6 3.2	31.3 3.3	34.1 2.1	34.0 2.3	35.5 2.7	40.8 1.8	41.9 2.1	39.9 2.0	39.3 2.8	29
V-51R	EP	20 2.2	23 2.2	25 2.3	29 1.8	35 2.0	38 2.5	39 2.3	38 3.3	39 2.8	24
Com-fit	EP	29.6 3.0	27.6 3.3	30.0 3.5	31.7 2.2	34.3 2.0	40.3 2.5	42.1 4.1	45.7 4.5	45.6 4.6	26
Silenta model 080	EM	11 3.3	15 2.3	23 2.1	33 2.9	35 2.3	40 3.3	41 2.6	38 2.5	37 2.4	20
Bilsom model 2318	EM	23 2.2	25 2.0	31 1.9	36 2.2	40 2.0	42 2.3	42 3.2	39 3.2	37 3.0	26
Caboflex	SA	22.5 3.1	22.3 2.7	23.4 2.3	27.8 2.4	32.2 2.8	37.2 3.3	39.5 3.6	41.1 4.8	41.5 4.9	22
Sound Ban	SA	25 2.6	24 2.1	22 2.0	24 1.8	36 2.4	46 2.5	47 3.5	48 4.7	46 3.9	22

[a] EP, earplug, EM, earmuff, SA, semiaural.
[b] For devices with multiple potential wear positions, the lowest NRR is reported. Therefore, the data shown for muffs and semiaurals represent the under-the-chin wear position.

information for comparing the ultimate protective capabilities of various HPDs.

A casual review of the attenuation data presented in Table 6.2 indicates that the protection provided by HPDs generally increases with test frequency. The attenuation roughly doubles from the 0.125 kHz band to the 4–8 kHz bands. Therefore, the wearer's exposure under the HPD depends on the spectral characteristics of the noise environment as well as the overall sound level.

These attenuation data also contradict the common assumption that earmuffs provide greater attenuation than earplugs. Earplugs typically list more attenuation than muffs at 0.25 kHz and below, but less attenuation at 0.5–2 kHz. Because both plugs and muffs provide sufficient protection at high frequencies for most industrial environments, the low and midfrequency attenuation is more important in HPD selection. However, real-world studies (7) indicate that the relative real-world attenuation of HPDs may vary from the ranking suggested by manufacturers' data.

NIOSH Method No. 1

Although the ANSI standard provides mean real-ear attenuation data and associated standard deviations for HPDs at individual frequencies, these data cannot be interpreted easily to indicate the wearer's overall level of protection. A single-number indicator of protection is desirable for ease of understanding, just as the TWA provides a single-number indicator of the employee's daily noise dose.

The most accurate way to estimate a single-number indicator of HPD attenuation is the National Institute for Occupational Safety and Health (NIOSH) method No. 1 (19). This method utilizes the octave band sound pressure levels for the employee's work environment and the real-ear attenuation data to calculate the R factor, which is the estimated reduction in the A-weighted sound pressure level provided by the HPD. This procedure is illustrated by the computational steps presented as Table 6.3.

NIOSH method No. 1 requires the user to determine the A-weighted sound pres-

Table 6.3.
Sample calculation of the R factor by NIOSH method No. 1, dB

Step	Octave band center frequency, kHz						
	0.125	0.25	0.5	1	2	4	8
(1) Noise spectrum	87	85	89	93	98	103	103
(2) Mean attenuation[a]	11	15	23	33	35	41	38
(3) Standard deviation[a]	3.3	2.3	2.1	2.9	2.3	2.9	2.4
(4) 2 × (3)	6.6	4.6	4.2	5.8	4.6	5.8	4.8
(5) A-weighting[b]	−16.1	−8.6	−3.2	0	+1.2	+1.0	−1.1
(6) (2) − (5) − (4)	20.5	19.0	22.0	27.2	29.2	34.2	34.3
(7) (1) − (6)	67.5	66.0	67.0	65.8	68.8	68.8	68.7

(8) $S = (10^{(67.5/10)} + 10^{(66.0/10)} + 10^{(67.0/10)} + 10^{(65.8/10)} + 10^{(68.8/10)} + 10^{(68.8/10)} + 10^{(68.7/10)}) = 39,846,328$

(9) R = A-weighted sound pressure level = 10 log S

(10) The measured A-weighted sound pressure level is 107 dB, so R = 107 dB − 76 = 31 dB

If the A-weighted sound pressure level measurement is not available, it may be calculated by the following steps.

| (11) (1) + (5) | 71.9 | 76.4 | 85.8 | 93.0 | 99.2 | 104 | 101.9 |

(12) $C = +10^{(71.9/10)} + 10^{(76.4/10)} + 10^{(85.8/10)} + 10^{(93.0/10)} + 10^{(99.2/10)} + 10^{(104/10)} + 10^{(101.9/10)}) = 51,359,260,000.$

(13) A-weighted sound pressure level = 10 log C = 107.1 dB.

[a] The values for the 4 and 8 kHz bands are the numerical averages of the values at 3.2 and 4 kHz, and at 6.3 and 8 kHz, respectively.
[b] For an explanation of the A-weighting values, see Ref. 6.

sure level for the employee's exposure. If a direct measurement of the A-weighted sound pressure level is not available, or if the user wants to check the measurement, the level may be calculated as shown by the extra steps at the end of Table 6.3.

If the octave band data used in computing the R factor (step 1) are representative of the daily exposure for an individual worker, then the resulting R may be used to estimate the employee's effective protected exposure by subtracting the R value from the A-weighted sound pressure level or, alternately, from the TWA.

Noise Reduction Rating (NRR)

Although NIOSH method No. 1 provides the most accurate estimate of the protection provided by HPDs, for many industries a simpler approach is desirable because staff members lack the acoustic instrumentation and training needed to obtain octave band sound pressure level data. To meet the need for simpler procedures, at least 11 attempts have been made to develop a single number rating scheme (20). The procedure which has emerged is the NRR (21), a modified version of NIOSH method No. 2 (19) which was proposed by the Environmental Protection Agency (EPA).

Manufacturers must publish the NRRs for their products on the packaging. When multiple-wear positions are possible for an HPD, such as placing an earmuff band under the chin or behind the neck rather than over the head, the manufacturer must list the poorest NRR from the values for various positions. Although the NRR is furnished, it is important to understand the procedures followed and the assumptions made in its determination. Sample calculations are shown as Table 6.4.

The starting point for NRR calculations is an assumed pink noise spectrum (6) of arbitrary level, as shown in step 1. C-

Table 6.4.
Sample calculation of the NRR for a HPD, dB

Step	\multicolumn{7}{c}{Octave band center frequency, kHz}
	0.125	0.25	0.5	1	2	4	8
(1) Assumed spectrum	100.0	100.0	100.0	100.0	100.0	100.0	100.0
(2) C-weighting[a]	99.8	100.0	100.0	100.0	99.8	99.2	97.0
(3) Overall C-weighted sound level = 108 dB (obtained by applying steps 8 and 9 of Table 6.3 to (2))							
(4) A-weighting[a]	83.9	91.4	96.8	100.0	101.2	101.0	98.9
(5) Mean attenuation[b]	20	23	25	29	35	38	39
(6) 2 × standard deviation[b]	4.4	4.4	4.6	3.6	4.0	4.8	6.0
(7) Protected A-weighted octave band sound pressure levels = step (4) − [step (5) + step (6)]							
	68.3	72.8	76.4	74.6	70.2	67.8	65.9
(8) Overall protected A-weighted sound level = 80.7 dB (obtained by applying steps 8 and 9 of Table 6.3 to step (7) above.)							
(9) NRR = step (3) − step (8) − 3 dB[c], or NRR = 108.0 − 80.7 − 3 = 24.3 dB.							

[a] For explanations of the C- and A-weighting values, see Ref. 6.
[b] The values for the 4 and 8 kHz bands are the numerical averages of the values at 3.2 and 4 kHz and at 6.3 and 8 kHz, respectively.
[c] 3 dB is a correction for spectral variability and uncertainty.

weighting corrections are applied to the assumed octave band sound pressure levels (step 2), and the overall C-weighted sound pressure level is determined (step 3). Next, the assumed pink noise spectrum octave band sound pressure levels are A-weighted, as indicated by step 4. Steps 5 and 6 list the HPD's mean real-ear attenuation and associated standard deviation values. The effective protected exposure levels are obtained in step 7 by subtracting the HPD's mean attenuation values (step 5), minus two standard deviations (step 6), from the A-weighted octave band sound pressure levels (step 4). Next, the overall A-weighted sound level under the protector is determined (step 8). Finally, the NRR is calculated by subtracting the predicted protected A-weighted sound level (step 8) from the C-weighted sound level (step 3), as shown in step 9. Note that step 9 also requires subtraction of an additional 3 dB, which is a safety factor to account for uncertainty about the spectral characteristics of the noise environments sampled to develop the NRR. For the example shown in Table 6.4, using attenuation data for the V-51R earplug, the calculated NRR is 24.3 dB.

In complying with the OSHA Hearing Conservation Amendment, the employee's protected exposure may be estimated by subtracting the NRR from the unprotected C-weighted sound pressure level measurement to yield an A-weighted sound pressure level for the employee's effective exposure under the HPD (5). The following equation summarizes the use of the NRR when C-weighted noise measurements are available:

Effective exposure, dB(A) (or TWA)

= noise level, dB(C) − NRR (or TWA).

One problem encountered in attempting to use this equation is that sound surveys are often conducted without determining the C-weighted sound pressure levels. Since the typical industrial noise spectrum includes more acoustic energy in the lower frequencies (22), the measured C-weighted sound pressure level is usually several dB higher than the measured A-weighted sound pressure level for the same environment. In order to account for this difference it is necessary to utilize an additional safety factor. Recall that the attenuation provided by HPDs is less at the lower frequencies than at the higher frequencies. Therefore, the OSHA regulations require that if only A-weighted sound pressure levels are available, or if the employee's TWA was established using A-weighting, then the HPD's published NRR must be reduced by an additional 7 dB, as follows:

Effective exposure, dB(A)
(or TWA)

= noise level, dB(A) − NRR − 7 dB
(or TWA).

An additional problem is encountered in using the NRR to predict an employee's effective exposure when the sound surveys are conducted using a dosimeter that establishes noise dose using A-weighting. The 7 dB correction to the HPD's NRR may be applied, but another option is to use available sound survey instrumentation to sample the general work area in order to establish the typical difference between C-weighted and A-weighted sound levels (C − A value). This measured C − A correction may then be applied to the NRR instead of the 7 dB correction factor that otherwise would be required. However, care should be exercised, since using the mean value of the difference could significantly underestimate the effective exposure for some HPD wearers.

Sample Calculations

In order to illustrate the effects of the environment's spectral characteristics, plus the potential variations in estimates of HPD effectiveness using C- and A-weighted sound measurements, sample calculations are given in Table 6.5 for the Com-fit and E-A-R earplugs, and the Silenta earmuff as used in noise spectra from two industrial environments. The attenuation data and NRRs were obtained from Table 6.2.

As the data in Table 6.5 indicate, the estimates of effective protection vary significantly depending upon the type of

Table 6.5.

Sample results for predicting the adequacy of three HPDs for use in two noise environments using NIOSH method No. 1 and the NRR, dB

Spectrum	Measured sound pressure levels for two environments								
	Weighting		Octave band center frequencies, kHz						
	C	A	0.125	0.25	0.5	1	2	4	8
(1)	104	97	95	102	98	85	78	71	64
(2)	106	107	87	85	89	93	98	103	103

Effective protection levels predicted by three methods

HPD	NRR	NRR-7	R	NRR with C-weighting	NRR with A-weighting	R, NIOSH method No. 1
Spectrum 1						
Com-fit	26	19	22	78[a]	78[b]	75[c]
E-A-R	29	22	26	75	75	71
Silenta	20	13	13	84	84	84
Spectrum 2						
Com-fit	26	19	33	80	88	74
E-A-R	29	22	34	77	85	73
Silenta	20	13	31	86	94	76

[a] C-weighted level − NRR = 104 − 26 = 78 dB
[b] A-weighted level − (NRR − 7) = 97 − (26 − 7) = 97 − 19 = 78 dB
[c] A-weighted level − R = 97 − 22 = 75 dB

sound survey data available as well as the predictive procedure utilized. The largest differences are obtained for spectrum 2, which exhibits a strong positive slope with increasing frequency. Based on A-weighted sound pressure level measurements, the Silenta muff would not be considered an adequate HPD for this environment. However, based on octave band data and NIOSH method No. 1, the Silenta would be considered acceptable for use in this spectrum.

Real-World Estimates of HPD Effectiveness

The previous sections have dealt with the sound reduction capabilities of HPDs as predicted using data generated by testing subjects in an idealistic laboratory setting. In this section we will review findings of studies that have attempted to establish the attenuation provided by HPDs in real-world environments.

Several different approaches have been used to evaluate the effectiveness of HPDs as used by employees day-to-day. Wearers have been pulled off the job and given threshold tests before and after removal of their HPDs (23, 24). Employees have been tested for potential temporary threshold shifts (TTS) by giving them audiograms at the beginning and end of the work shift (25–27). Physical attenuation measurements have been made by placing microphones immediately outside and inside of the wearer's HPD (28). Hearing trends over time for HPD wearers have been evaluated by analyzing the audiometric data base for groups of employees wearing different HPDs (1, 27, 29).

Summary of Real-Ear Studies

Berger (7) has presented a thorough review of real-ear attenuation studies of HPDs as worn by employees in industry. He summarized 10 studies that included data for over 50 different industrial plants with a total of 1551 subjects. The results of this review are presented as Figure 6.11, which pools attenuation estimates from studies including at least 10 subjects. Berger assumed that industries which agreed to participate in field studies would be more likely to have well managed hearing conservation programs; therefore, he reasoned that these data overestimate the protection actually provided by HPDs to wearers in general industry.

In Figure 6.11 the manufacturers' published attenuation data, which use a correction of −2 SD, are compared to the field attenuation data, which use a correction of −1 SD. Berger argued that a 1-SD correction is appropriate for real-world data because the standard deviations are larger in field studies than in lab studies. In fact, subtraction of 2 SD from field data would result in negative attenuation values, implying that the distribution is not normal and that HPDs sometimes amplify sound.

Amplification has been documented for some earmuff and earplug designs (30, 31). However, amplification by HPDs is not typical.

When the data presented as Figure 6.11 are averaged across the earplug users (1241 subjects) and earmuff users (310 subjects), the data shown as Table 6.6 are obtained. The field data support the argument that HPD designs which minimize potential misuse by wearers generally provide the greatest protection as used in real-world environments. The summary data indicate that, overall, earmuffs provide more protection than most earplugs.

The most effective earplugs are the foam, Com-fit and custom-molded plugs. Expanding foam plugs tend to provide a seal even if the employee inserts the device only part way into the ear canal. Likewise, it is difficult to wear a custom-molded plug improperly because the plug tends to fall out if not inserted fully. Com-fit plugs do depend upon the degree of insertion and tightness of fit; however, the three-flange design might be expected to produce more attenuation with partial insertion than a plug with only one or two flanges.

Temporary Threshold Shift (TTS) Studies

In contrast to real-ear threshold shift measurements at a single point in time, the TTS method estimates HPD effectiveness over the course of an entire workday by detecting any TTS incurred by employees while wearing HPDs in noise environments. We (25–27) have conducted in-plant studies to compare the prevention of measurable TTS by different types of HPDs as worn by employees. Each of these studies was initiated after analysis of the audiometric data base for exposed workers indicated potentially inadequate hearing protection for some employees.

One TTS study (27) investigated the ability of the Silenta earmuff and Com-fit and E-A-R earplugs to prevent measurable TTS in employees at a production

LABELED NRRs VS. FIELD PERFORMANCE

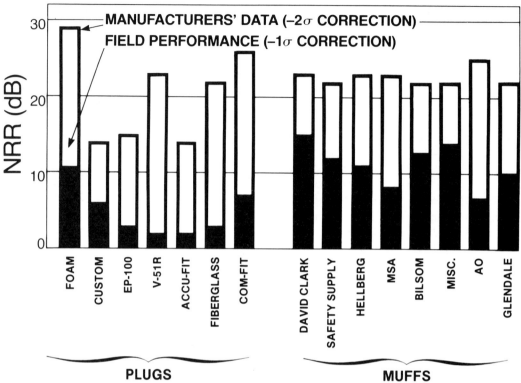

Figure 6.11. Manufacturers' labeled NRRs versus real-world attenuation data for various HPDs. (From Berger EH: Using the NRR to estimate the real world performance of hearing protectors. *Sound and Vibration* 17(1):12, 1983 (7).)

Table 6.6.
Summary of the average performance for earplugs and earmuffs based on labeled data versus real-world data, and the difference between the two types of data, based on data from review by Berger (7)

HPD type	Number of subjects	Labeled NRR 98 (−2 SD)	Real-world NRR 84 (−1 SD)	Labeled real-world
Earplugs	1241	20	5	15
Earmuffs	310	23	12	11
Total	1551	22	9	13

facility where the TWA was 107 dB (described as spectrum 2 in Table 6.5). Statistical analyses indicated that the E-A-R plug provided significantly better protection than the Com-fit plug at 0.5–4 kHz, and significantly better protection than the Silenta muff at 0.5, 3 and 4 kHz. The Silenta provided significantly better protection than the Com-fit at 1–2 kHz.

The three HPDs compared in this study had all been in use at this plant for at least 3 yr prior to the investigation, and annual audiometric data were available for all subjects. Therefore, the TTS findings could be compared with results from audiometric data base analyses to detect any correlation between the short- and long-term methods of estimating HPD effectiveness. The last four annual audiograms for each TTS subject were evaluated for threshold variability by using the %BWs statistic (sequential percent better or worse) described by the authors (1, 8, 29). High values of this statistic indicate unacceptable variability in hearing threshold level (HTL) measurements for successive annual audiograms. The findings presented as Figure 6.12 show that the E-A-R wearers exhibited an accepta-

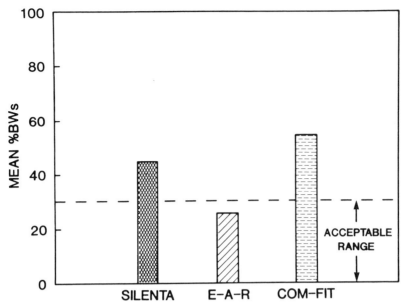

Figure 6.12. Mean values of the %BWs (sequential percent better or worse statistic over the preceding three annual audiograms for groups of employees wearing three HPDs in a TWA of 107 dB. Royster LH, Royster JD, Cecich TF: An evaluation of the effectiveness of three hearing protection devices at an industrial facility with a TWA of 107 dB. (Royster et al: *Journal of the Acoustical Society of America* 76(2):485–497, 1984, (27).)

ble mean %BWs value of 26%. However, the Silenta wearers and Com-fit wearers exhibited unacceptably high mean %BWs values of 45% and 53%, respectively.

This TTS study has three major implications. First, the rank order of the effectiveness of the three HPDs based on daily TTS measurements agreed with the ranking based on audiometric data covering a period of 3 yr. Short-term test procedures for evaluating the real-world effectiveness of HPDs have been criticized as being unrepresentative of wearers' habitual utilization patterns. The agreement between short- and long-term indicators in this study supports the validity of short-term methods. Second, the results suggest that data-base analysis procedures can potentially indicate the relative effectiveness of HPDs based on as few as two or three annual audiometric evaluations. Third, the potential effectiveness of HPDs for use in an environment cannot be judged solely by the manufacturers' published attenuation data or NRRs. As shown by

the data for spectrum 2 in Table 6.5, an estimate of the potential effectiveness of these three HPDs based on laboratory attenuation data would have predicted better protection from the Com-fit than from the Silenta using the NRR, or equal protection from each using NIOSH method No. 1. The actual findings from the TTS study and data base analysis support the recommendation in Table 6.1 that the selection of HPDs available to wearers exposed to TWAs of 100 dB or above be limited to devices which are difficult to misuse, such as foam plugs and earmuffs.

Earplugs Plus Earmuffs

Industrial HPD fitters who are concerned about employees with extremely high noise exposures often suggest that these workers wear earplugs under muffs to increase their degree of protection. However, the gain in attenuation from double protection is less than one might expect intuitively.

Berger (16) conducted a laboratory

study of the attenuation provided by different combinations of plugs plus muffs. Partial results are shown as Figure 6.13, which presents real-ear attenuation data for a small-volume earmuff in combination with a fiberglass down plug, a premolded plug and a foam plug worn with either a partial insertion, a standard insertion or a deep insertion. At the lower frequencies the measured net attenuation depended upon the choice of plug. In contrast, above 2 kHz, the attenuation measured for double protection was equivalent regardless of which earplug was chosen, and the net attenuation was limited by bone conduction transmission. The attenuation gain from double HPDs, compared to the small-volume muff alone,

was about 10 dB at 4–8 kHz for all plugs. At 0.125–1 kHz, the attenuation gain ranged from about 10–30 dB, depending on the particular earplug worn under the muff. Berger also tested the effects of adding different muffs over selected earplugs. In this case the particular choice of earmuff made little difference in the net attenuation once an earplug had been selected.

This study indicates that, for configurations of earplugs plus earmuffs, the major determinant of the net attenuation is the selection of the earplug. Employees exposed to extreme noise levels may benefit from double protection if the spectrum is dominated by low frequency energy. However, double protection would

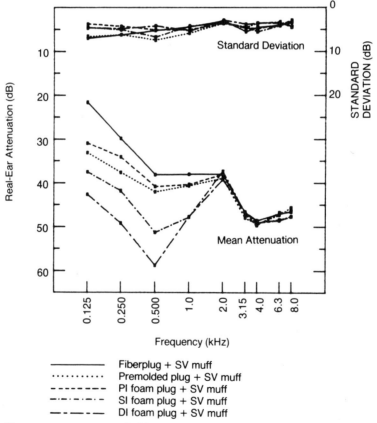

Figure 6.13. Net attenuation provided by a small volume (SV) earmuff in combination with a fiberglass down plug, a premolded plug, and a foam plug worn with either partial insertion (PI), standard insertion (SI), or deep insertion (DI) (From Berger EH: Laboratory attenuation of earmuffs and earplugs both singly and in combination. *American Industrial Hygiene Association Journal* 44:321, 1983, (16).)

be of little advantage in spectra with pre-dominant energy at 2 kHz and above, compared to a single HPD worn properly. Nevertheless, for real-world environments which pose a critical risk of NIPTS, double protection could minimize the possibility of inadequate attenuation due to poorly fitted or improperly worn HPDs.

Recommendations for Derating HPD Attenuation Data

The available estimates of the real-world protection provided by HPDs indicate that industrial wearers attain much less attenuation than test subjects in laboratory situations. Although the current real-world data are probably representative of the attenuation typically achieved by employees, the authors consider this to be less than what *can* be achieved in industrial situations. The data reflect two main shortcomings in HPD utilization. First, in most industries, management has not established or supported adequate procedures for HPD selection, issuing and reissuing; the training of wearers; or the enforcement of proper HPD utilization (3). Second, even in HCPs which are adequately administered, the wearers often fail to fulfill their responsibility to properly wear, maintain and care for the HPDs provided to them (3). These shortcomings are found across the spectrum of United States industry. They are observed equally as often at corporations with extensive medical facilities as at plants with very limited financial and personnel resources.

Derating recommendations should reflect the degree of HPD effectiveness which can be practically achieved in real-world environments. The authors believe that the level of protection indicated by the data presented as Table 6.6 and Figure 6.11 could be improved by 5 dB if industrial personnel would follow the guidelines for HPD utilization procedures outlined in this chapter.

We recommend that the manufacturer's published NRR be derated by 10 dB before estimating the wearer's protected exposure level or TWA.

After the NRR has been derated, HPDs should be selected to achieve a predicted effective A-weighted TWA under the protector of 85 dB or less. Note that the recommended derating is in addition to the 7 dB correction that must be subtracted from the NRR if A-weighted rather than C-weighted sound pressure level data are used. Therefore, the previously given equations for predicting the wearer's effective exposure should be modified as follows:

Effective exposure, dB(A)
    (TWA)

    = noise level, dB(C) − NRR − 10 dB.
      (TWA)

Effective exposure, dB(A)
    (TWA)

      = noise level, dB(A)
        (TWA)

          − NRR − 10 dB − 7 dB.

Similarly, the manufacturer's published attenuation data should be derated by 10 dB at each octave band center frequency before proceeding with NIOSH method No. 1 calculations.

This derating procedure is recommended only for the purpose of permitting the user to judge the potential effectiveness of HPDs in different sound environments using data which would correspond more closely to the actual attenuation which might be attained by industrial employees on the job. In recommending a derating factor of 10 dB, we are assuming that the industry would establish a five-phase HCP, including a complete hearing protection phase as outlined herein. If these conditions were not met, a larger derating factor would be required.

This derating scheme should not be assumed to provide an accurate estimate of the long-term effectiveness of a given HPD as used in a particular environment. The actual protection provided by a HPD can only be effectively judged by an appropriate analysis of the audiometric data base.

SELECTING, ISSUING AND REISSUING HPDs

Limitations of Guidelines

The following sections present recommendations which a hearing conservationist may follow to begin HPD utilization in a plant or to judge the adequacy of procedures already in use. Neither these guidelines nor any others should be interpreted as the final authority for a particular industrial environment; the hearing conservationist should treat practical experiences as an equally valuable source of information. Some HPD issuers we have observed relied exclusively on published materials in deciding how to respond to wearers' complaints. Perhaps because they lacked confidence in their own experiences, they ignored evidence from their situations which could have helped them solve the problems. The HPD fitter should be creative in dealing with such situations.

Selection Guidelines

Types of HPDs

In order to satisfy the varied requirements of wearers, physical environments and job tasks, the choice of HPDs in stock should include a minimum of three earplugs, two earmuffs and one semiaural HPD. The choice for individual wearers may have to be restricted based on the TWA, as shown in Table 6.1, but each wearer should always be offered a selection of at least three HPDs.

The earplugs offered should differ in style in order to fit various ear canal shapes. A good combination would include a foam plug such as the E-A-R (E-A-R Division, Cabot Corporation) or Decidamp (Siebe Norton), a plug with five sizes such as the V-51R (sold under numerous brand names), and a multiflanged plug such as the Com-fit (Siebe Norton) or the EP-100 (Willson). Each earplug should be offered with and without at-

tached strings. A complete listing of all HPD manufacturers is given annually in *Sound and Vibration*.

The company should offer one large volume muff, such as the Bilsom 2318, and one small volume muff, such as the Silenta 080. Large-volume muffs, which offer better attenuation at low frequencies, typically provide sufficient protection for TWAs of 100 dB or above. However, some wearers may object to the bulkier cup and greater headband tension necessary to attain this protection. Small volume muffs generally offer adequate attenuation for TWAs below 100 dB. In noise spectra with acoustic energy mainly above 2 kHz, a small-volume muff may be satisfactory for higher TWAs (27). The small-volume muff is lighter, less bulky and exhibits less headband tension.

At least one semiaural HPD should be available, such as the Sound Ban (Willson) or Caboflex (E-A-R Division, Cabot Corporation). Semiaurals are an attractive option for use in intermittent noise because they can be put on and removed quickly, and carried around the neck when not needed.

Basic Stock Requirements

Employees in most environments settle on a fairly typical selection distribution which provides a basis for initial HPD purchases. Generally only 2–10% of employees select earmuffs or semiaural HPDs. In our sample of industries in the southeastern United States, 2% of workers preferred earmuffs (3), probably due to the discomfort of wearing muffs in a hot, humid climate. Special environments were exceptions: workers in cold storage rooms and production areas with controlled humidity accepted earmuffs. In arid or colder states a higher percentage of workers prefer muffs, especially for outdoor jobs.

In industries which offer the three styles of plugs recommended above, roughly equal numbers of wearers prefer each type. For sized plugs, the distribution of sizes which should be ordered will depend upon the make-up of the worker population to be fitted. Ear canal sizes vary by sex and race, with women typically having smaller canals than men, and blacks typically having smaller canals than whites. Presented as Figure 6.14 is the size distribution of V-51R plugs issued at one industrial facility to black and white females and males. Note that the percentages of plugs needed in each size would vary for employee populations with different proportions of workers in each sex/race group. Initially the two sizes of the Willson EP-100 plug should be purchased in equal numbers. For the Com-fit plug, the initial purchase should contain 20% large, 50% medium and 30% small sizes. Of course, these recommended initial size distributions should be modified to reflect the sex and race characteristics of the users.

When purchasing earplugs initially, the fitter should retain the option to exchange excess unused HPD brands and sizes within 6 months of the purchase date to readjust for the users' preferences.

Special HPD Needs

Even with five HPDs in stock, the fitter will encounter a few wearers whom these HPDs may not satisfy. For example, conical ear canals tend to expel insert HPDs; if muffs or semiaurals are unacceptable, then custom-molded plugs may be the best choice. Persons with allergies may require HPDs in different materials. In environments where high sound levels preclude required vocal communication between wearers, it may be necessary to purchase a limited number of earmuffs with electronic microphones and receivers.

Fitting Factors Which Influence HPD Acceptance

Attitude and Experience of the Fitter

Employees quickly detect the fitter's degree of sincerity as well as his/her familiarity with the HPDs, the work envi-

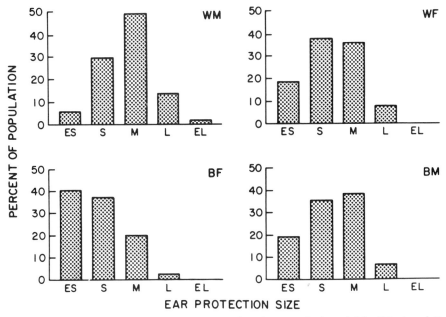

Figure 6.14.   The percentages of V-51R earplugs fitted in one industrial facility to white males (*WM*), white females (*WF*), black males (*BM*), and black females (*BF*), showing differences in ear canal size distributions. (From Royster LH, Holder SR: Personal hearing protection: problems associated with the hearing protection phase of the hearing conservation program. In Alberti PW (ed): *Personal Hearing Protection in Industry*, New York, Raven Press, 1982, (35).)

ronment, and potential problems in using HPDs. For firsthand experience, the fitter should wear each of the available HPDs for a trial of at least 4 hours out in the work environment, not back in the office. Collecting pros and cons about each HPD from workers who wear a variety of styles will help the fitter understand why individuals prefer different types. The fitter should maintain an objective attitude about the styles offered rather than developing prejudices. The goal is to find the HPD which is best for each individual rather than to steer all workers toward any particular style. Most important, the fitter must convey a positive attitude toward HPD utilization. Irreparable damage is done if the fitter tells an employee "these things are a pain" or "you gotta wear the dumb things," as some have admitted doing.

Planning and Scheduling Considerations

If a plant population is being fitted for the first time, then a little political planning is appropriate. Managers and supervisors should be fitted initially and required to start wearing their HPDs immediately. This procedure demonstrates to employees that HPD utilization is important to the company since the leaders are taking the initiative in wearing HPDs to make sure that the styles selected are appropriate for the work environments. Leaders are thereby forced to play an image-making role which will commit them publicly to the enforcement of a strong HPD policy.

After the HPDs have been issued to managers and supervisors and any problems in the issuing procedures ironed out, it is time to fit hourly workers. In each department, it is recommended that the first employees fitted be the most highly respected employees, who can contribute their natural leadership in establishing HPD utilization as a group norm. The employees in the departments with the highest TWA exposures should be fitted

first because they need protection the most and will appreciate the benefits of wearing HPDs most quickly. Hopefully they will make positive comments about HPDs to workers in other departments. It would be counterproductive to fit minimally exposed employees first because they are least likely to perceive benefits and most likely to complain about being required to use HPDs. The fitter must be aware of how the political influence of management, union officers and wearer groups will affect HPD utilization and exploit these factors to attain a high percentage of *proper* HPD utilization.

The fitter should seek the suggestions and cooperation of supervisors in scheduling fitting appointments for the workers in their departments so that production will not be interrupted more than necessary. A 10- to 15-min appointment is needed with each employee. Whenever practical, the worker should be fitted at the start of the shift, then report to his/her work station wearing the newly issued HPDs. By removing the HPDs after entering the noise, he/she can hear how much louder the noise sounds without them. Obviously, if the worker has already incurred TTS that day, this demonstration will have less impact.

Preparation for the Fitting Session
Gathering Information Before Fitting

The fitter can shorten the time off the job to fit an employee by gathering relevant information from the worker's record beforehand. For new hires, the fitter will probably obtain the information by interviewing the employee. Information to be recorded includes the amount of previous experience wearing HPDs, prior noise exposure history, audiometric records, auditory history for pathologies, accidents, and nonoccupational hearing hazards, and the employee's current or anticipated job assignment and TWA.

Audiometric results will alert the fitter to consider potential communication problems while wearing HPDs for individuals with preexisting significant hearing loss. Workers with beginning or advanced NIPTS need extra counseling about wearing HPDs to prevent additional loss.

Medical factors may limit the choice of HPDs. For example, active otitis precludes the insertion of earplugs, and earmuffs might also aggravate otitis by closing off the canal. If the worker has had fungus in the ear canals in the past, HPDs may encourage the problem to recur. Allergies may make one HPD material preferable to another.

The characteristics of the employee's work environment affect HPD selection not only with respect to attenuation, but also physical convenience for the job situation. Earplugs should have attached cords for wearers producing food products or other sensitive items which would be contaminated by lost plugs, and plug color should contrast with the product. Employees who handle irritating substances need attached cords for plugs so that they will not have to touch the plugs with dirty hands to remove them. Earmuffs or semiaurals are also good choices for these situations.

Setting up the Fitting Facility

The fitting facility should be a private room where the employee being fitted will not be observed by other workers, because many individuals are reluctant to ask questions or self-conscious about following instructions, and embarrassed about the fitting process. The waiting area adjacent to the fitting room is ideal to display samples of the various HPDs available for selection so workers can begin to consider the choices. Inside the fitting room there should be a work table, with chairs, where the fitter can arrange the needed materials for easy accessibility. The following items are needed:

1. Samples of all HPDs for the employee to examine
2. Soapy water or disinfectant for cleaning trial HPDs
3. A cup of clean water to lubricate trial plugs

4. An otoscope or other light source with a washable tip
5. A sizing tool for estimating ear canal size
6. Cotton swabs and balls, with alcohol for cleaning tools
7. Paper towels or cloths for drying purposes

Fitting Procedures

Educational Orientation

Before actually fitting the HPDs, the fitter should summarize the company's policies regarding HPD utilization, including the responsibilities of both the company and the employee, and the penalties for failure to wear HPDs. The fitter should explain why HPDs are needed in the employee's work environment and state the short- and long-term benefits the employee will gain by wearing HPDs. This orientation should be more detailed for newly hired employees, but the information should also be reviewed for veteran workers.

Otoscopic Examination

Both ear canals must be inspected prior to fitting any HPDs to detect signs of medical pathologies or excess cerumen which would need treatment before HPDs could be worn. Observing the shape of each canal will also help in selecting an appropriate plug. The physician or audiologist who oversees the HCP should teach the fitter what to observe and how to use the otoscope or similar light source safely, bracing against sudden movements.

If excess wax is present, it must be removed prior to inserting an earplug to prevent the plug from impacting the wax and closing off the canal, producing an immediate conductive hearing loss. Excess wax should be removed only by a physician or by a nurse under the supervision of a physician.

Choosing an Appropriate HPD

The wearer should be allowed to select the type of HPD desired from the options which provide adequate attenuation for the TWA. If the wearer has no preference, he/she may ask what HPD most workers use, allowing the fitter to suggest the most appropriate style. Physical characteristics may reduce the worker's ability to use some styles of HPDs (32, 33); examples include missing fingers, weak finger strength, arthritis of the hands or shoulders, fingers too large to insert plugs correctly, pinnas too large to fit under muff cups, and hearing impairment which affects communication. If the wearer selects a HPD which might be impractical, the fitter should resist the impulse to pressure the worker to change his/her selection. Personal choice is important to the employee's motivation to wear HPDs, and the most effective HPD is the one which the worker will wear properly and constantly. A high attenuation HPD may be less protective than a lower attenuation device if the wearer removes it even for brief periods of time, as shown in Figure 6.10. Therefore, the fitter should attempt to obtain a proper fit with the wearer's selected protector. If this attempt demonstrates that the employee's chosen HPD does not achieve an adequate fit, then the worker will be more willing to accept the fitter's recommendation. The wearer should be told to return for refitting if the initial HPD proves unsatisfactory after a trial period of 1–2 weeks.

Fitting the HPD

The fitter should follow the procedures recommended by the manufacturers of particular HPDs unless experience has shown that a modified fitting procedure provides better results for wearers. The following paragraphs outline general fitting procedures for categories of HPDs.

Premolded Earplugs

Some industrial personnel simply ask the workers what size plugs they would like to have. This is unacceptable even for those who have worn HPDs for years, because wearers tend to select plugs in a smaller size than they actually need (34).

Measuring tools are most helpful to inexperienced fitters, while experienced fitters often rely on their visual judgment of the size and shape of each canal. About 5–10% of employees will require a different size of plug for each ear canal. The goal is simply to decide which size to try first; it is often still necessary to adjust the size through trial and error.

Trial earplug insertions during the fitting process should be made as comfortable as possible. One way to minimize friction against the ear canal lining is to straighten the canal by pulling the pinna outward and upward, as shown in Figure 6.15, or as appropriate for the individual. It also helps to moisten the plug by dipping it into water, then shaking off the excess.

The size plug tried first should be too large rather than too small. If the first size inserted is too large, then the next smaller size will feel better to the wearer. However, if the first plug inserted is very comfortable because it is too small, the wearer will think that the correct, larger size feels worse. While evaluating the fit, the fitter should tell the employee what the criteria are for judging whether the plug fits correctly. For example, with a flanged plug like the Com-fit, the outer flange should close off the entrance to the ear canal (Fig. 6.15). The seal of the plug against the canal walls can be estimated by pulling gently on the handle of the inserted plug to see if there is sufficient resistance or suction.

The employee's exclamations about discomfort cannot always be taken at face value by the inexperienced fitter. Some workers will exaggerate their reactions to obtain a smaller size. Individuals who have not worn earplugs before will normally experience some discomfort. The fitter should explain to the employee that the earplug has to fit snugly in order to achieve significant attenuation, firmly stressing that the correct size is critical.

After determining the correct size plug for each ear canal, the fitter should repeat

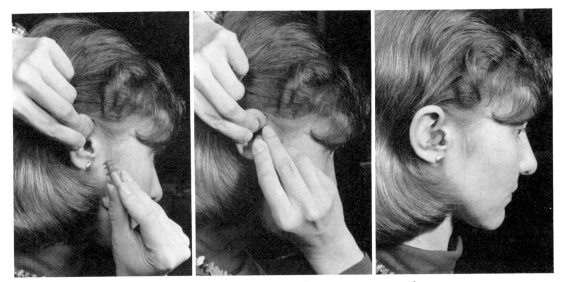

Figure 6.15.   Sequenced steps for inserting an earplug.

the insertion process again while explaining each step. Next, the fitter should demonstrate and explain proper plug removal. With premolded HPDs, it is possible to create a significant vacuum if the plug is removed too rapidly, and jerking the plug out may actually injure the eardrum. Manufacturers usually suggest twisting the plug slightly and/or pulling it downward by the handle to break the seal before it is removed.

After demonstrating and explaining the procedures, the fitter should coach the employee in practicing earplug insertion and removal until satisfied that the employee is able to follow the correct procedures independently. It may help to guide the employee's arm in reaching over the head to pull the opposite pinna (Fig. 6.15). Even if the employee has worn plugs before, the fitter should give full instructions and watch the employee practice. Many wearers have never received any instructions regarding plug insertion, so they may have formed incorrect habits which need to be unlearned.

If a sound source is available in the fitting room, the fitter can use it to teach the employee how to achieve the best fit by adjusting the earplugs until the greatest attenuation is attained. Alternately, the employee can adjust the plugs while listening to the noise in the work area. This process helps the worker understand that the fit of the earplugs is critical in providing protection. Another technique for teaching the employee how to attain an acoustic seal is to use the occlusion effect as an indicator of an adequate seal. When a plug is properly seated, the wearer normally perceives his/her own voice as louder in the occluded ear than in the open ear. Earplugs need to be reseated periodically during use to maintain a seal.

Formable Earplugs

Fitting procedures for formable plugs are less demanding, but fitting is still necessary. These plugs will fit a broader range of ear canal shapes than premolded styles, but formable HPDs will not fit everyone equally well, and employees require instruction to use them properly. The fitter's task is to make sure that the plug achieves an adequate seal for the individual. A few persons have ear canals too large to be fitted with expandable foam, down or large premolded plugs; elastomeric or custom-molded plugs might be alternatives. Some individuals, mostly females, may have canals too small to use foam HPDs easily. Encased down plugs must tightly fill the ear canal to provide significant protection.

It is just as important to demonstrate the correct procedures for inserting formable plugs as for premolded plugs. Manufacturers of formable plugs typically provide well illustrated instructions for using their products. The fitter should observe the employee inserting and removing the selected HPDs twice, or more, if needed, to teach the methods. One way the fitter can judge the adequacy of the worker's insertion technique is to observe the shape of foam, waxed cotton, and elastomeric plugs after they are removed. If the plug has been inserted deeply enough, it will usually show an indentation from the first bend of the ear canal.

Semiaurals and Earmuffs

Contrary to common belief, muffs and semiaurals also must be checked for proper fit and suitability for the wearer. Prominent cheekbones prevent muff cushions from achieving a seal across the temple area. Some individuals have pinnas that are too large to be placed within the muff cups comfortably. The depth of the skull may be too short or too long for the adjustment range of the muffs. Persons with narrow skulls will not receive adequate tension from the muff headband, while those with wide skulls will not be able to make the muffs reach both ears. Extremely thick hair and beards may interfere with the seal. If eyeglasses are uncomfortable with muffs or prevent a good seal, adaptor pads may be used.

Semiaural HPDs do not have as many fitting constraints as muffs, but skull width may be too narrow for proper tension. Wearers with shorter neck length may find semiaurals unacceptable because the band interferes with head movements. A few potential wearers have ear canal entrance shapes which cannot be sealed adequately by certain semiaural

pod or cap designs. After the fitter has determined that the selected muff or semiaural will fit the wearer and has demonstrated placement methods, the employee should be observed placing and removing the HPD at least twice, and coached if needed.

Custom Molded Earplugs

The skill and care of the fitter are critical in determining the quality of fit and the resulting attenuation achieved with custom-molded plugs (34). The fitter should be trained by the manufacturer's representative or a highly experienced fitter before attempting to make custom molds. The mold impression must completely fill the concha and the canal extension should reach to the first bend of the canal. The custom-molded plug does perform consistently once it has been made, since the wearer cannot easily wear it incorrectly. Although the published attenuation for custom molds is less than for some other HPDs, the custom mold may be a good choice if the wearer likes it and will wear it. The major drawbacks of this type of HPD are its initial cost and the time necessary for fitting (3).

Final Instructions

Hygiene

The fitter should not overemphasize the need to clean HPDs out of fear that wearers will develop external otitis from infrequently washed HPDs. Fitters we interviewed mainly in the southeastern states (3) estimated that the rates of otitis among HPD wearers were no higher than reported for the general population (4). We have collected used HPDs which were filthy, yet the wearers at these plants did not exhibit a high incidence of ear canal irritations or otitis. The fitter would lose credibility if he/she stressed hygiene beyond practical limits. For example, mechanics typically cannot use earplugs without getting grease on them, and it would be counterproductive to urge them to wash their plugs several times per day. However, the fitter should recommend extra hygiene care in environments where employees handle potentially irritating substances to prevent transfer of the irritants into the ear canals.

In normal environments, wearers should be instructed to wash their plugs daily in warm soapy water, although most employees will actually wash them only once or twice a week. To encourage HPD hygiene, it is a good idea to issue two pairs of plugs so the worker can wear one and wash the other. Muff cushions and semiaural caps should be wiped clean with a damp rough cloth or soft brush at least every week to prevent dirt and oil from building up on their surface. The foam insert inside the muff cup can be removed for washing, but it must be replaced since it is critical for the muffs' overall attenuation.

Storage

Earplug wearers should always be issued storage containers for their plugs to reduce damage and loss and to provide convenience. The container should be compatible with the employees' environments and work clothes. The convenience or hassle of daily HPD storage can affect employees' attitudes toward using earplugs. Employees who wear semiaurals or earmuffs should be provided a safe place to store their HPDs.

Replacement HPDs

The fitter should tell the employee how often to return for replacement HPDs to prevent them from becoming too worn. Recommended replacement schedules for several common types of HPDs are shown in Table 6.7, based on the durability estimates made by industrial fitters (3). Estimated effective-use periods are attainable for most industrial situations, but use duration will vary with environmental factors.

Wearers should be cautioned to replace their HPDs whenever they show signs of

Table 6.7.
Recommended durations of use before automatic replacement of several common types of HPDs

Device	Use before replacement
E-A-R, Decidamp	3 days–3 weeks
V-51R	2–6 months
Com-fit	6–18 months
Earmuffs	1–2 yr[a]
Semiaurals	6–12 months[b]

[a] Cushions may need replacement every 3–6 months.
[b] This recommendation is based on a limited sample size.

wear, such as hardening, cracks or chips, shrinkage, or failure of foams to come clean or to regain their original dimensions after expansion (35). Several worn plugs are shown in Figure 6.16. Muff wearers should obtain replacement cushions if they crack or harden. Cushions which have conformed to the contours of the user's head and/or eyeglass frames do not require replacement if they are still comfortable, because attenuation is not usually reduced (36). However, loss of headband tension for muffs or semiaurals requires new HPDs.

Responding to Questions

Throughout the fitting session, the fitter should encourage the employee to ask questions and answer those that are raised. Seemingly odd-ball problems may be very important to the wearer. For example, during an educational program a male worker asked one of us:

> "Will wearing hearing protectors affect my sex life?"

When asked later to explain his concern, he expressed fear that wearing plugs at work might decrease his responsiveness at home when his wife blew in his ear. The fitter must handle such personal concerns with sensitivity and sincerity, yet stand firm when workers make complaints in an attempt to be exempted from wearing HPDs. Most fitters we have considered to be indifferent to employee problems were those who seldom wore HPDs themselves or rarely entered the

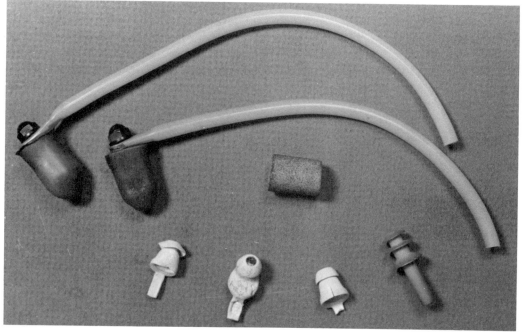

Figure 6.16.   Examples of worn HPDs, illustrating cracks from material deterioration, breakage from material fatigue, dirt and discoloration, and toothmark indentations.

production environment. If the fitter is uninformed or insensitive, the employee may simply decide not to wear the HPDs. Several compilations of questions employees commonly ask, with corresponding answers, are available for reference (14, 37–39).

Record Keeping

All pertinent information obtained during the fitting session should be recorded in the employee's medical file. A separate record card should be kept to document the type of HPD, size issued (if appropriate), employee training in HPD use and care, and reissues. For earplugs, the sizes for each canal should be recorded separately. The fitting information (style and sizes) should be updated when HPDs are checked at the time of the annual audiogram, and anytime when the worker is refitted.

In addition to listing the fitting information, the record card should indicate the frequency of HPD replacements for each user. This information documents

the adequacy of the hearing protection phase of the HCP.

Reissuing Procedures

In many industrial HCPs the effort expended on careful fitting, issuing, and employee training regarding HPD utilization is wasted because reissuing is not controlled. Unmonitored employees may obtain and wear HPDs which are too small or otherwise inadequate for their TWAs. Simple replacements of the exact type and size of HPDs issued by the fitter can safely be handled by a supply room clerk. However, this person must have a copy of the fitting record card and must be carefully trained not to deviate from the type and size of HPD designated for each worker. Each reissue date should be recorded for sized HPDs.

All employees who wish to change their style or size of HPD should return to the fitter for refitting. During this refitting session the fitter should ask the wearer to describe any sources of dissatisfaction and attempt to prevent their recurrence by issuing another HPD and/or reeducating the employee. The fitter should note the reported difficulties on the HPD record card, as well as designating the new type of protection issued. The reissuing session can provide the fitter with valuable feedback regarding the effectiveness of the HPDs as employees are using them. This information may show a need to modify training procedures, fitting recommendations or other aspects of the HCP.

In addition to replacing worn or lost HPDs upon request, the company should establish a regular schedule for mandatory HPD replacements to control the use of HPDs which are worn, damaged or abused.

PROBLEMS ASSOCIATED WITH HPD USE

Employees typically make numerous complaints about wearing HPDs, and managers may cite these objections as a reason for not enforcing HPD use. Although occasional difficulties are inevitable, many sources of employee dissatisfaction can be eliminated by following intelligent procedures for HPD selection, fitting and use. The most common problems are summarized below, and measures are suggested to prevent or minimize their occurrence.

Discomfort

Authors who have reported the relative frequency of HPD complaints agree that employees' most common objection to HPDs is discomfort (3, 35, 40, 41). Sometimes the personnel who fit HPDs discount this complaint by stating that a little discomfort is necessary for adequate attenuation, and that employees will get used to it after an adjustment period. Although these remarks are valid, comfort must be a primary consideration in HPD fitting because employees will not accept devices which create pain or annoyance.

In our ongoing nationwide interviews with HPD issuers (3), they have described numerous types of discomfort. Workers say that plugs are too large or too tight, creating a sensation of fullness or stopped-up ears. Custom-molded plugs which fit too snugly may cause pain down the side of the neck. The "echo chamber" sensation caused by occluding the ear canal is annoying, as is the "popping" sensation which occurs when the plug's seal is broken by jaw movements. Many employees experience itching in their ear canals when they begin wearing plugs, probably because the canal becomes dry when cerumen, its natural lubricant, is removed. A similar condition has been attributed to scraping the canal with cotton swabs (42).

Employees find earmuffs too heavy and too tight, causing headaches, especially if worn with glasses. Earmuffs are too hot in warm climates; in high humidity the muff cups can accumulate perspiration, requiring the employee to empty and dry the cups. Absorbent cotton pads worn between the cushion and the skin may increase user acceptance. Consistent with employees' comments, studies in which subjects rated the comfort of muff models have found that an excessive clamping force against the head and uneven distribution of force by the cushions are related to discomfort. In contrast to workers' comments, some studies have found no correlation of earmuff weight with acceptability (43–45), perhaps because each wearer judged only one muff. When employees rank multiple muffs they do discriminate their relative weight, and weight is related to acceptability (46). The employees' comfort depends on the total weight of all headgear, so lightweight muffs are essential if other headgear is also required.

Careful HPD selection and fitting will minimize discomfort.

Communication and Signal Interference

Numerous investigations have been summarized (47, 48) regarding the potential for HPD wearers to experience increased interference with voice communication and detection of other sounds such as warning signals and changes in machine noise. Many workers, especially those with preexisting hearing loss, are reluctant to wear HPDs because they believe that the attenuation provided will increase their safety risks, or because they rely on machine sounds to perform their jobs (3, 11, 40). Earmuffs do severely reduce sound localization ability (49, 50), but earplugs have less effect since the pinna is uncovered (51). Of course, noise itself masks all kinds of signals, so intentional warning sounds such as sirens or bells should be at least 15 dB above their marked threshold in the noise environment and should be selected to be distinctive from other environmental sounds (52). However, vital incidental sounds such as changes in machine noise or underground mine creaks may not be distinguished easily from the variable background noise. For normal hearing listeners, wearing HPDs does not interfere with perception of intentional warning signals, but detection of incidental sounds may be reduced (53–55). Hearing-impaired listeners wearing HPDs usually hear distinctive warning signals, but they may not perceive incidental sounds (53, 55).

Vocal communication in the work setting is important both for shouting safety warnings and exchanging routine information. Speech understanding is improved or unchanged when normal hearing listeners wear HPDs in noise above 85 dB, A-weighted sound pressure level, (56–63) but comprehension is significantly reduced for hearing impaired listeners (58, 60–62, 64–68). In familiar situations, a limited message set and visual cues help the impaired listener to compensate, making recognition easier (59). The worker who is new on a job has more communication difficulty because of unfamiliarity with the relevant cues. However, facilitative cues are usually irrelevant in danger situations, when the worker needs to perceive unexpected warning shouts or novel messages. In such cases, wearing HPDs can pose a safety risk to all workers, regardless of hearing status.

In speech communication situations, the voice signal itself is less intense if the speaker is wearing HPDs. Due to the occlusion effect, the speaker perceives his own voice more loudly and reflexively decreases vocal intensity (56, 59, 68). This reduction in the signal adds to the communication difficulty of the listener. Employees must be taught to increase their perceived vocal intensity when they are wearing HPDs. Female voices are especially difficult to understand because their voice range includes higher frequencies that are more easily masked by the background noise and attenuated by the listener's HPDs and/or NIPTS.

Unfortunately, many industrial personnel who issue HPDs or enforce their wear have been taught that HPDs do not degrade auditory perception for wearers, regardless of their hearing status. Based on this misinformation, they tell workers with hearing loss that they can hear just as well with HPDs as without them. The employees know better; consequently they lose confidence in the responsible individual and in the HCP as a whole. The workers may stop wearing HPDs, or alter them by drilling holes or otherwise reducing their attenuation. To avoid these unwanted consequences, the issuer must consider the employee's audiogram when suggesting suitable HPDs. For those workers who have already incurred substantial loss which appears to be stable, we recommend a HPD with the minimum necessary attenuation so that speech and signal detection ability will be retained as much as possible.

Industrial personnel have told us that older workers, especially those employed before HPDs were introduced, are the most resistive to wearing HPDs. Communication and signal detection problems are probably the primary reason for this resistance, since older workers have poorer hearing due to age effects (69, 70) and NIPTS. Fitters also report that the majority of employees who prefer earmuffs to earplugs are older workers, and we have observed this trend ourselves (27). We speculate that this preference is related to communication. Earmuff cups can be lifted when the wearer needs to listen, and some muffs have less low frequency attenuation than some plugs.

Design Problems and Environmental Incompatibility

Some HPDs exhibit design deficiencies or material defects that limit their effectiveness in some environments. Material problems include deterioration and breakage. The V-51R earplug is made from a soft vinyl, but it tends to harden with use, shrink and crack (35), as shown in Figure 6.16. For some individuals, this hardening may occur within 2 weeks of use, apparently due to ear canal chemistry. Occasionally V-51R plugs may become sticky if they have been stored for a long time in a sealed container; if this occurs they may be washed and used normally.

The cords attached to earplugs often separate from the plugs (3, 35). This may be only an inconvenience unless cords are used to prevent plugs from falling into a sensitive product, such as food. HPD manufacturers typically design cords to detach under sudden force, so that if the strings become caught in machinery they will fail rather than jerking the plug out of the wearer's canal. Some cord designs enable employees to detach and replace the cords; this makes cord separation easier because the end becomes greasy, causing the cord to slip out during wear.

Earplug removal may be an occasional problem. Waxed cotton plugs may break off in the canal, especially if a hot environment softens the wax. In a few cases, nurses have reported that the central shaft of flanged plastic plugs can break off in the wearer's canal, requiring removal with tweezers. Frequently the tabs or handles designed to facilitate plug removal separate from the body of the plug.

For formable, encased silicone plugs, the handles detach much sooner if the user habitually pulls the sheath to lengthen the plug for insertion, rather than rolling it between the fingers.

Fiberglass down material should only be used if purchased as plugs encased in solid plastic, not as swatches of loose down or plugs with a perforated casing. Individual glass fibers have become lodged in the ear canal, requiring surgical removal (3). In some instances infection may result.

For custom-molded plugs, the fitter should purchase molding kits which allow the material for each ear to be mixed separately. If the impression material for both ears is mixed simultaneously, it may begin to harden before the second impression has been made (3). Custom-molded plugs also vary in their durability and tendency to shrink. Since these HPDs are expensive, the fitter should try out a small number of any brand before purchasing a large quantity.

For semiaural HPDs and earmuffs, the fitter should select a brand for which replacement parts are readily available. The canal caps of semiaurals and the cushions of earmuffs may need replacement before the bands show wear or loss of tension.

Certain environmental conditions promote material deterioration. Extreme heat and cold may increase cracking and breakage of plastic parts. Humidity may adversely affect polyurethane foam plugs by increasing their expansion rate to the point that the plug will not remain compressed long enough to be inserted into the canal. Plugs with an internal air bubble may swell up in extreme heat, so that they no longer fit the wearer.

Environmental factors may make some HPDs a better choice than others. Earmuffs may be selected over plugs to keep sparks out of workers' ears. The material of HPDs should not attract or hold airborne particles, such as sawdust or carbon dust. In lumber mills, earmuffs left overnight on hooks on the wall may fill up with sawdust, or a spider may make his home in the muff cups.

Task demands also limit HPD selection. Large volume earmuffs may be too heavy and/or bulky to be practical, especially with welding hoods, respirators, hard hats, goggles, or glasses. Workers whose hands get very dirty, especially with potentially irritating substances, need plugs with attached cords to minimize touching the plugs during removal. Foam plugs may be impractical for those workers unless they have facilities to wash their hands before reinsertion.

Thoughtful HPD selection and attentive employee training will reduce problems resulting from incompatibility of HPD design with environmental constraints.

HPD Misuse and Abuse

Employees frequently use HPDs incorrectly (33). In some cases workers have never received adequate training because the issuers themselves cannot demonstrate proper use techniques. In other cases fitters point out with exasperation that workers who have been trained and retrained will persist in wearing HPDs incorrectly or intentionally altering HPDs to reduce their effectiveness.

Deficiencies in HPD placement techniques include partial plug insertion, reversed orientation of plugs and semiaurals which are directional, failure to place the pinna completely within muff cups, and incorrect orientation of muff cups. Occasionally employees with large ear canals will insert foam plugs too deeply, requiring them to be removed with tweezers. Abusive HPD alterations include cutting off flanges or drilling holes through plugs to prevent them from sealing, clipping off portions of custom-molded plugs, removal of the canal caps from semiaural devices, drilling holes in earmuff cups, and bending earmuff headbands to reduce tension. Workers may heat plastic HPD bands with a cigarette lighter in order to stretch or bend them for greater comfort, as shown in Figure 6.17.

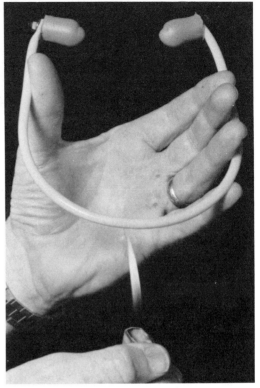

Figure 6.17. Demonstration of how a cigarette lighter may be used to stretch the plastic band of a semiaural HPD.

Sometimes the offending employee does not realize that he is defeating the purpose of HPD wear. Careful employee training is needed to teach workers that modifications such as ventilation holes or headband stretching, which increase the comfort of HPDs, also destroy their protectiveness. Of course, some offenders *do* understand this, but they do not believe that they will incur hearing damage. The importance of education is obvious here as well. A need to express individuality may inspire employees to paint earmuff cups, a harmless decoration. However, if a worker with medium-size ear canals wants to wear size extra-small earplugs because fewer people have plugs in that particular color, then the wearer would attain essentially no protection.

Inadequate education also allows employees to believe that any object placed in their ears will protect them from hazardous noise. Interviewees have told us that employees use numerous items besides the traditional cotton wads as substitutes for commercial HPDs, including cigarette filters, cartridge shells, wads of plastic food wrap, and beeswax. Figure 6.18 illustrates a substitute HPD which an employee made by attaching bits of non-attenuating packing foam to Com-fit cords. The worker did not realize that his invention was inferior to purchased foam HPDs until the safety director found the substitute plugs during a routine HPD monitoring check. Sometimes employees' inventions may be fairly effective: the nurses who discovered plastic wrap and beeswax being used as HPDs tested their attenuation by audiometer and reported that they appeared to provide adequate protection. However, their use was forbidden because these substances did not have an official NRR, and one homemade HPD would lead to another.

Canal Irritation and External Otitis

The occurrence of external otitis related to wearing earplugs appears to be rare. Ear canal inserts might contribute to external otitis through elimination of ventilation in the canal, introduction of foreign substances if the plug is dirty, and potential abrasion of the skin of the canal and/or removal of normal cerumen. In a theoretical discussion of factors contributing to diffuse external otitis, Senturia et al. (71) named elevated humidity, high temperature, skin maceration due to

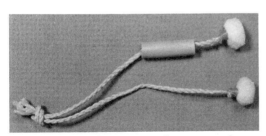

Figure 6.18. Substitute earplugs an employee made by attaching packing foam to the cords from Com-fit plugs, as discovered during a routine check of HPD condition (courtesy Igloo Corporation, Houston).

moisture, contamination of the canal by exogenous bacteria or fungi, trauma to the skin by insertion of a foreign object, and removal of the lipid surface film and cerumen which normally lubricate and protect the skin of the meatus. One could infer from this discussion that earplug use might promote external otitis if a tightly fitting plug were worn in hot, humid conditions. We collected one description of frequent otitis externa among underground miners working in a warm environment with 100% humidity. Interestingly, the safety director who reported this problem said that it decreased when foam plugs were introduced to the mine. He speculated that the foam plugs allow more ventilation around their edges than vinyl plugs.

Our interviews with industrial personnel have revealed very few descriptions of external otitis, and most interviewees believed that plug use aggravated a preexisting condition rather than contributing to a new pathology. For example, numerous personnel have told us that veterans who served in the South Pacific, Korea and Vietnam contracted fungus infections of the ear canal which flare up if earplugs are used. Although earmuffs also reduce ventilation and increase humidity around the ear, nurses tell us that muffs do not aggrevate these conditions as much as plugs.

Contact dermatitis of the ear can occur due to irritants or allergic reactions (71). We have received reports of inflammations which appeared to be related to the introduction of environmental contaminants into the meatus by careless plug use. In one facility in Idaho, employees who used a caustic solution to remove potato skins were required to wear gloves to protect their hands from the solution, but they failed to remove their gloves before handling their earplugs. A similar situation in Montana involved employees who used a caustic bath to remove hair from hog carcasses. In North Carolina, workers on an assembly line producing hydraulic pump components developed inflammation when the hydraulic fluid got into their ears via plug insertion. The problem was eliminated by issuing these employees plugs with attached cords, so that they could remove the HPDs without touching them, and by training the workers to wash their hands before plug insertion.

Allergic reactions to HPD materials have been mentioned only a few times during our industrial interviews. In these instances the plastic of muff cushions or cords attached to plugs was described as causing redness or a rash around the external ear and where the cords touch the face and neck.

Interviewees also described various irritations of the ear canal, including redness, rashes, dryness, and soreness of the skin lining the meatus. We do not know whether these conditions result from allergic reactions, contact dermatitis, cerumen removal, or other causes unrelated to earplug use. Some nurses described abrasions or lacerations of the ear canal caused when substances such as dirt, sawdust, or metal filings adhering to an earplug damaged the skin. However, the ear canal appears to be very resistant to irritation by foreign materials, judging by the dirty condition of many earplugs we have collected in industrial sites. Reasonable cleaning routines should be sufficient to prevent canal irritation.

The Canadian military has conducted a study (11) to determine whether there was increased fungus or bacteria in the ear canals of soldiers wearing triple flange plugs, foam plugs washed after each wearing or foam plugs washed once a week. During 8 weeks of observation, no fungus was found. The groups showed equivalent occurrences of positive bacterial cultures (25%), but no clinically significant otitis externa. The flight surgeon in charge of the study concluded that foam plugs did not cause a greater hygiene problem than flanged plugs. This result contradicts the common belief that foam plugs absorb contaminants and create a greater damage of otitis than other plugs. Actually, vinyl alloy foam plugs cannot absorb anything far below the surface because the foam is made of closed cells. Polyurethane foam plugs can absorb water.

In environments where toxic chemicals are used, interviewees typically expressed the view that disposable earplugs are preferable to reusable ones because they are "cheap insurance" against problems due to contaminants. Rather than relying on employees to carry out frequent washing procedures, these personnel instructed workers to use plugs once and discard them.

Other Problems in HPD Use

Some persons who have large amounts of cerumen may repeatedly impact the wax toward the eardrum by inserting earplugs. These individuals may benefit from regular use of over-the-counter softening agents to facilitate wax drainage. They may need the company nurse to examine their ear canals regularly to detect wax build-up before it blocks the canal.

A few persons experience a coughing reflex when earplugs are inserted. The coughing impulse may subside once the plug is seated for some employees, or it may continue as long as the plug remains in the canal (32, 72). If an affected employee cannot learn to insert plugs without triggering the coughs, the alternative is to wear muffs or canal caps. Some employees experience dizziness or imbalance as a result of earplug insertion (3, 73). We have never obtained a detailed description of the exact nature of this sensation or its duration. One experienced nurse attributed the dizziness to wearing a plug too large for the ear canal. Hypothetically, the insertion of a premolded plug could slightly compress the air between the plug and the eardrum, and the compression could be transmitted to the cochlea via the ossicular chain. For individuals with a fistula in the otic capsule, and perhaps for a few other sensitive persons, the increased pressure could trigger dizziness.

Cosmetic appearance is very important to many employees. Women may dislike styles of HPDs which "mess up your hair" or "look ugly." Custom-molded plugs may be rejected because "they look like bubble gum stuck in your ears." Young men may resist any conspicuous HPDs which interfere with their macho image.

In other situations, conspicuous HPDs are desirable. Employees may prefer earplugs of particular colors for reasons of group identification: they want the same color as other members of their ethnic group, or the team color of their favorite ball club. The issuer must ensure that the employee can attain an adequate fit with the style or size of HPD desired for its color.

Inconvenience discourages workers from using HPDs, so the issuer should suggest styles which are appropriate for task demands. If a worker loses his earplugs frequently, attached cords are helpful. Obtaining replacement HPDs should be reasonably convenient for the worker; therefore, the reissuing location(s) should be as close to the production areas as practical. Employees who enter and exit noise hazard areas frequently will appreciate plugs on strings or semiaural HPDs which can be hung around the neck in quiet areas. Durable carrying cases in shapes which fit into pockets are necessary for all reusable plugs. Some interviewees have actually purchased HPDs expressly for their cases, thrown away the plugs, and used the cases for the plugs they prefer.

The HPD issuer must be thoroughly familar with the work environment and must listen to employees' comments to choose the HPDs which would best meet job-related constraints and make HPD wear as trouble-free as possible.

GETTING THE MAXIMUM USE OUT OF HPDS

Developing an In-House Expert

We have been struck with the lack of knowledge exhibited by some industrial personnel responsible for the fitting, issuing and utilization of HPDs. No company can expect the hearing protection phase of its HCP to succeed without allowing the responsible individual to acquire the needed expertise. In some cases the HPD fitter may be the key individual in charge of the entire HCP, but this is not necessarily so. If audiometric testing is performed in-house, we strongly recommend that the same person be assigned as both HPD fitter and audiometric technician so that he/she can inspect HPDs at the time of the annual audiogram and relate hearing changes to the adequacy of the HPDs as worn. A nurse, safety technician or secretary without heavy administrative duties will have more time and energy to devote to the HCP than a safety, medical or personnel director who is already bogged down. If audiometric testing is done by an external service, HPD fitting and employee counseling should still be performed by an internal staff member.

If the company is willing to provide training and to designate HPDs and audiometry as a primary responsibility for this person, then an individual without prior experience or knowledge can maintain these two phases of the HCP. Once the staff person has been selected, formal training is the first step. A certification course sponsored by CAOHC (Council for Accreditation in Occupational Hearing Conservation) provides basic information and fulfills OSHA requirements. However, additional knowledge must be acquired from reference books, appropriate journals, professional meetings, and special seminars.

Education

Hearing conservation is a *benefit* to employees: the reduced exposures achieved through engineering or administrative noise control and personal HPD utilization decrease the worker's risk of losing his/her vital auditory sensitivity, and audiometric evaluations detect hearing changes due to pathology and off-the-job causes as well as work-related noise exposure. However, benefits may be forgotten by managers and supervisors who become absorbed with achieving regulatory compliance. They may perceive making workers wear HPDs as their hardest task. Workers may perceive the requirement to wear HPDs as one of the most annoying demands by management. Both management and employees need education to appreciate the value of hearing protection and take responsibility for HPD utilization (74). Educational programs should occur *before* HPDs are fitted and issued.

Management

Management must be educated first to generate their active support. Nominal support is typical: the company's written plan for hearing conservation is filed away, and the key individual would get no backing if the written procedures were actually applied. Education for management should familiarize them with the effects of noise on employee health and work efficiency plus the company's legal obligations in hearing conservation, describe the cost-benefit analysis of an effective HCP, and show how firm guidelines for HCP procedures will minimize the incidence of potential problems. Benefits of an effective HCP include lower absenteeism, reduced accident rates, increased productivity, improved job interest and concentration, and less worker fatigue and irritability (75–77), as well as reduced potential liability for compensation claims both currently (8) and in the future.

The key individual will generate managerial interest if the appeal is to the company pocketbook. Because the OSHA Hearing Conservation Amendment requires that all the elements of an HCP be implemented, it costs no more to establish a successful HCP which brings back returns to the company than a half-hearted one. We have observed no correlation between resources invested (large medical staffs, expensive monitoring equipment,

etc.) and program quality. Most HCPs we have considered to be effective were administered by a single staff member who was genuinely concerned about employees' hearing and who had the backing of management (2).

Managers must understand that universal enforcement of HPDs is the crux of an effective HCP. They typically fear that real enforcement of HPD wear would result in confrontations, dismissal of resistive workers, possible unionization of the plant, and worsening of employer-employee relations. The key individual can help overcome these fears by citing successes in other firms, or arranging for a conference between influential managers and a representative of a company which has enforced HPD utilization without bad repercussions.

To familiarize managers with the HPDs offered by the company, the educational program should include a demonstration of each type. After the presentation, each manager should be fitted with HPDs and reminded that the rule that HPDs must be worn will not be taken seriously by workers unless it also applies to the VIPs. Managers may appreciate the value of HPDs better if they use them for off-the-job recreational activities, so giving them an extra pair of plugs for home use is a good investment.

In annual updates for managers, the key individual can report on the status of the HCP. Supporting statements about achievements and deficiencies with results from audiometric data base analysis (1, 8, 27, 29, 78, 79) will increase the credibility of this presentation. Audiometric data can show superior hearing trends for departments where supervisors strictly enforce HPD wear than for areas where supervisors are lax. The variability in HTLs from year to year is also reduced when effective HPDs are worn consistently. The potential compensation costs and productivity costs associated with nonwear can be used to convince managers that HPD utilization should be included as an item in personnel performance evaluation.

Supervision

Next, supervisors should be educated together so that they can be uninhibited about asking questions and voicing concerns. Supervisors need more information about HPDs than either managers or employees in order to answer workers' questions and support the need to wear HPDs with facts rather than orders (80, 81). It is critical to elicit supervisors' support for HPD utilization because they are responsible for daily enforcement, and they influence employees through their own attitudes and behavior.

If the HCP is new, supervisors should be fitted with HPDs before employees are fitted. Supervisors can try out their new HPDs on the job for a few days to get used to them, troubleshoot for any constraints which would make certain HPDs more practical, arouse employees' interest, and demonstrate the company's care in planning the HPD phase. A second supervisory meeting should be held after the trial to collect comments and suggestions, correct problems and address any objections to HPD use.

Employees

Finally 30-min presentations should be made for all employees who regularly or occasionally wear HPDs. Sessions should be held for groups of 20–30 employees to encourage questions. The program should cover the advantages and disadvantages of the types of HPDs available, their use and care, and company policy for enforcing HPD utilization. The presentation should stress the importance of proper fit for comfort and attenuation, and the need to wear HPDs during the entire exposure time to receive full benefit.

Other Relevant Individuals

If replacement HPDs are obtained from the attendant in charge of the supply room or tool crib, this person must understand that the effectiveness of HPDs depends on the appropriate style and size being worn, so that he/she will not succumb to workers' requests for different HPDs. External consultants must be informed of the HCP policies which the company has selected and must understand their role in the HCP. For example, the physicians and audiologists to whom employees with suspected pathologies or extreme threshold shifts are referred may need to be familiarized with HPD utilization in industry. The key individual should specify the type of report needed about the clinical findings and reach an agreement with the consultants as to whether recommendations about HPDs will be made directly to the employee or discussed first with the company personnel. These precautions will prevent potential conflicts such as a physician telling an employee with mild ear pathology not to wear HPDs, without realizing that the worker would have to transfer to another job to follow this recommendation.

Motivational Concepts and Techniques

Educational programs are useful for informing supervisors and employees of the facts about noise-induced hearing loss and why the company has established the HCP for their protection, but the risk of future hearing impairment is too distant to convince many workers to wear HPDs day after day. Effective motivational techniques bring the rather abstract concept of gradual hearing damage down to a more concrete and immediate level by focusing on measured hearing changes in the employee's own audiogram and emphasizing short-term benefits of wearing HPDs. The HPD fitter can generate worker motivation by demonstrating the company's sincere interest in hearing conservation and establishing HPD utilization as a group norm so that peer influence will reward wearers.

Annual Audiogram Results

For workers who do not have an important reason (such as communication) *not* to wear HPDs, the strategy is to show them important reasons *to* do so. By far the most effective tool for this purpose is the worker's own audiogram. Brief personal counseling with the employee following his/her annual audiogram and personalized written feedback about hearing changes bring the vague threat of hearing loss closer. A recent time series field study (82) confirmed that audiometry increases workers' motivation to wear HPDs, as others have previously suggested (2, 81, 83). Explaining audiogram results to the employee and counseling him/her about using HPDs to prevent additional hearing loss is the most effective strategy in approaching resistive employees. The technician must have enough time in the testing schedule to give the worker a summary of his/her hearing status in relation to the thresholds expected for the worker's age, sex and race (69, 70) and the amount of hearing threshold change shown over time. If audiometric testing is performed by a mobile testing service, the company may request that the mobile service provide on-the-spot employee feedback when an appropriate professional is available to interpret results. Written notification of results to employees is valuable, but the personal contact with the worker at the time of testing should not be sacrificed. In reality this may not always be practical with a mobile testing program, but the in-house HPD fitter can also counsel employees about their audiometric results even if testing is performed by someone else.

In counseling employees about their audiograms, it is important to contradict commonly held misconceptions about hearing loss. Many workers ask whether they "passed the test," apparently believing that there is a magic cutoff for normal or useful hearing. A related belief is that normal declines in hearing with age will create "failing" results eventually, so

wearing HPDs merely postpones the inevitable. The technician should show the worker on an audiogram chart what the average thresholds are for his/her current age and for retirement age, based on NIOSH norms (84) or nonindustrial noise-exposed reference populations (69, 70), or presbycusis control populations (85). The technician should then contrast these mild age effect threshold patterns with potentially severe NIPTS curves. It is especially effective to use anonymous audiograms from actual employees at the plant as illustrations for NIPTS, pointing out that the loss was developed in the worker's own noise environment. If the employee has already acquired a significant loss, the technician must refute any impression that it is too late to do any good by wearing HPDs from now on. The technician should stress that saving the remaining hearing will help the employee in social interaction and the enjoyment of music and other auditory pleasures.

Industrial personnel we have interviewed state that older male employees are typically most resistive to wearing HPDs, followed by very young males. Direct worker surveys (86, 87) confirmed this impression. We suggest that older workers reject HPDs because wearing them compounds the communication problems associated with preexisting hearing losses. This difficulty can be minimized by offering such workers the HPD with the lowest acceptable attenuation at frequencies below 2 kHz. Personal counseling with these individuals can increase their motivation to preserve their remaining hearing by wearing HPDs.

Special Audiometric Techniques

Audiometry can also be used for demonstrations of daily TTS as a motivational technique. Zohar, et al. (88) graphed pre-work and postwork audiograms for employees on one day when HPDs were worn and one day when no protection was used. Pairs of audiograms (without names) were posted on bulletin boards to show the contrast between the substantial TTS acquired without HPDs and the absence of TTS while wearing HPDs. The percentage of employees wearing HPDs increased immediately and continued to rise for at least 5 months after TTS demonstrations ended.

Occupational hearing conservationists who have used daily TTS as a motivational technique for individual employees have reported good success in convincing resistive workers that HPDs work. This method is recommended, especially if unidentified audiograms can be posted or discussed in safety meetings to influence large numbers of employees without spending the time to perform prework and postwork audiograms on each one.

Another audiometric technique for employee motivation is to give employees audiograms with their earplugs inserted and without them to demonstrate that poorly fitted or inserted plugs provide little attenuation. This method does not provide a laboratory equivalent estimate of HPD attenuation, but it does show when one insertion position is better than another and gives a reasonable estimate of the real-world attenuation provided by the HPDs that may be evaluated using this procedure. Harvey (89) reported that employees who received these demonstrations learned to obtain significantly greater attenuation, either by better insertion of their old earplugs or selection of a different type and/or size of HPD. This type of individual demonstration appears to be a viable motivational technique, although the time involved would make it feasible only for employees who show threshold shifts.

Behavioral Techniques

A few attempts to apply behavioral methodology to increase HPD acceptance have been reported. An essentially punitive overcorrection technique (90) produced only temporary gains in the percentage of wearers, but positive reinforcement methods have yielded longer lasting improvements. Zohar (91) summarized two industrial studies in which token economies were established to reward workers for wearing HPDs. In both sites, utilization rose to 90% and remained at that level after tokens were discontinued, suggesting that a new group norm had been established. Others (92) have proposed that token economies work because employees induced to wear HPDs for a trial period become accustomed to their extra-auditory benefits, such as reduced fatigue, irritability, tinnitus, and headaches.

Sincere Concern

The techniques used to approach HPD utilization may be less important than the projection of sincerity by the company personnel involved in eliciting employees' cooperation. The key individuals responsible for the HCP must truly care about protecting employees. Otherwise, workers may discount their motives on the basis that the company simply wants to avoid OSHA citations, fines or compensation costs. The HPD fitter can demonstrate sincerity by sharing information honestly. For example, workers should be cautioned to expect a certain amount of mild discomfort until they become accustomed to wearing HPDs. However, the fitter should encourage employees who experience severe discomfort to return for refitting. Experienced fitters report that the personal attention they give to complaining employees is worth at least as much as the improved comfort achieved by refitting. The company can also demonstrate the sincerity of its HCP by encouraging workers to take a pair of HPDs home for hobby noise exposures, and by providing HPDs to employees who experience noise annoyance without being technically overexposed.

Coordination among all the company personnel involved in administering HPD utilization is another aspect of corporate sincerity. Contributing departments such as safety, medical, environmental, hygiene, etc., must maintain active communication to ensure that everyone is aware of their own roles and the complementary roles of other staff members. We have visited firms, especially large corporations, in which representatives of different disciplines gave contradictory descriptions of the procedures for HPD fitting, reissuing and utilization enforcement. In one case the nurses who fitted sized earplugs did not know that safety personnel were issuing formable plugs and earmuffs to the same employee population. Because the nurses never ventured into the production areas, they were unaware of what HPDs were actually being worn. The safety and hygiene staff were familiar with the plant environment and the HPDs in use, but they had no access to audiometric results. This example illustrates the need for active communication not only between the administrators running the HCP, but also between the administrators and the hourly workers. Personnel who genuinely try to protect employees will seek out information by regularly visiting the production areas to observe, ask for comments, and do spot checks of HPD utilization. Consequently, we have observed that HPD issuers who spend time in production areas report more problems associated with HPD utilization because they are familiar with the problems which do exist. Even remote administrators can obtain this type of knowledge *if* they assign plant HPD fitters the responsibility of collecting worker feedback, then hold regular meetings of all fitters to share the information and discuss needs for any changes. Regular conferences among the staff who oversee the HCP are necessary to communicate perceived problems and coordinate efforts to solve them.

Peer Group Influence

In companies where the HCP is effective, safety and health awareness is part of the plant atmosphere and part of the workers' image of themselves as employees. The key individual and supervisors cultivate group identification with safety consciousness.

Written information is often used to remind workers about HPD utilization, but it must be carefully selected to have a large impact. Cartoon posters are too impersonal, but appealing photographs can be meaningful if they depict emotional interpersonal contexts such as parent-child or husband-wife interactions which depend on auditory communications. Posters which invite the reader to make personal comparisons are also effective; for example, a poster can present normal age effect hearing levels as a way for the worker to check his own hearing against the norms. Posters of audiometric trends or HPD utilization percentages for departments can be used to stimulate healthy competition and peer pressure regarding HPD utilization. Competition among supervisors is especially useful since they influence their own departments (93). Hearing conservation articles in company newsletters may be useful if personnel can write genuinely interesting stories which contribute to group pride in hearing conservation.

In general, safety meetings are a better way to reinforce HPD utilization than posters or articles. One successful safety director distributed samples of new brands of HPDs at safety meetings and asked the wearers to report back to the group at the next meeting regarding their acceptability. He was willing to order any brands which employees preferred as long as the attentuation was adequate. Workers knew that they could ask questions or voice valid complaints in these meetings and get an attentive response.

Natural group leaders are another important resource which can be tapped to contribute to HPD utilization if the company is sincere. The HPD fitter or the key individual may approach respected employees to compare brands of HPDs for potential purchase, or to initiate HPD use in their departments. If there is an older worker with NIPTS from past exposure who is willing to describe his own experiences with hearing loss to other workers, such a personal testimonial can be extremely influential in convincing other workers of the value of wearing HPDs. Informal group leaders cannot inspire HPD utilization unless the company's formal leaders enforce HPD use uniformly. Luz et al. (94) demonstrated that when US Army drill instructors did not wear HPDs on the firing range, significantly more new recruits ignored instructions to wear them.

Enforcing HPD Utilization

Policy

The rule at the foundation of every successful HCP we know of is simple: everyone who enters a designated noise area must wear HPDs, no matter how brief the visit. In plants where this rule is in effect, production workers feel free to inform executives to go get HPDs, and plant managers take time to pick hourly workers off the line for nonwear. The policy is absolute. It costs little. It works.

Of course, first-time violators should not be fired. A strict enforcement policy must be backed by genuine concern and a willingness to work with employees who have problems with their HPDs. The response to an initial violation should be counseling and HPD refitting, if necessary. Subsequent violations should be dealt with through a graduated series of steps from verbal warnings and written warnings to time off without pay, transfer to a less desirable job out of the noise area, or eventual termination. Where such policies exist, very few workers ever actually have to be dismissed, but the company must be willing to do so if pushed. The disciplinary policy should be written as part of the HCP plan and given as a condition of employment during the hiring process. In unionized companies, the policy should be included in the union contract. Although such a strict policy

may sound punitive or harsh, it can be implemented in a firm, humane manner.

Industrial personnel we have interviewed agree that a firm policy is mandatory because a minority of employees will not respond to educational or persuasive attempts to achieve compliance. This conventional wisdom was supported by results of a study by Hager et al. (95), who compared audiometric results for workers employed at a site during periods of voluntary HPD wear and mandatory enforcement. Mean hearing thresholds after specified years of employment were better for employees subject to mandatory HPD utilization than for workers subject to voluntary wear policies. Furthermore, the data for individuals who had worked during both policy periods showed the benefit of requiring persons with preexisting hearing loss to start wearing HPDs to prevent additional loss.

Monitoring

Several ways are available to monitor actual utilization. Obviously, unannounced checks should be conducted periodically to determine compliance percentages by departments. Wear checks should be made by different people and at different times of day, so that they are not predictable. The resulting HPD utilization percentages can be posted, discussed during safety meetings, and presented to supervisors. Managers should hold supervisors accountable for the performance of their departments by including HPD utilization as part of job performance reviews.

It is just as important to check *what* HPDs employees are wearing as to see whether they are wearing any at all, so separate HPD condition checks are needed in addition to wear checks. Workers may trade around to obtain HPDs other than those issued to them. In addition to controlling this problem through reissuing records, it is good to monitor utilization between HPD reissuing times by checking whether the types and sizes being worn match the fitting records. The checker should ask randomly selected employees to remove their HPDs to look for wear, abuse or substitution. As shown in Figure 6.18, the objects on the ends of earplug cords may not be standard plugs. Other alterations which are not apparent to the observing supervisor include cutting foam plugs in half or drilling holes in plugs or muffs. Periodic HPD condition checks will detect these problems before the audiometric technician finds hearing threshold shifts resulting from modified HPDs at the time of the next annual audiogram.

The HPD purchase orders are another useful source of information about what protection is being worn. If the number of plugs ordered in small sizes significantly exceeds those ordered in larger sizes, the technician should suspect that the reissuing procedures have broken down, unless the worker population is mostly female or black. The reorders submitted over the course of a year should reflect the same distribution of HPD brands and sizes as the fitting records.

FUNCTION OF HEARING PROTECTION IN HEARING CONSERVATION

During the protracted process of developing regulations for industrial hearing conservation in the United States, one central question has been whether the utilization of HPDs is an acceptable substitute for engineering and/or administrative noise controls. The high initial cost of noise reduction and the impracticality of administrative controls for many environments have resulted in increasing emphasis on reducing employees' exposures by HPD utilization rather than by direct hazard elimination. Although feasible engineering controls are required by the noise regulation (96) when the employee's TWA equals or exceeds 90 dB, it has been suggested that noise controls be required only if the TWA is 95 dB or above. In future debates concerning the best trade-off between engineering controls and per-

sonal hearing protection, the issue will continue to be whether HPD utilization is capable of protecting employees from occupational NIPTS.

The OSHA Hearing Conservation Amendment contains numerous provisions concerning the ways in which suitable HPDs are to be selected and fitted, plus specifications that the employer must train employees in the use and care of HPDs and supervise workers in using them correctly. These provisions indicate OSHA's recognition that employees will not be protected if HPDs are simply provided. However, the current regulation does not go far enough in specifying strict requirements for HPD utilization.

One severe shortcoming of the Amendment is its failure to recognize that the manufacturers' published HPD attenuation data are idealistic figures which can not be attained in general industrial environments. Therefore, as recommended in this chapter, the published attenuation data should be derated by 10 dB in order to reflect more accurately the real-world protection afforded to wearers. It is especially important to acknowledge the real-world attenuation of HPDs when they are used as a substitute for 14 hr of quiet preceding audiometric evaluations. If employees incur TTS while wearing inadequate HPDs prior to their baseline and annual tests, then monitoring audiograms will be less effective in detecting threshold shifts. The authors support the use of HPDs prior to audiometric testing (97), but only under the condition that the HPDs used are capable of preventing TTS based on real-world estimates of attenuation.

Another major deficiency of the Amendment is its failure to require that industry evaluate the effectiveness of HCPs against performance criteria, so that both the employer and the enforcing agency can determine whether employees are being protected. OSHA did express interest in methods for evaluating industrial HCPs (98), but the agency concluded that currently available methods were not yet fully enough developed to require their use (5). We (97) support the use of audiometric data base analysis as a method for evaluating HCP success, especially regarding HPD effectiveness (1, 8, 27, 78). The evaluation of HCPs is discussed in Chapter 10.

SUMMARY

The data presented in this chapter indicate that HPDs can protect employees from NIPTS if worn correctly within the context of an ongoing HCP. However, their protectiveness is less than indicated by the published attenuation data and NRRs. Results from TTS studies and audiometric data base analyses show that a few types of HPDs can provide adequate protection for workers exposed to TWAs of up to 107 dB, at least for noise spectra with high frequency emphasis. However, the majority of HPD types presently being used in industry offer sufficient protection only for TWAs of up to about 95 dB.

Although HPDs *can* be effective within these limits, this degree of protection can only be attained if industry expends the effort to control the use of HPDs very carefully. National survey results show that most industries currently do not follow acceptable procedures for implementing HPD utilization; therefore, improvements are badly needed. The recommendations outlined in this chapter provide a guide for achieving an effective hearing protection phase of the HCP (2).

References

1. Royster LH, Royster JD: Methods of evaluating hearing conservation program audiometric data bases. In Alberti PW (ed): *Personal Hearing Protection in Industry*. New York, Raven Press, 1982.
2. Royster LH, Royster JD, Berger EH: Guidelines for developing an effective hearing conservation program. *Sound Vibration* 16(1):22, 1982.
3. Royster JD, Royster LH: *Hearing Protection Devices as Used in Real World Environments*. Final report submitted to OSHA. Submission number 501-2 to docket OSH-011. Washington, DC, U.S. Department of Labor, 1982.
4. Singer JD, Tomberlin TJ, Smith JM, Schrier AJ: *Hearing Status in the United States and the Auditory and Nonauditory Correlates of Occupational Noise Exposure*. Contract report number 68-01-6264. Washington, DC, Environmental Protection Agency, 1982.
5. Occupational Safety and Health Administration: Occupational noise exposure: hearing conservation amendment. *Federal Register* 48:9738, 1983.
6. Irwin JD, Graf ER: *Industrial Noise and Vibration Control*. Englewood Cliffs, N.J., Prentice-Hall, 1979.
7. Berger EH: Using the NRR to estimate the real world performance of hearing protectors. *Sound Vibration* 17(1):12, 1983.
8. Royster LH, Royster JD: Making the most out of the audiometric data base. *Sound Vibration*, 18(5):18–24, 1984.
9. International Organization for Standardization: *Acoustics—Determination of Occupational Noise Exposure and Estimation of Noise-Induced Hearing Impairment*. Draft, International Standard ISO/DIS 1999, 1982.
10. Occupational Safety and Health Administration. Occupational noise exposure: hearing conservation amendment. *Federal Register* 46:4078, 1981.
11. Forshaw SE, Cruchley JI: Hearing protector problems in military operations. In Alberti PW (ed): *Personal Hearing Protection in Industry*. New York, Raven Press, 1982.
12. Durkin J: *Effect of Electronic Hearing Protectors on Speech Intelligibility*. Report number 8358. Washington, DC, U.S. Department of the Interior, Bureau of Mines, 1979.
13. Karmy SJ: The fact upon the acoustic attenuation provided by ear muffs of the simultaneous use of other items of safety equipment. In *Proceedings of the 10th International Congress on Acoustics*, vol. 2: B-15.2, 1980.
14. Berger EH: *EARlog 9: Responses to Questions and Complaints Regarding Hearing and Hearing Protection (Part II)*. Indianapolis, E-A-R Division, Cabot Corporation, 1982.
15. Zwislocki J: In search of the bone conduction threshold in a free sound field. *J Acoust Soc Am* 29:795, 1957.
16. Berger EH: Laboratory attenuation of earmuffs and earplugs both singly and in combination. *Am Ind Hyg Assoc J* 44:321, 1983.
17. Else D: A note on the protection afforded by hearing protectors: implications of the energy principle. *Ann Occup Hyg* 16:81, 1973.
18. ANSI: S3.19-1974: Method for the measurement of real-ear protection of hearing protectors and physical attenuation of earmuffs. New York, American National Standards Institute, 1974.
19. National Institute for Occupational Safety and Health: *List of Personal Hearing Protectors and Attenuation Data*. Report number 76-120. Cincinnati, U.S. Department of Health, Education, and Welfare, 1975.
20. Johnson DL, Nixon CW: Simplified methods for estimating hearing protector performance. *Sound Vibration* 8(6):20, 1974.
21. Environmental Protection Agency: Noise labeling requirements for hearing protectors. *Federal Register* 42:56139, 1979.
22. Royster LH, Stephenson JE: Characteristics of

several industrial noise environments. *J Sound Vibration* 47:313, 1976.

23. Edwards RG, Hauser WP, Moiseev NA, Broderson AB, Green WW: Effectiveness of earplugs as worn in the workplace. *Sound Vibration* 12(1):12, 1978.
24. Edwards RG, Broderson AB, Green WW, Lempert BL: A second study of the effectiveness of earplugs as worn in the workplace. *Noise Control Engineering* 20(1):6, 1983.
25. Royster LH: Effectiveness of three different types of ear protectors in preventing TTS. *J Acoust Soc Am* 66(Suppl 1):S62, 1979.
26. Royster LH: An evaluation of the effectiveness of two different insert types of ear protection in preventing TTS in an industrial environment. *Am Ind Hyg Assoc J* 41:161, 1980.
27. Royster LH, Royster JD, Cecich TF: An evaluation of the effectiveness of three hearing protection devices at an industrial facility with a TWA of 107 dB. *J Acoust Soc Am* 76(2):485–497, 1984.
28. Goff RJ, Blank WJ: A field evaluation of muff-type hearing protection devices. *Sound Vibration* 18(10):16, 1984.
29. Chung DY, Hardie R, Gannon RP: The performance of circumaural hearing protectors by dosimetry. *J Occup Med* 25:279, 1983.
30. Royster JD, Royster LH: Evaluating the effectiveness of hearing conservation programs by analyzing group audiometric data. Seminar presented at the convention of the American Speech-Language-Hearing Association, Toronto, November 1982.
31. Johnson DL: (Personal communication) 1983.
32. Berger EH: (Personal communication) 1983.
33. Guild E: Personal protection. In *Industrial Noise Manual*, ed. 2. American Industrial Hygiene Association, 1966.
34. Riko K, Alberti PW: How ear protectors fail: a practical guide. In Alberti PW (ed): *Personal Hearing Protection in Industry*. New York, Raven Press, 1982.
35. Franzen RL, Stein L: Influence of the fitter on earplug performance. *Sound Vibration* 8(1):25, 1974.
36. Royster LH, Holder SR: Personal hearing protection: problems associated with the hearing protection phase of the hearing conservation program. In Alberti PW (ed): *Personal Hearing Protection in Industry*. New York, Raven Press, 1982.
37. Carroll C, Crolley N, Holder SR: A panel discussion of observed problems associated with the wearing of hearing protection devices by employees in industrial environments. In Royster LH (ed): *The Evaluation and Utilization of Hearing Protection Devices in Industry*. Proceedings of session at the spring 1980 meeting of the N.C. Regional Chapter, Acoustical Society of America. Available from Raleigh, NC, D. H. Hill Library.
38. Berger EH. *EARlog 8: Responses to Questions and Complaints Regarding Hearing and Hearing Protection (Part I)*. Indianapolis, E-A-R Division, Cabot Corporation, 1982.
39. Berger EH: *EARlog 10: Responses to Questions and Complaints Regarding Hearing and Hearing*

Protection *(Part III)*. Indianapolis, E-A-R Division, Cabot Corporation, 1983.

40. Karmy SJ, Coles RRA: Hearing protection: factors affecting its use. In Rossi G, Vigone M (eds): *Man and Noise*. Torino, Italy, Edizioni Minerva Medica, 1976.
41. Angell BJ: Personal attributes affecting the use of hearing protection in industry. (M.S. thesis submitted to North Carolina State University, Raleigh, 1982.)
42. Rettinger G: (Cleansing of the ear canal with cotton swabs—sense or nonsense?). *Deutches Arzteblatt* 76:1747, 1979.
43. Acton WI, Lee GL, Smith DJ: Effect of head band forces and pressure on comfort of ear muffs. *Ann Occup Hyg* 19:357, 1976.
44. Lheude EP: Ear muff acceptance among sawmill workers. *Ergonomics* 23:1161, 1980.
45. Damongeot A, Tisserand M, Kkrawsky G, Grosdemange J, Lievin D: Evaluation of the comfort of personal hearing protectors. In Alberti PW (ed): *Personal Hearing Protection in Industry*. New York, Raven Press, 1982.
46. Ivergard TBK, Nicholl AGMcK: User tests of ear defenders. *Am Ind Hyg Assoc J* 37:139, 1976.
47. Wilkins PA, Martin AM: *The Effect of Hearing Protectors on the Perception of Warning and Indicator Sounds—A General Review*. Technical report 98. Southampton, England, Institute of Sound and Vibration Research, 1978.
48. Wilkins PA, Acton WI: Noise and accidents—a review. *Ann Occup Hyg* 25:249, 1982.
49. Noble WG: Earmuffs, exploratory head movements, and horizontal and vertical sound localization. *J Aud Res* 21:1, 1981.
50. Russell G: Limits to behavioral compensation for auditory localization in earmuff listening conditions. *J Acoust Soc Am* 61:219, 1977.
51. Russell G: Effects of earmuffs and earplugs on azimuthal changes in spectral patterns: implications for theories of sound localization. *J Aud Res* 16:193, 1976.
52. Wilkins PA: Assessing the effectiveness of auditory warnings. *Br J Audiol* 15:263, 1981.
53. Wilkins PA: *A Field Study to Assess the Effects of Wearing Hearing Protectors on the Perception of Warning Sounds in an Industrial Environment*. Contract report number 80/18. Southampton, England, Institute of Sound and Vibration Research, 1980.
54. Wilkins PA, Martin AM: The effects of wearing hearing protection on the perception of warning sounds. In Alberti PW (ed): *Personal Hearing Protection in Industry*. New York, Raven Press, 1982.
55. Abel SM, Kunov H, Pichora-Fuller KM, Alberti PW: The effect of hearing protection on narrowband signal detection in industrial noise. *J Otolaryngol* 12:83, 1983.
56. Kryter KD: Effects of ear protective devices on the intelligibility of speech in noise. *J Acoust Soc Am* 18:413, 1946.
57. Coles RRA, Rice CG: Letter to the editor: earplugs and impaired hearing. *J Sound Vibration* 3:521, 1965.
58. Williams CE, Forstall JR, Parsons WC: Effect of

earplugs on passenger speech reception in rotary-wing aircraft. *Aerospace Med* 42:750, 1971.

59. Martin AM, Howell K, Lower MC: Hearing protection and communication in noise. In Stephens SDG (ed): *Disorders of Auditory Function II*. New York, Academic Press, 1976.

60. Chung DY, Gannon RP: The effect of ear protectors on word discrimination in subjects with normal hearing and subjects with noise-induced hearing loss. *J Am Audit Soc* 5:11, 1979.

61. Rink TL: Hearing protection and speech discrimination in hearing-impaired persons. *Sound Vibration* 13(1): 22, 1979.

62. Frohlich GR: The effects of ear protectors and hearing loss on sentence intelligibility in aircraft noise. In Money KE (ed): *AGARD Conference Proceedings No. 311, Aural Communication in Aviation*. Advisory Group for Aerospace Research and Development, 1981.

63. Padilla M: Why some workers resent wearing earplugs. *Occup Health Saf* 50(1): 6, 1981.

64. Pollack I: Speech communication at high noise levels: the roles of an automatic gain control system and hearing protection. *J Acoust Soc Am* 29:1324, 1957.

65. Michael PL: Ear protectors: their usefulness and limitations. *Arch Environ Health* 10:612, 1965.

66. Lindeman HE: Speech intelligibility and the use of hearing protectors. *Audiology* 15:348, 1976.

67. Howell K, Martin AM: An investigation of the effects of hearing protectors on vocal communication in noise. *J Sound Vibration* 41:181, 1975.

68. Abel SM, Alberti PW, Haythornthwaite C, Riko K: Speech intelligibility in noise: with and without ear protectors. In Alberti PW (ed): *Personal Hearing Protection in Industry*. New York, Raven Press, 1982.

69. Royster LH, Thomas WG: Age effect hearing levels for a white nonindustrial noise exposed population (NINEP) and their use in evaluating industrial hearing conservation programs. *Am Ind Hyg Assoc J* 40:504, 1979.

70. Royster LH, Driscoll DP, Thomas WG, Royster JD: Age effect hearing levels for a black, nonindustrial noise-exposed population (NINEP). *Am Ind Hyg Assoc J* 41:113, 1980.

71. Senturia BH, Marcus MD, Lucente FE: *Diseases of the External Ear*, ed 2. New York, Grune & Stratton, 1980.

72. Ohlin D: User training and problems. In Royster LH, Hart FD, Stewart ND (eds): *Proceedings of Noise-Con 81*. Poughkeepsie, NY, Noise Control Foundation, 1981.

73. Imbus HR: Medical aspects of hearing conservation. In Crocker MJ (ed): *Inter-Noise 72 Proceedings*. Poughkeepsie, NY, Institute of Noise Control Engineering, 1972.

74. Lewine JF, Driscoll DP: Providing a uniform training program on hearing conservation for a large corporation. In Royster LH (ed): *Hearing Conservation Programs—The Educational Phase*. Proceedings of special session at the fall 1981 meeting of the N.C. Regional Chapter of the Acoustical Society of America. Available from Raleigh, NC, D. H. Hill Library.

75. Schmidt JW, Royster LH, Pearson RG: Impact of an industrial hearing conservation program on occupational injuries. *Sound Vibration* 16(1):16, 1982.

76. Lofgreen H: The human and economic benefits of hearing protection in the plant. *Can Occup Saf* 20:2, 1982.

77. Staples N: Hearing conservation: is management shortchanging those at risk? *Noise Vibration Control Worldwide* 12:236, 1981.

78. Royster JD, Royster LH: Judging the effectiveness of hearing protection devices by evaluating the audiometric data base. In Royster LH, Hart FD, Stewart ND (eds): *Proceedings of Noise-Con 81*. Poughkeepsie, NY, Noise Control Foundation, 1981.

79. Royster LH, Lilley DP, Thomas WG: Recommended criteria for evaluating the effectiveness of hearing conservation programs. *Am Ind Hyg Assoc J* 41:40, 1980.

80. Stapleton L, Royster LH: Educational programs for hearing conservation. In Royster LH, Hart FD, Stewart ND (eds): *Proceedings of Noise-Con 81*. Poughkeepsie, NY, Noise Control Foundation, 1981.

81. Stapleton L, Royster LH: Educational programs. In Royster LH (ed): *Hearing Conservation Programs—The Educational Phase*. Proceedings of special session at the fall 1981 meeting of the N.C. Regional Chapter of the Acoustical Society of America. Available from Raleigh, NC, D. H. Hill Library.

82. Karmy SJ, Martin AM: Employee attitudes towards hearing protection as affected by serial audiometry. In Alberti PW (ed): *Personal Hearing Protection in Industry*. New York, Raven Press, 1982.

83. Maas RB: Compliance with OSHA on hearing conservation. *Environ Contr Saf Manag* 142(6):11, 1971.

84. National Institute for Occupational Safety and Health. *Criteria for a Recommended Standard . . . Occupational Exposure to Noise*. Report number HSM 73-11001. Cincinnati, Ohio, U.S. Department of Health Education and Welfare, 1973.

85. Robinson DW, Sutton GJ: *A Comparative Analysis of Data on the Relation of Pure-Tone Audiometric Thresholds to Age*. Report number AC 84. Teddington, England, National Physical Laboratory, 1978.

86. Chung DY, Gannon RP, Roberts ME, Mason K: Hearing conservation based on hearing protectors: a provincial report. In Alberti PW (ed): *Personal Hearing Protection in Industry*. New York, Raven Press, 1982.

87. Foster A: Hearing protection and the role of health education. *Occup Health* 35:155, 1983.

88. Zohar D, Cohen A, Azar N: Promoting increased use of ear protectors in noise through information feedback. *Hum Factors* 22:69, 1980.

89. Harvey DG: A method to increase the effectiveness of ear protection. *Sound Vibration* 15(5):24, 1981.

90. Sadler OW, Montgomery GM: The application of positive practice overcorrection to the use of hearing protection. *Am Ind Hyg Assoc J* 43:451, 1982.

91. Zohar D: Promoting the use of personal protec-

tive equipment by behavior modification techniques. *J Saf Res* 12:78, 1980.

92. Lofgreen H, Holm M, Tengling R: How to motivate people in the use of their hearing protectors. In Alberti PW (ed): *Personal Hearing Protection in Industry.* New York, Raven Press, 1982.

93. Carroll BJ: An effective safety program without top management support. *Prof Saf* 27(7):20, 1982.

94. Luz GA, Decatur RA, Thompson RL: *Psychological Factors Related to the Voluntary Use of Hearing Protection in Hazardous Noise Environments.* Medical Research Laboratory report number 1066, Fort Knox, KY, U.S. Army, 1973.

95. Hager WL, Hoyle ER, Hermann ER: Efficacy of enforcement in an industrial hearing conservation program. *Am Ind Hyg Assoc J* 43:455, 1982.

96. Occupational Safety and Health Administration: Occupational Safety and Health Standards; occupational noise exposure; CFR 1910.95. *Federal Register* 36:10518, 1971.

97. Royster JD, Royster LH: *Response to the U.S. Department of Labor's Request for Comments Concerning the Noise Regulation.* Submitted to OSHA docket OSH-011. Washington, DC, U.S. Department of Labor, 1981.

98. Occupational Safety and Health Administration. Occupational noise exposure, hearing conservation amendment. *Federal Register* 46:42622, 1981.

CHAPTER 7

Training Programs in Occupational Hearing Conservation

CHARLES T. GRIMES

INTRODUCTION

The problem of hearing loss associated with long-term noise exposure has been on record for approximately 150 years (1). Sadly enough, the millions of industrial workers who have endured the lifelong consequences of noise exposure, suffer from a completely preventable impairment. In the absence of complete control of noise at the source, prevention of hearing loss due to industrial or other long-term noise exposure may be achieved through the implementation of, and consistent adherence to, the principles of hearing conservation. The various components of a hearing conservation program are usually identified as: (a) noise level and exposure documentation; (b) noise control, either at the source or by interrupting the sound transmission paths to the listener; (c) audiometric baseline and periodic monitoring with associated professional review; (d) Personal hearing protection devices; (e) education regarding the harmful effect of long-term noise exposure and the benefits of self-protection.

In this chapter we will look at the history of training programs for the occupational hearing conservationist (OHC) and the current curriculum and requirements of the Council for Accreditation in Occupational Hearing Conservation (CAOHC) for certification of OHC's and Course Directors (CD).

HISTORY

The audiometric testing component of hearing conservation has been an area of major concern due to the many different types of equipment, personnel and methodologies available to perform the tests. In the early 1960s, The American Association of Industrial Nurses (AAIN) now the American Association of Occupational Health Nurses (AAOHN) recognized a need to provide specific training for industrial nurses in the administration of pure-tone air conduction hearing tests. With the goal of developing a course syllabus, the nursing association in conjunction with the American Speech and Hearing Association, now the American Speech-Language-Hearing Association (ASHA), and representatives of several other national organizations formed the Intersociety Committee on Audiometric Technician Training. This group published the Guide for Training Audiometric Technicians in Industry in 1965 (2).

The Guide contained a course outline, resource materials and course objectives. It provided an organizational framework for teaching the methods and procedures for conducting air conduction threshold tests in industry. The first training courses to utilize this Guide were sponsored by the Association of Industrial Nurses of the State of New Jersey. It is estimated that over 1000 nurses were trained in various courses during the later 1960s.

Spurred by the efforts of the U.S. Department of Labor to formulate the hearing conservation regulations mandated by the Occupational Safety and Health Act of 1970, the Intersociety Committee met several times to formalize a plan for the training and certification of industrial audiometric technicians, a title that was later changed to OHC. The outgrowth of these meetings was the CAOHC which was established in 1973. The CAOHC has evolved into a 16-member multidisciplinary council made up of two representatives from each of eight member organizations. The member organizations are: The American Academy of Occupational Medicine, The American Academy of Otolaryngology—Head and Neck Surgery, The American Association of Occupational Health Nurses, The American Industrial Hygiene Association, The American Occupational Medical Association, The American Speech-Language-Hearing Association, the National Safety Council, and the Military Audiology and Speech Pathology Society. This latter group was added in the Fall of 1984. The CAOHC's by-laws specify the purposes as: the establishment of standards for CDs and OHCs and the certification of those who meet the standards; to maintain a roster of certified individuals; to stimulate and develop improved teaching methods and programs; and to elevate and maintain the quality of hearing conservation.

TRAINING PROGRAMS

Course Director Certification

The CAOHC has taken a two-pronged approach to the training and certification of OHCs. The first is to specify the content and duration of the training courses (this will be discussed in detail later). The second is to require that the training courses be organized by a course director who has been certified by the CAOHC on the basis of educational and experiential prerequisites.

One must meet certain requirements to be eligible to become a CD. First, it is necessary to demonstrate an adequate ed-

ucational background by holding or being eligible for certification by one of the certifying boards of the CAOHC member organizations. With the exception of the National Safety Council all other member organizations have certifying programs. Second, the CD must also be actively engaged in hearing conservation work by either being employed full-time in hearing conservation for a period of 1 yr or part-time for a period of 3 yr. The experience requirement may also be met by having previously participated in four CAOHC-approved OHC courses as a faculty member. An application documenting fulfillment of the educational and experience requirements must be filed for review and approval by the CAOHC board. Finally, the applicant must complete an 8-hr orientation course before becoming a certified CD.

The content of the CD orientation course includes:

1. A section on the organizational and operational aspects of giving an OHC training course including such topics as personnel, teaching methods, audiovisual and reference materials, practicum instrumentation, and follow-up of trainees after the course
2. A section on technical information such as instrumentation and procedures for noise analysis, audiometric equipment, personal hearing protective devices (HPD), and procedures for quantifying the effectiveness of hearing conservation programs
3. A section on current legal and administrative aspects of conservation programs such as OSHA field directives and worker compensation plans
4. A section on review of the areas of medical considerations regarding HPDs, referral criteria, and management of ear disease in a noise-exposed worker population
5. A section on the effects of noise exposure both auditory and nonauditory
6. A discussion section on issues in hearing conservation that may be of particular concern to the course participants

Recertification of CDs is required every 5 yr. Recertification is accomplished by either attendance and completion of another orientation course or by documenting performance as a CD for at least one OHC course for each of the previous 5 yr. In the spring of 1984, there were approximately 700 certified CDs. About 75% of these CDs were audiologists with the remaining 25% comprised of physicians, nurses and industrial hygienists. These CDs organize OHC training courses throughout the United States. The courses may be publicly offered by CDs who are private practice consultants, members of commercial enterprises or university faculty members. Courses are also frequently conducted as in-house projects by the military and by large companies that must train a number of their own personnel for OHC duties.

Certification as an Occupational Hearing Conservationist

Certification by the CAOHC as an OHC is awarded following the successful completion of a 20-hr training course that meets several criteria. The course must: follow the CAOHC course outline, including practical and written examinations; be preapproved by the CAOHC; and be organized and conducted by a CAOHC-certified CD. After completion of the course, OHC certification is awarded on the basis of written application to the CAOHC. OHCs must recertify every 5 yr by completing an 8-hr, CAOHC-approved refresher course.

The curriculum for the OHC training course is specified by the CAOHC in the OHC Training Manual (3). The second edition of the training manual should be available by the time this book is published. The manual is available for a small fee, from the CAOHC. The course outline is reproduced below.

The following topics shall be covered. The time allocations are minimum times with the remainder, up to a minimum of 20 hr, to be allocated among other areas at the discretion of the course instructor.

A. Topic: Hearing Conservation in Noise (60 min)
  a. Overview of Industrial Noise as a Problem
  b. Effects of Noise on People
  c. Social, Economic and Legal Ramifications Including Community Noise
  d. Objectives of Training Program
    1) Valid Baseline and Monitoring Audiograms
    2) Effective Ear Protection Program
    3) Identification and Referral
    4) Employee Education Program
    5) Other Areas
  e. Responsibilities and Limitations of Occupational Hearing Conservationists
B. Topic: Anatomy, Physiology and Pathology of the Human Ear (60 min)
  a. Structure and Function—Lecture
  b. Visual Inspection of the Ear—What to Look For
  c. Causes and Types of Hearing Loss
C. Topic: Sound, Psychophysics and Audition (60 min)
  a. Parameters of Sound and Definitions
    1) Pure and Complex Signals
    2) Frequency
    3) The decibel
    4) Audiometric Standards
    5) Other Definitions—HL vs SPL, etc.
D. Topic: Federal and State Industrial Noise Regulations (60 min)
  a. OSHA and Other Federal Regulations
  b. Compensation
  c. State Labor Department
  d. Environmental Noise
E. Topic: The Audiometer (90 min)
  a. Description and Demonstration of Instruments
  b. Operation of the Audiometer
  c. Audiometer Performance Check
  d. Methods of Calibration
  e. Review of Terminology
F. Topic: Audiometric Techniques (60 min)
  a. Instructions to Subject
  b. Test Procedure—Demonstration
  c. Special Situations
  d. Audiometric Records
  e. Testing Environment
G. Topic: The Audiogram (30 min)
H. Topic: Review—Questions and Answers (60 min)
I. Topic: Supervised Audiometric Testing (150 min)
  a. Self-Recording Audiometer
  b. Manual Audiometer
  c. Other Types of Audiometers
  d. Testing of Persons With Both Normal Hearing and Hearing Loss
J. Topic: Review of Audiometric Techniques (60 min)
  a. Additional Practicum

K. Topic: Principles of Noise Analysis (60 min)
   a. Description of Instrumentation
   b. Procedures and Demonstration of Noise Measurement
L. Topic: The OHC in the Industrial Setting (60 min)
   a. Responsibility to Employees
   b. Role in Plant Educational Program
   c. Role in Overall Hearing Conservation Program
   d. Referral Criteria
M. Topic: Personal Ear Protection (90 min)
   a. Attenuation Characteristics of Ear Protection
   b. Earmuffs, Plugs
   c. Practicum in Fitting and Counseling Procedures
N. Topic: Record Keeping (60 min)
   a. History
   b. Audiograms
   c. Calibrations
O. Topic: Review of Hearing Conservation Program (60 min)
   a. Summary of Total Program
   b. Question and Answer Program
P. Topic: Examination (60 min)
   a. Practical and Written

There are additional requirements such as a student-faculty ratio of 6 to 1 for the audiometric practicum with at least one audiometer for every three students. Students should obtain practice using a variety of types of audiometric equipment e.g., manual, self-recording and microprocessor based. The course faculty must include instructors drawn from at least three of the professional disciplines represented on the CAOHC Board.

The OHC training course is clearly an ambitious undertaking for a 20-hr endeavor. The content areas specified in the outline could be developed into several semester-length courses if the intent was to establish full appreciation of the topics in the context of hearing conservation. The intent however, is to provide a very broad-based exposure to the complexities of a total hearing conservation effort while focusing in depth on the front line areas, i.e. audiometry, HPDs and employee education. In order to avoid confusing the student about the ultimate nature of their role, it is recommended that, throughout the course, appropriate em-

phasis should be placed on those tasks that the OHC is NOT qualified to perform on the basis of OHC training. These include: teaching other OHCs; interpreting audiograms; diagnosing hearing loss; recommending noise control measures; performing noise analysis and taking the administrative responsibility for the hearing conservation program.

There are approximately 12,000 CAOHC certified OHCs at this time. The majority are occupational health nurses but the number of non-nursing trained individuals taking OHC courses is growing rapidly. These days it is not at all uncommon for OHC courses to draw students otherwise employed in the areas of personnel, safety and clerical support positions.

OSHA TRAINING REQUIREMENTS FOR OHC

The OSHA Noise Amendment specifies two methods for becoming an OHC (4). These are through completion of the CAOHC training course discussed above and by on the job training or the apprenticeship method. In the latter case the OHC must demonstrate, to the supervisors satisfaction, the achievement of competence in administering audiometric tests, obtaining valid audiograms, and properly using, maintaining and checking calibration and proper function of the audiometer being used. On-the-job training of an OHC can be more or less successful depending on the characteristics of the individual and the supervisor. The inherent weakness in that approach is exactly the reason that the CAOHC course includes so much information in the curriculum. It is important that the OHC perceive hearing conservation as a total process consisting of several individual components and not just as an audiometric test. The success and competence of the OHC is, in part, determined by the overall perspective the individual brings to bear on their specific responsibilities. For example, the hearing test itself, and the personal contact with the employee at the time of the hearing test, may present invaluable opportunities to further the educational component of the program and to gain insights into the overall success of the hearing conservation effort. An OHC who has been relatively narrowly trained (or even worse, untrained) only in the use and care of audiometers and the administration of audiometric tests is not likely to appreciate the breadth of hearing conservation opportunities that the hearing test presents.

Microprocessor audiometers are specifically identified in the OSHA Hearing Conservation Amendment as not needing a certified operator (see Appendix I). While the language of the amendment is not completely clear, the intent appears to be that, since microprocessor based audiometers run themselves, the operator does not need any particular knowledge. This, of course, is nonsense. While the underlying technology of the microprocessor-based audiometer is different, in all practical respects, the microprocessor-based audiometer is similar to the self-recording audiometer. With both types of equipment there will be some industrial workers who, for whatever reason, cannot produce a valid audiogram. When this occurs, the test will have to be administered with a manual audiometer by a trained OHC.

SUMMARY

In this chapter I have presented in detail the training requirements for OHCs

and CDs as specified by the CAOHC. These requirements have been developed and modified over approximately a 10-yr period. This represents the determined effort of the CAOHC to bring constancy and structure to the training of OHCs. The purpose of this effort is to develop a national, and perhaps international, corps of OHCs who have not only the necessary training and experience to obtain valid audiometric results but who also have insight and appreciation for the total process of hearing conservation. The trained OHC understands that industrial noise-induced permanent threshold shift is completely preventable and appreciates the various components of industrial hearing conservation that must be integrated to produce a successful program. The work of the CAOHC is exemplified in the OSHA Hearing Conservation Amendment as the only recognized formal OHC training program.

References

1. Fosbroke J: Practical Observations on the Pathology and Treatment of Deafness. No 11. *Lancet* (1):645–648, 1830–1831.
2. Sittner, MA: CAOHC Update. Occup Health Nurs. 35–36: September 1983.
3. CAOHC: *Council for Accreditation in Occupational Hearing Conservation Manual.* Cherry Hill, NJ CAOHC, 1978.
4. Occupational Safety and Health Administration: Occupational noise exposure: Hearing Conservation Ammendment. *Federal Register.* 48:9738, 1983.

CHAPTER 8

Employee Training Programs in Occupational Hearing Conservation

ALAN S. FELDMAN and CHARLES T. GRIMES

NEED FOR EDUCATIONAL PROGRAMS

The threat to worker health and safety is well recognized in the industrial setting. It occurs as a consequence of exposure to a wide range of noxious stimuli and other hazards. Measures to counteract the threat have only been implemented gradually. Workers' compensation has been one way of attempting to attack this problem. On the one hand it financially compensates the worker for loss or damage to bodily function while on the other hand it motivates employers through financial penalty to structure health and safety programs geared toward the reduction of hazards and the prevention of injury or illness.

In today's workplace the three "E"s of health and safety: Engineering, Enforcement, and Education, constitute another approach. When feasible, the elimination or reduction of health and safety hazards through engineering is desirable, but this is not always possible. Consequently rules relating to the use of personal protective equipment such as safety glasses, hard hats and hearing protective devices (HPDs) are established and enforced with varying degrees of success. Worker compliance is often a direct consequence of the third facet—education.

Recognition of the value of education as a means of promoting health and safety in the workplace has led to the inclusion of training requirements in a large number of regulations established by the Occupational Safety and Health Administration (OSHA).

The goal of employee training programs is to influence employee behavior in a manner which counteracts the workplace hazards by increasing the sense of importance of self-protection on the part of the worker. It also provides the worker with an understanding of the potential hazards to safety and health, as well as a knowledge of appropriate preventive measures. This is particularly relevant when the potential damage is insidious, such as is the case with hearing loss or asbestosis. Cohen et al. (1) stress that the most important method of effecting self-protection against workplace health and safety hazards is through employee education.

The OSHA has published proposed guidelines, the purpose of which is to provide employers with a model for designing, conducting, evaluating and revising training programs (2). These guidelines set forth a model consisting of: (a) the identification of training needs; (b) the determination of content; (c) the preparation of instructional objectives; (d) the development of learning activities; (e) the provision of training; (f) the evaluation of program effectiveness, and (g) the improvement of the program.

In the context of occupational noise, the fundamental content of training programs has been established in regulation (3). This presumes that the training needs are identified, but such is probably not the case. The fundamental need for employee information relates to a general disregard for the potential hazard to hearing posed by noise exposure. This, in turn, is related to the limited appreciation of the effect of hearing loss on one's life. It is far too easy to externalize the communication problems consequent to the invisible handicap we know as hearing loss.

The limited information base and minimal value placed on good hearing, as well as the insidious nature of hearing loss, all lead to a limited voluntary participation on the part of workers who are exposed to noise. Presently, there are even a substantial number of employees who will refuse to participate in an annual hearing testing program. Good hearing health is not a high priority with many workers.

Training needs for employees exposed to hazardous noise must be based on a need to modify attitude and motivation as well as a broadening of the knowledge base about the ear, hearing, hearing loss, and the effects of noise, with the ultimate goal being the prevention of hearing loss. To expect voluntary participation on the part of employees in the use of hearing protection is usually a mistake. There is a need for a change in worker attitude and goals. In order to change employee behavior, the negatives of hearing loss must be understood and appreciated by the employee. This can be achieved, in part, through education.

EDUCATING MANAGEMENT ABOUT OCCUPATIONAL HEARING CONSERVATION

It follows that the more important an issue is to management, the more concern there will be about developing effective programs to deal with those issues. In general, it is reasonable to assume that upper and middle level management is not much better informed or sensitive about hearing loss or the effects of noise on hearing than is the workforce. Society as a whole tends to be rather naive in that regard.

It is imperative that education about occupational noise and hearing conservation programs begin with management. Top level management must be informed and supportive of why and what is going on in the development of a hearing conservation program (HCP). As is often the case, enlisting support for such programs is accomplished through familiarizing management with the potential costs of not having effective programs. Management will offer many excuses why it is difficult to incorporate training programs into the HCP. Most commonly, the excuses involve time and money, two factors that are not independent. While it is true that good educational programs cost money, they will, at the same time, save the company money. Ultimately such programs will lower worker compensation liability, improve productivity, contribute to OSHA compliance, and result in a healthier workforce. These all are positive factors in cost containment.

Participation within the program at symbolic levels is another way management can instill confidence and trust of the workforce, thereby enhancing worker cooperation with the HCP. For example, ideally all levels of management should participate in the annual hearing testing program. This would label the program more as a health benefit than as a mandated measure, and employees tend to respond more favorably toward the former. Furthermore, even though exposure would not reach action level time-weighted averages (TWAs), any time management moves around in noisy areas HPDs should be visibly worn. This presents a "do as I do, not only as I say" message. It demonstrates an understanding of the importance of HPD use by the worker. These actions by management are a form of education and go a long way toward establishing an employment climate which is viewed as positive by the worker. As such the actions will contribute toward minimizing negative attitudes about the HCP.

RECRUITING UNION SUPPORT

In every respect, soliciting the support of unions is as critical to the success of health and safety programs as is the support of management. The education of labor leaders about the hazards of noise and the importance of compliance with HCPs as a means of preventing hearing loss is an important move in that direction.

Unions are sometimes placed in awkward positions in dealing with health and safety issues. On the one hand they must do everything possible to encourage the health and safety of their membership, but at the same time they must be concerned about such things as job security and upward mobility. These latter could conceivably be jeopardized if, for example, hearing loss adversely impacted communication skills considered necessary for promotion to a position for which an employee was in line. Also, unions must support compliance requirements and noncompliance penalties. This support is easier to enlist when knowledge and understanding of the problem is present. The union must concur with the goal of prevention of hearing loss and it must support the procedures necessary to achieve that goal.

It is good practice to have separate educational programs on hearing conservation for management, shop and production supervisors, and union representatives prior to initiating such programs for the production workforce. It provides these groups with a knowledge base from which to draw in response to employee reaction.

Educational programs should include a clear and open statement from management concerning what the company is doing about the noise in the workplace and about company policy concerning all phases of the HCP. Openness and honesty is an important component of any educational program.

EDUCATIONAL PROGRAM AND WORKFORCE

Efficient manufacturing operations cannot tolerate too many people off a production line for significant periods of time. Employees may also offer resistance to being taken off line, especially when earnings are related to productivity. The educational component of HCPs must be structured to avoid such resistance. There must be some flexibility built into the initial and annual training program that is appropriate for individual work operations. Flexibility is inherent in the OSHA regulations on training requirements, since nothing is mandated beyond certain content areas and that a program be provided on an annual basis. It is possible, for example, to spread the program over time by discussing each content area on a separate occasion rather than covering all content areas in one long presentation.

TRAINING PROGRAM SPECIFICATIONS

The training program specifications in OSHA 1910.95 require that all employees who are exposed to a TWA of 85 dB or greater must receive an annual training program. This program should include, but not be limited to, a consideration of: (a) the effects of noise on hearing; (b) the purpose of HPDs—the advantages and disadvantages of different types, as well as information about HPD attenuation, selection, fitting, use and care; and (c) the purpose of audiometric tests and the procedures pertaining to them.

Other related information would include an open discussion about the noise standard, a copy of which must be posted in the workplace. The information about noise effects should include an orientation about the normal ear and hearing as well as the effects of hearing loss on communication. This latter is implicit rather than explicit in the standard.

GOAL OF TRAINING PROGRAMS

The fundamental goal of training programs in hearing conservation is to inform the workers about the potential consequences of noise exposure and to motivate them toward hearing conservation, both on the job and off it. The basis for this goal is self-evident. Millions of workers suffer from hearing loss as a consequence of occupational noise exposure. It is important that off the job noise also be identified as carrying the same threat to hearing as does noise at the workplace. Ideally, a by-product of this program will be an elevated sense of importance of good hearing. The intangible impact of hearing loss initially contributes much to the poor attitude of workers toward a program of hearing conservation.

To achieve the training goals, educational programs must contain some essential features that are geared toward changing worker attitudes about hearing loss. Behavior is a consequence of one's attitude, knowledge and skills. Training programs can expand a knowledge base, but the effect of attitude or their motivational appeal deserves some direct attention and will really determine how well the educational objectives are achieved.

Evidence

Learning is enhanced when the student (worker) can relate facts to experience. Unfortunately, experiencing hearing loss is difficult at best and, once the facts become reality, the problem is not reversible. We are therefore forced to teach consequences of behavior that cannot be made concrete for the worker until it is too late. Additionally, most of us are trying to teach abstractions that we ourselves have not personally experienced. We are confident that we know of what we speak by having spent hundreds or maybe thousands of hours attempting to help others who have acquired hearing loss from various causes and who have, through personal confrontation, convinced us of the serious nature of a hearing handicap.

We must begin from the premise that most people are motivated by a basic instinct for self-preservation. In fact, survival should be one of the strongest of motivational forces. Approached from this point of view, the role of the senses

with regard to survival, can be related to everyone's experience. Hearing as one of the senses, can be shown to play a central role in the process of survival within the context of our social structure. Cultural values tend to support the independence of each individual. At the same time, awareness of the vulnerability of the organism continues to be heightened by the explosion of information in the health-related areas. Noise-induced hearing loss presents a natural opportunity to tie these areas together—immortality is a myth; everyone is susceptible to noise-induced permanent threshold shift (NIPTS); and, once acquired, hearing loss presents, at the least, a challenge and, at the worst, a threat to independence. Cast in this perspective, the employee must be provided with substantive evidence that noise has a negative impact on hearing and that hearing loss can and should be prevented. The creative nature of the presentation is the key here. It is essential that the program provide insight into difficult concepts such as the distinction between poor hearing and poor speech discrimination, auditory background/foreground problems, and so forth. The effects of noise on hearing must be understood and appreciated by the employee.

Reasoning

The success of reasoning is very dependent on whether or not the change in behavior that is sought is perceived as positive or negative by the worker. In this regard, it is difficult to convey your message about the use of HPDs when you do not accept the validity of worker complaints about discomfort or impaired communication that may accompany the wearing of these devices. For example, complaints about headache, nausea and other discomfort with ear plugs could be very real. Some people may experience a bizarre autonomic nervous system response to stimulation of Arnold's nerve, which is a branch of the vagus nerve. Insertion of a HPD into the ear canal can result in such stimulation and subsequent complaints. It is as important to listen to the concerns of the employee as it is to convey your message. By helping overcome misconceptions, biases and fears about HPDs, it becomes easier to achieve success with the HPD program.

TRAINING PROGRAM OBJECTIVES

The success of the occupational noise standard really hinges on the proper use of HPDs and close monitoring of hearing levels and changes as well as counseling and/or professional follow-up of changes in hearing. One objective of the training program, consequently, would be to promote consistent compliance with on-the-job HPD usage and voluntary usage off the job when engaged in noisy activities such as the use of chain saws and when hunting. Employees must know how and when to properly use HPDs. Their motivation to protect their hearing can be elevated through the training program, and that is a primary program objective.

Proper counseling about observed changes in hearing must follow professional review of audiograms and identification of a standard threshold shift (STS). This counseling should be viewed as a component of the annual training program because its relevance to the individual is very great, and it will, therefore, be more meaningful than would an abstract discussion of hearing loss. Proper counseling will lead to the objective of greater insight and understanding of the hazard by the employee.

Another important objective is to increase the likelihood of the employee seeking further professional evaluation when so advised if indicated by professional review of audiograms. When hearing tests are performed on an annual basis, small, but relevant, changes in hearing may be detected. We are well aware that factors other than noise can contribute to a developing hearing loss. Consequently, good hearing conservation is predicated on early detection and management of possible medically related problems whose first symptom may be a change in hearing. The annual training program can help develop a hearing health orientation. Nonmedical factors, such as impaired communication skills due to the hearing loss should be viewed as in need of management by the employee. Awareness of this can be promoted in the annual training program.

WHEN SHOULD TRAINING PROGRAMS BE PROVIDED

The noise standard is performance oriented with regard to the details of packaging the annual training program. Beyond specifying minimal content there is little in the way of specifics. As a matter of fact, there is considerable merit to fragmenting the program over the year. It is well known that spaced learning is more effective than mass learning.

It is reasonable to expect that at the onset of new programs a more lengthy and detailed orientation would be advisable. This is the phase at which management at all levels and union representatives should also receive training. As noted earlier, this training should ideally precede the employee program. Both programs should be reasonably sequenced with the initiation of a clearly stated HPD compliance policy and the onset of audiometric testing. This initial program should have sufficient time built in to afford the employees an opportunity to ask questions and receive answers.

Following the general training program, opportunities for reinforcement come with (a) counseling centered around individual selection and fitting of the HPD, and (b) counseling concerning the outcome of audiometric testing and possible recommended course of action as a consequence of professional review of the audiograms.

In subsequent years the formal presentation of an annual training program could be a brief session, such as a 10-min audiovisual presentation, but the HPD and audiometric outcome counseling opportunities also will continue to occur annually.

METHODS OF PRESENTATION

There are a variety of options available to management dealing with the method of presentation of the required training program. While no single approach is guaranteed to be successful, some are more likely to meet objectives than others.

Print Material

A popular approach is to provide employees with pamphlets or brochures. These are commercially available (4, 5) or may be specifically developed by an individual employer (6). The advantage of the latter is that company policy about the HCP may be directly addressed in the print material.

When the company relies strongly on print material as the means of providing the informational content of the annual training program, the likelihood of achieving the goal is small. First, there is no assurance the employee will read the material and, secondly, even when it is read there needs to be an opportunity for the employee to ask questions about the topic. Many employees may not read English and others may not be able to read any language. The advantage to the company is obvious. Print material presentation requires a minimum of time lost from the job.

This is not to say brochures should not be used. The use of print material can be a helpful reinforcement of programs also presented in other ways. Brochures also can be a way of reaching family members of the employee, thereby expanding the number of people to whom the information is made available.

Audiovisual Presentation

An increasingly popular technique for the presentation of the annual training program is the use of brief movies, videotapes and tape-slide presentations. Again, simply showing a film on the hazards of noise is not really a powerful teaching tool. It is true that the employee is more likely to attend to a film than to read a pamphlet, but unless there is an opportunity for interactive dialogue the strength or impact of the message can be seriously diluted.

A number of audiologists involved in the provision of hearing conservation services to industry now include their own audiovisual programs. These may be given in conjunction with the annual audiometric testing program, either when using mobile services or in-house services, or may be presented to larger groups of employees at periodic safety meetings.

One advantage of a tape-slide production is that it is relatively simple to tailor an audiovisual program to individual companies with the change of just a few slides. A disadvantage of any filmed production is that the same program cannot be repeated year in and year out without losing its ability to maintain the employee's interest.

Formal Lectures and Group Motivational Programs

Perhaps the potentially strongest type of educational program is one involving lectures that include some orientation toward motivational programming. Lectures will usually be enriched through the use of some filmed material, such as slides or movies, but there is greater flexibility in lectures due to the inherent opportunity for interactive dialogue.

Motivational programs essentially deal with value system modification. The job climate, peer pressures and management style all contribute to the level of motivation in any given work environment. The presentation of information alone will not contribute much toward a change in motivation. Nonmotivational environments may be expected to exhibit high job turnover, worker apathy, a cumbersome organizational ladder, fatigue, and poor safety records.

Workers are better motivated by work climates in which there is confidence and trust, interest in subordinates, an understanding of problems, approachability, recognition, information sharing, loyalty, and interesting work.

Motivational programs should convey a sense of concern about the employee perspective. It is not sufficient to "preach a lot, teach a lot and advertise a lot" in the workplace. In order to motivate, management must also listen a lot. Nor can management expect a complete change in attitude all at one time. There needs to be a broadening of latitude of acceptance from a point of disagreement toward agreement. Movement along the continuum should be the objective rather than a complete shift from rejection to acceptance.

TYPICAL CONTENT OF THE ANNUAL TRAINING PROGRAM

At the minimum, the annual training program is to be given to everyone exposed to a TWA of 85 dB or greater and must include those components previously identified as being specified in regulations. These latter were:

1. The effect of noise on hearing
2. HPD: the purpose of hearing protection, advantages, disadvantages and attenuation of different types, instruction in its selection, fitting and care
3. The purposes and procedures of audiometric testing

It has been noted that the nonspecificity of the standard allows for reinforcement of the educational programming throughout the year. It also would permit certain instructional components to occur at very appropriate times. For example, a discussion about the individual employee's hearing test outcome is more emphatic after professional review and at the time recommendations for follow-up are provided. This would make counseling about HPDs more pertinent for those employees exhibiting an STS. A sign-up sheet or ros-

ter of participants should be maintained for all training programs.

Table 8.1 offers an outline of topics to be covered in an annual training program. These can be covered by one or several people either in a single session, such as a safety meeting, or throughout the year. The list of topics is not all inclusive but may be expanded as desired. For example, one topic omitted that could be included is nonauditory effects of noise. When offered as a lecture type of program, slides could be used to reinforce some

Table 8.1
Hearing conservation program annual training program content areas

NOISE AS A HAZARD
  Definition of noise
  Workplace noise
  Environmental noise
  Hobbies

EFFECTS OF NOISE ON HEARING
  Hearing loss - temporary threshold shift
  Hearing loss - permanent threshold shift
  Tinnitus
  Insidious nature of noise-induced hearing loss
  Audiogram as a picture of hearing and hearing loss

HEARING LOSS EFFECTS ON COMMUNICATION
  Distinction between hearing and understanding speech
  Why people seem to mumble

ANNUAL HEARING TEST
  What the test is
  How to take the hearing test
  Why the hearing test is given

PREVENTION OF NOISE INDUCED HEARING LOSS
  Use of hearing protective devices
  Avoiding unnecessary exposure on and off the job

HEARING PROTECTIVE DEVICES (HPDs)
  Types of HPDs
  Advantages/disadvantages and attenuation of HPDs
  Instruction in use, care and fitting of HPDs

COMPANY POLICY
  Selection and replacement of HPDs
  Penalties for noncompliance
  Plans for noise and noise exposure reduction
  Monitoring of program

points and maintain interest. The entire program could be included in a relatively brief filmed (either movie, video tape or tape/slide) version. It could also be largely covered in print form. In order to maintain interest, some variation must be programmed. To repeat the same film from year-to-year for example, would greatly diminish its effectiveness. There are a great many resources available for training programs. Some suggestions for locating audiovisual or other types of material are included at the end of this chapter.

SUMMARY

The most critical time for HCP educational programs is now. This is the transitional time for industrial hearing conservation. By the time the next generation of industrial employees enters the workforce, HCPs will be well entrenched and accepted by most workers as an integral part of the job. Our task is to introduce hearing conservation as a relatively recent component of the industrial employment setting. Educating the present workforce about hearing loss and hearing conservation will not only require imparting specific knowledge on the topics, but will also require creativity and persistence in reshaping attitude and values.

In this chapter we have presented information concerning the content areas of the annual educational program and recommended several techniques to promote worker acceptance of HCPs through both direct and indirect educational experiences.

References

1. Cohen A, Smith MJ, Anger KW: Self-protective measures against workplace hazards, *J Safety Res* 11(3):129, 1979.
2. Occupational Safety and Health Administration: Training guidelines; request for comments and information, *Federal Register* 48:169, 39317–39323, 1983.
3. Occupational Safety and Health Administration: Occupational noise exposure; hearing conservation amendment; final rule, *Federal Register* 48:46, 9738–9785, 1983.
4. Hearing Conservation: *A Guide To Preventing Hearing Loss.* Daly City, Calif, Injury Prevention Library, PAS Publishing, 1983.
5. *Noise and You, The ABC's of Hearing Conservation*, Greenfield, Mass, Channing L. Bete Co, 1973.
6. Noise Reduction and Hearing Conservation: *Employee Information*, Syracuse, NY, Niagara Mohawk Power Corp,

Resources for HCP Educational Programs

1. Films for a Safer Tomorrow catalog—Safety and Training
   International Film Bureau Inc.
   332 South Michigan Avenue
   Chicago, Ill 60604
2. Audiovisual Resources in Occupational Safety and Health: an Evaluation Guide
   DHHS (NIOSH) Publication #82-102
   Department of Health & Human Services
   Public Health Service
   Centers for Disease Control, NIOSH
   4676/Columbia Parkway
   Cincinnati, Ohio 45226
3. Eastman Kodak Company
   Dept. 412-L
   Rochester, NY 14650
   A. Making Black and White or Colored Transparencies for Overhead Projection #S-7
   B. Effective Lecture Slides #S-22
   C. Slides With a Purpose #V1-15
4. Planning & Producing Slide Programs #S-30
   Eastman Kodak Company
   Dept. 454
   343 State Street
   Rochester, NY 14650
5. Industrial Training Systems Corp.
   823 East Gate Drive
   Mount Laurel, NJ 08054
6. Most manufacturers of HPDs have printed and/or audiovisual materials available. Two of these are:
   A. E.A.R. Corp.
   7911 Zionsville Road
   Indianapolis, Ind 46268
   B. Bilsom International, Inc.
   11800 Sunrise Valley Drive
   Reston, Va 22091

CHAPTER 9

Audiometric Testing, Review and Referral: Protocol and Problems

CHARLES T. GRIMES, ALAN S. FELDMAN and DONALD JOSEPH

INTRODUCTION

The widespread implementation of industrial hearing conservation programs (HCP) poses interesting problems for management and management consultants. Prior to the early 1970s, few industrial concerns had on-going, effective HCPs. The ones that did were, for the most part, large corporations that had a firm commitment to worker health and safety and had substantial financial resources to back such programs. The federal mandate for HCPs requires protection of workers from industrial noise exposure, and stable hearing as documented by an annual audiometric test. These tests are the validating criteria of program effectiveness.

Most of the companies now required to provide HCPs not only have no history of conducting such programs but also lack the in-house expertise for design and administration. On the surface, audiometric testing appears to be a relatively simple, straight forward task. However, valid audiometric tests require considerable behind-the-scenes effort to control background noise at the test site, maintain equipment calibration, train personnel to administer the tests, and organize the volumes of data that ultimately are created.

In this chapter we will discuss some of the "nuts and bolts" of audiometric tests and consider the management of the audiogram review and follow-up of the results. We will concentrate on review and interpretation of individual test data. The use of group data to evaluate HCP effectiveness is discussed in Chapter 10.

AUDIOMETRIC TESTING

Producing a valid, industrial audiometric test can be considered as a set of discrete tasks that, taken together, form the basis of the testing part of the HCP. These tasks are: control of background noise in the test environment; calibration of the audiometric equipment; case history information; obtaining pure-tone, air conduction thresholds; and considerations of the training of personnel to administer the tests (see Chapter 7).

Control of Background Noise Levels

The problem of controlling the level of background noise in the test location has presented a challenge to anyone who has ever tried to administer reliable hearing tests.

It is important to control background noise levels because the noise can mask the test signals. Should that occur, the testing program faces some very serious validity problems from the outset. In fact, the entire rationale for testing would be negated. It is a fact that if the background noise cannot be maintained at sufficiently low levels, valid hearing testing cannot be performed. As a result, many small but significant hearing losses may not be identified by the hearing testing program.

The intensity level of the background noise must be determined with certainty.

The only way to quantify noise level is to make octave band measurements centered at the test frequencies. This requires a sound level meter with an octave band analyzer. These measurements are necessary in each location where hearing tests will be administered. Table 9.1 indicates the octave band sound pressures that can be tolerated in the environment (see Hearing Conservation Amendment: Final Rule, in Appendix I).

It should be noted that the values of Table 9.1 are less stringent than the ANSI 1977 background noise standard (1) that is applied to most hearing test environments. This is an accommodation to industry which recognizes the substantial costs involved in controlling background noise at levels appropriate for obtaining zero decibel hearing level (0 dB HL) thresholds for clinical purposes. Even with this accomodation, background noise is difficult to maintain at specified values and will almost always require the use of a special sound shelter.

Demonstrable control of background noise in the test environment is not subject to negotiation or interpretation. The OSHA rules are clear on this point. The stated levels must be maintained or the entire audiometric test program is jeopardized.

Equipment Calibration

Calibration of the audiometer is performed initially when the unit is manufactured. Like all other types of electronic equipment, however, the instrument is subject to the stresses of temperature, humidity and mechanical shock as a consequence of being moved from place to place. In addition, the audiometer must be calibrated to the earphones with which it will be used since no two earphones are exactly the same. The earphones are probably the weakest link in the calibration chain because they are subject to the greatest physical abuse. It is necessary to regularly check the calibration of the instrument.

The audiometer calibration check is accomplished in several ways. The first is termed *functional* or *biological* calibration. This refers to a method of determining if the calibration has changed by testing the thresholds of one or more persons each day that the instrument is to be used. The person or persons tested should have known stable thresholds of sensitivity that are less than 25 dB HL. Persons with conductive hearing loss, even of very mild magnitude, are not acceptable. Records of these threshold tests should be kept for comparison to each new set of thresholds. In this way, a change in audiometer calibration can be identified immediately, thereby avoiding the possibility of producing several days or weeks of invalid hearing tests. In addition to the threshold hearing check, the instrument should also have a listening check to identify the presence of inappropriate earphone, attenuator, interrupter, and frequency selector background sounds such as static, clicks and intermittent or distorted signals. This listening check should also be done each day.

An increasingly popular instrument being used for biological calibration is a type of artificial ear. Earphones from the audiometer can be coupled to this bioacoustic simulator permitting the audiometer output levels to be validated quickly and objectively. Some models will also monitor background noise levels. The listening check mentioned above is also necessary when these devices are used to check calibration.

Table 9.1.
Maximum allowable sound pressure levels in dB re: 20 μPa

Test frequency	Octave band levels: ears covered with earphones
Hz	
500	40
1000	40
2000	47
4000	57
8000	62

Once each year, or sooner if a change of 10 dB or more is noted on biological calibration, the audiometer must have an *acoustic* calibration (see Appendix I). Since the earphones and the audiometer must be calibrated together, the earphones must be returned with the audiometer whenever it is sent for recalibration or repair.

In addition, audiometric equipment must have an *exhaustive* calibration every 2 yr. Exhaustive calibration must meet the requirements of the ANSI specification for audiometers (2). As with control of background noise levels, equipment calibration is not subject to interpretation. If audiometers are not demonstrated to be calibrated to specifications, hearing test data are not valid.

Case History

Whenever any bodily function is evaluated, a knowledge of past events which might have affected that function is essential. The possible causes of hearing loss are too numerous and varied to be considered by the occupational hearing conservationist (OHC). However, it is most helpful for the OHC to know if the employee has a known or suspected hearing loss. New employees entering the hearing conservation program should complete some type of personal questionnaire prior to their baseline testing. Many programs develop their own questionnaire; however, one similar to that shown in Figure 9.1 is adequate. A quick glance at the history sheet will identify those employees who might produce abnormal audiograms.

PREVIOUS EMPLOYERS	YEARS SERVICE	DUTIES	NOISE EXPOSURE YES	NOISE EXPOSURE NO	EAR PROTECTION YES	EAR PROTECTION NO

1. HAVE YOU EVER SERVED IN THE MILITARY OR AN EQUIVALENT SERVICE: ☐ YES ☐ NO
 •IF YES, WERE YOU EXPOSED TO NOISE BEYOND YOUR BASIC TRAINING: ☐ YES ☐ NO

2. HAVE YOU EVER HAD ANY OF THE FOLLOWING:

YES	NO		IF YES, WHICH EAR LEFT	RIGHT	BOTH
•☐	☐	HEARING LOSS	☐	☐	☐
☐	☐	EAR SURGERY	☐	☐	☐
☐	☐	EAR INJURY	☐	☐	☐
☐	☐	EAR ACHES	☐	☐	☐
☐	☐	EAR INFECTIONS	☐	☐	☐
☐	☐	RINGING EARS	☐	☐	☐
☐	☐	EAR PRESSURE	☐	☐	☐

YES	NO	
☐	☐	DIABETES
☐	☐	MUMPS, SCARLET FEVER, MEASLES (UNDER-LINE)
☐	☐	SINUS PROBLEMS
☐	☐	ALLERGIES
☐	☐	HIGH BLOOD PRESSURE
•☐	☐	HEAD INJURIES
☐	☐	HIGH FEVER DISEASES
☐	☐	DIZZINESS

3. HAVE YOU EVER HAD ROUTINE EXPOSURE TO ANY OF THE FOLLOWING NON-OCCUPATIONAL NOISE SOURCES:

YES	NO		YES	NO	
☐	☐	SNOWMOBILES/MOTORCYCLES	☐	☐	TRAP, SKEET, OR TARGET SHOOTING
☐	☐	POWERTOOLS	☐	☐	MUSIC (DRUMS, ROCK & ROLL)
☐	☐	CHAIN SAWS	☐	☐	OTHER________

4. •HAVE YOU SEEN A DOCTOR ABOUT YOUR EARS IN THE PAST YEAR: ☐ YES ☐ NO EVER: ☐ YES ☐ NO
 •DO YOU HAVE TROUBLE UNDERSTANDING CERTAIN WORDS: ☐ YES ☐ NO
 •DOES ANY MEMBER OF YOUR FAMILY HAVE A HEARING LOSS: ☐ YES ☐ NO
 HOW WOULD YOU EVALUATE YOUR OWN HEARING: ☐ GOOD ☐ FAIR ☐ POOR
 WHICH EAR DO YOU HEAR BEST FROM: ☐ BOTH THE SAME ☐ LEFT ☐ RIGHT
 •HAVE YOU EVER HAD YOUR HEARING TESTED BEFORE: ☐ YES ☐ NO

EMPLOYEE'S SIGNATURE

•INTERVIEWER'S REMARKS

Figure 9.1. Sample employee history questionnaire. The audiogram and identifying information are on the reverse side.

When a previous professional evaluation of the employee's hearing is reported in the history, the OHC should ask additional questions. Who performed the evaluation? Was a hearing test performed? When was the evaluation done? Was a diagnosis made and, if so, what was the employee told? A visit to the family physician for wax removal does not constitute an evaluation.

If the HCP does not utilize such a history sheet, or the employee has not yet completed it, the OHC must at least ask whether the individual thinks he or she has a hearing loss and, if so, in which ear.

Subsequent annual audiograms require another brief glance at the updated history sheet to determine whether any conditions might have developed or been recalled since the last examination to cause the employee to believe a hearing loss may exist. An essential question is whether the employee believes his or her hearing has changed since the last hearing test. History information should always be signed by the employee because it may at sometime in the future be relevant to compensation considerations.

It must be remembered that audiograms are important written medical records. Comments written on an audiogram sheet by the examiner should consist of only factual data, with one exception. The OHC should indicate on the sheet whether he or she feels that the test is reliable and valid. An employee who is ill, fatigued, worried, or nervous may give poor or inconsistent responses. Some employees may be slow learners or have short attention spans. Others may have language problems or be poorly motivated to concentrate on performing well.

There are a great many reasons why a baseline or annual audiogram may be abnormal. Some may be medical or physical reasons and many of these will be evident by the employee's history sheet. Draining ears or sudden hearing loss or dizziness will be obvious to the employee and will merit referral to a physician if such an examination has not already taken place. Other reasons may not be as obvious to the employee or the examiner. Individuals with upper respiratory infections or allergies may have "plugged-up ears" which, to them, are not unusual or severe enough to mention, but that may cause a significant decrease in hearing sensitivity. A recent flight in an aircraft may produce an identical situation.

Ears that itch are not uncommon, and a low grade otitis externa may result in an accumulation of epithelial debris in the ear canal which may result in decreased hearing. This debris accumulation, like cerumen, may build up so slowly and gradually that it may be ignored. In addition, an employee with otitis externa may not be able to tolerate hearing protective plugs or muffs. Indeed, he or she may not be able to tolerate the testing earphones and may need medical referral for treatment of the condition before the hearing test can be completed. If the ears are infected and draining the earphones should not be contaminated. To prevent this, thin gauze can be placed over the ears (under the earphones) when the test is done. The earphone cushions should then be disinfected after the test. In most cases however, the test can be performed.

Temporary threshold shifts may follow noisy hobbies or off-the-job activities which were not listed on the history sheet, and thus not recalled by the employee. Tinnitus may also result. Likewise, many medications contain ingredients which may affect hearing, or cause tinnitus, or act as a sedative. Any such variables have the potential for affecting the hearing test and many have immediate relevance for appropriate review and follow-up. Any such existing condition should be noted in the employee's history.

Otoscopic Examination

An otoscopic examination is usually considered appropriate prior to audiometric testing. The appropriateness of such an examination by OHCs or technicians is, however, questionable. Beyond the identification of an earplug in the ear canal or profuse discharge, the validity of other observations tends to be poor. Otoscopic examination is just not that simple for the nonprofessional. Even many professionals, including audiologists, nurses and general physicians, cannot always make valid interpretations of otoscopic examinations in many ears.

Furthermore, if there is obstructive cerumen or pathology it will be revealed by the audiometric test. It is the test and the case history which should act as the criteria for referral, not a technician's judgment of whether or not there is obstructive cerumen in the ear canal. Even an inspection by the OHC or technician which suggests that a collapsed canal under the earphone might be contributing to an abnormal audiometric result, has little value in the review and referral paradigm. Ultimately the referral decision must be made by the program professionals. The audiogram and/or history remains the basis for these decisions.

In addition to the lack of validity of otoscopic inspections by OHCs or technicians, there is an implied liability assumed by the supervising professional for such actions. Relating visual otoscopic findings to test results is interpretative and diagnostic and is beyond the scope of a technician's role. Conversely, simply reporting otoscopic observations can lead to over-referral as well as the failure to identify real problems. The only real place for otoscopic inspection in the HCP is when the condition and size of the ear canal must be checked for the fitting of a hearing protective device (HPD).

Audiometric Test Procedure

Each employee exposed to workplace noise of 85 dBA or greater must be provided with a baseline and annual audiometric test at the employer's expense. The employee hearing test must be preceded by 14 hr of quiet. Quiet in this context is defined as "without exposure to workplace noise." This requirement may be met by the use of HPDs if the employee is to be on the job immediately prior to the test. Since practicality dictates against testing everyone prior to the beginning of the work shift, the use of HPDs to achieve quiet is widely practiced.

There are three types of audiometric equipment available for the determination of pure-tone, air-conduction thresholds: (a) the manual audiometer; (b) the self-recording or automatic (Bekesy type) audiometer; and (c) the microprocessor-controlled audiometer. The procedure for giving the test will vary somewhat depending on the type of audiometer.

The employee should be seated in a sound-controlled environment and instructed that a series of sounds will be heard in one ear and then the other, to which a response is required even if the sound is very faint. The response will usually be finger raising or button pushing in the case of manual audiometry, or definitely button pushing for either self-recording or microprocessor audiometry. The variations of acceptable responses for manual air-conduction audiometry are infinite. We recommend that the response begin when the tone is first perceived and continue until the tone stops. If the response is finger raising, the worker should use the hand on the side being tested. These are internal validity checks that are helpful to the OHC. The earphones should then be put in place by the examiner after requesting that eyeglasses, large earrings, wigs, or another object that would prevent the earphone cushions from resting snugly against the external ear be removed. Earphones should also be removed by the examiner at the conclusion of the test.

Determining Thresholds Manually

The procedure recommended for determining thresholds manually is:

1. Begin at 1000 Hz in either the right ear

or better ear, as determined by the case history

2. Start with the attenuator at 0 dB HL, turn the tone on, and slowly decrease attenuation (make the tone louder) until the first response is obtained
3. Verify the first response level by repeating the tone to obtain a second response (the use of pulsed tones is recommended)
4. Increase the attenuation (decrease the HL) by 10 dB and present again. From this point on the tone presentation level will always be determined by the previous response. That is, each time the employee responds to a tone, the level should be decreased 10 dB and, conversely, when no response is obtained, the level should be increased 5 dB.
5. This ascending bracketing procedure should be continued until the lowest response level is obtained on two out of three trials.
6. When the threshold for 1000 Hz is established, the identical procedure should be followed to obtain thresholds at 2000, 3000, 4000, 6000, and 500 Hz in the first ear. A recheck of the 1000 Hz threshold should be performed on the first side tested. The frequencies stated are required. Other frequencies may be tested at the discretion of the program administrator. Most often, 8000 Hz is included because of its contribution to the typical noise-induced hearing loss configuration.
7. The same procedure is then used to obtain thresholds for the second ear except that the recheck at 1000 Hz is optional.

Self-Recorded Thresholds

Obtaining self-recorded thresholds is relatively simple. The instructions may vary only in that the response button must be held down until the tone is completely inaudible. The examiner must, however, monitor the progress of the test closely. While the audiometer is designed to sequentially obtain all necessary thresholds, a tracing that does not cross one of the horizontal divisions of the audiogram form at least six times is not valid (Fig. 9.2). Failure to demonstrate six crossings may occur for a number of reasons. One frequent cause is confusion between the test-tone and head noises in the higher frequencies if the employee has a ringing type tinnitus.

Thresholds with Microprocessor-Controlled Equipment

Similar to self-recorded audiometry, microprocessor-controlled equipment has been preprogrammed to test the appropriate frequencies. In this case, however, the adjustments of the dB HL of the test tones is also controlled by the audiometer based on the response pattern of the employee. The threshold levels are established according to predetermined response criteria and the threshold values are then either recorded manually or, if equipped with a printer, produced as hard copy by the machine.

Regardless of the type of audiometric equipment used, it is the responsibility of the examiner to monitor the reliability and validity of the employee's responses. It may be necessary to stop the test to repeat the instructions if the validity of the test results is questioned. Any of the three types of audiometers is quite acceptable as long as the data are valid. In any group of industrial employees, however, it is likely that a few will be unable to produce acceptable results with the self-recording and/or microprocessor equipment and will ultimately have to be tested manually.

It should also be indicated that the type of audiometric testing done in most industrial hearing conservation programs will identify only the presence of a hearing loss. The usual test is of air-conduction sensitivity for pure tones, and precludes an evaluation of the many other facets of the communication process. In spite of this limitation, this test is a valuable tool for screening purposes. All industries do not limit their program strictly to the OSHA regulations; some test additional frequencies and some even do bone-conduction testing and speech reception and discrimination testing, although this is not common. The number of employees as well as the number and qualifications of the hearing conservation team may result in a wide range of variation of test protocols.

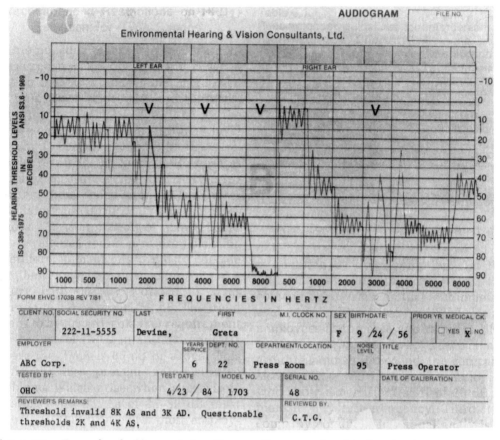

Figure 9.2. Example of self-recorded audiogram. Note questionable thresholds indicated by V. Right ear 3000 Hz threshold is not valid due to lack of six crossings at any HL.

Medical Considerations

Screening audiometry performed in the early school years results in referrals which usually diagnose predominantly conductive hearing losses due to otitis media. On the other hand, threshold audiometry in industry results in referrals which usually diagnose predominantly sensorineural hearing losses. The primary purpose for testing hearing in industry is well understood. There are, however, other benefits that result from these tests, among them is the identification of hearing loss that is not noise related. Some of the causes of such hearing loss are serious, possibly life threatening, medical disorders.

In a recent study, 107 referrals from industry resulted in the identification of 53% of those referred who had otologic diagnoses other than noise-induced hearing loss (3). If the employee indicates on the history sheet or complains of earache, drainage, severe persistent tinnitus, unilateral hearing loss, sudden or fluctuating hearing loss, dizziness or a feeling of pressure or fullness in the ears, either at the time of the baseline or the annual test, he or she should be referred for evaluation if one has not been performed.

An audiogram which may be typical of noise-induced hearing loss may also be found in employees with presbycusis, viral-induced hearing loss, ototoxicity, genetic factors and other medical problems. In addition, pure-tone audiometry and subsequent referral may lead to identification of chronic otitis, Ménière's disease, early acoustic neurinoma, nasopharyngeal tumor, syphilis, and many more conditions which are amenable to medical or surgical therapy. There are some otologic diseases which can be overlooked since they may cause few if any complaints. Two of these might be serous otitis media with minimal hearing loss or cholesteatoma which may have scant or nondetectable drainage and minimal or no hearing loss.

Hearing monitoring programs may not detect all ear disease, but they will identify a significant number of employees who will benefit from referral, and such programs will, overall, help to prevent pain, suffering, disability, and hours off the job. In addition, they will provide for an appreciation by the employee of the concerns for his or her health by the employer. In this sense the HCP is more than an OSHA compliance program, it is a hearing health benefit program.

DEVELOPING CRITERIA FOR AUDIOGRAM INTERPRETATION

As the federal occupational safety and health, as well as most state compensation, regulations are currently constituted, preemployment baseline and periodic follow-up hearing tests have inherent value to both the employer and employee. The cornerstone of most industrial HCPs is an identification or preemployment audiogram. The document is essential for several reasons. It serves to identify preexisting hearing loss prior to placement in a work environment having noise levels that may damage hearing. As such, it functions to protect the employer against the responsibility for preexisting hearing loss which could lead to a considerable saving in compensation liability. In addition, the initial audiogram obtained on any employee serves to establish a baseline against which future hearing tests are compared. This aspect of HCPs is vital because it is the only proven way of assuring that the techniques for control of noise exposure are effective in preventing hearing impairment. The potential value of the identification or baseline and follow-up audiograms extends far beyond

the usual industrial and compensation frame of reference when appropriate professional measures are used to review and evaluate the data.

The purposes of baseline and monitoring audiometry in industry are: to identify hearing loss, to identify medically significant problems that may be revealed by the presence of hearing loss, the audiometric test can be used as an educational tool to enhance the workers appreciation for the hazards of noise exposure and the benefits of hearing conservation, and to identify those workers whose hearing is changing due to noise exposure or other causes.

Framework for Review and Interpretation

In order to achieve the intended purposes of an audiometric testing program, a system for interpreting the audiograms must be implemented along with the guidelines necessary to make reasonable decisions concerning referral and follow-up.

The sheer volume of audiometric data generated by even small companies over the period of a few years, makes manual interpretation systems difficult. Ideally, all problem audiograms will receive individual attention by a qualified professional. Much of the data, however, can and probably should be managed by automated processes that have been designed by the program professionals or reputable consultants. Many well designed computerized systems for categorizing audiometric data are currently available. An example of one such system is provided in Table 9.2.

The category system shown in Table 9.2 has been developed and refined over a period of more than 10 yr (4). All test results are initially categorized by computer on the basis of the audiometric configuration. The program makes comparisons both among frequencies monaurally and within frequencies binaurally. A category designation, e.g. 2 is assigned on the basis of these comparisons. All problem

Table 9.2.
What the categories mean[a]

Category (1) (Normal hearing)	**Hearing thresholds are within limits established for normal hearing;** i.e. no worse than 25 dB at any frequency
Category (2) (Mild to moderate high frequency loss)	**Hearing for communication purposes is essentially unimpaired.** There is hearing loss present in the high frequencies. Category 2A denotes no loss greater than 25 dB at 500, 1000, 2000 Hz, and no worse than 50 dB in the higher frequencies. Category 2B exceeds 50 dB at 4000, 6000, and/or 8000 Hz, Very few losses in category 2A or 2B will be compensable
Category (3) (Moderate to severe high frequency loss)	**Provisional Pass. Significant hearing loss exists.** The adequacy of hearing for communication purposes is questionable and the individual is borderline for aural rehabilitation. There is no threshold worse than 25 dB at 500, 1000 and/or 2000 Hz, but it is 55 dB or more at 3000 Hz. Most losses in this category will be minimally compensable
Category (4) (Possibly medically related hearing loss)	**Fail. Significant hearing loss exists of undetermined type and origin.** The individual should be referred for complete examination. Thresholds exceed 25 dB at 500, 1000 or 2000 Hz. This category has a high potential for compensation if not identified prior to employment
Category (5) (Inconsistent test)	**Test responses inconsistent.** A retest is indicated since better test results are necessary for the reviewer to make reliable interpretations
Category (6) (Previously professionally evaluated hearing loss)	**Significant hearing loss exists which is known to the individual.** The employee has seen a professional about the hearing status. A copy of the professional's (physician/audiologist) report should be obtained for the employee's record
Category (7A)[b] (STS: further professional evaluation optional)	**Significant change from baseline audiogram; no referral needed.** Additional professional evaluation is not likely to provide further helpful information. If exposed to noise on the job, employee should be rechecked and reoriented about hearing protection use
Category (7B)[b] (STS: further professional evaluation is advised)	**Significant change from baseline. Should be referred for further professional evaluation.** This change is likely to be other than noise related. If exposed to noise on the job, employee needs to be rechecked and reoriented about hearing protection use
Category (8) (No change)	**No significant change from baseline audiogram.** Original designation still applies

[a] Reproduced by courtesy of Environmental Hearing and Vision Consultants Ltd., E. Syracuse, NY.
[b] Criteria for category 7A and 7B are 10 dB or more (average) loss at 2000, 3000 and 4000 Hz, and/or 25 dB or more at any frequency.

categories (3; 4; 5; 6; 7A; 7B) are then reviewed by an appropriate professional. The second review is the point at which decisions are made concerning referral for additional evaluation and follow-up. Category classifications may be revised at this time at the discretion of the professional reviewer.

This system has proved to be sufficiently flexible to meet the demands of widely diverse industrial concerns. Major revisions have not been necessary with each of the changes in the OSHA Regulations. We have found this system to be especially valuable when the contracting company chooses to also adopt the system of explanatory letters to employees that accompany each category. It is not intended that the categories themselves be divulged to the employee, since the system is proprietary and the numbers would have no meaning to hearing professionals and other interested parties without an explanation. Figure 9.3 shows a hypothetical, individual test report which identifies the employee's results as category 2A. Figure 9.4 is the letter that would be given to the employee as a report of the hearing test. The letter is usually printed on the employer's letterhead. Such a system insures that the employee gets adequate feedback on the results of the test and provides an opportunity for the company to promote the HCP not only as a government mandate but as an integral part of the company's overall health and safety effort.

Problems Associated with Referral Criteria

Cost-Benefit Factors

The benefits inherent in preventing noise-induced hearing loss are obvious. OSHA estimates that HCPs for all employees will eliminate over 200,000 cases of material impairment in 10 yr, and more than 600,000 after 30 yr. But HCPs, in themselves, are costly to industry. The necessary instruments and equipment for monitoring noise and audiometric testing are delicate, sensitive and expensive. Qualified personnel to conduct the now-mandatory examinations must be employed. Time away from the job is nonproductive but inevitable if employees are to be tested, educated and counseled.

When employees fail to comply with OSHA standards there are several avenues of approach. In-house procedures or

INDIVIDUAL REPORT • HEARING CONSERVATION PROGRAM

EMPLOYEE NAME	EMPLOYEE NO.	SEX	BIRTHDATE
David M Harrison	109525454	M	08/30/58

AUDIOGRAM

TEST DATE	LEFT EAR 500	1000	2000	3000	4000	6000	8000	RIGHT EAR 500	1000	2000	3000	4000	6000	8000	CATEGORY	TEST
04/23/84	10	05	15	20	20	45	30	05	05	15	20	15	25	15		ORIGINAL
																PREVIOUS
04/23/84	10	05	15	20	20	45	30	05	05	15	20	15	25	15		BASELINE
04/23/84	10	05	15	20	20	45	30	05	05	15	20	15	25	15	2A	CURRENT
FREQUENCY IN HERTZ	500	1000	2000	3000	4000	6000	8000	500	1000	2000	3000	4000	6000	8000		

CLIENT NAME
A.B.C Corporation
Campbell Plant

Environmental Hearing & Vision Consultants

FORM 1122

Figure 9.3. Individual audiometric report. The current test is categorized 2A (see Table 9.2).

```
                              A.B.C. Corporation
                              8600 Main Street
                              Campbell, NY 14821

                         Dear David Harrison:

                             Your recent audiometric
          screening conducted as part of A.B.C. Corporation's Hearing
          Conservation Program indicated that when compared to the normal
          population, you have a hearing loss of which you may or may not be
          aware.  The greater part of the loss occurs in the higher
          frequencies, but it may interfere with routine communication.  It
          is not possible from this test alone to establish the cause of the
          loss.  You may wish to consult an audiologist or ear physician,
          especially if speech sounds unclear or you have other ear or
          hearing complaints.  Our consultants recommend that you see a
          specialist if any change occurs in your hearing prior to your next
          regularly scheduled audiometric screening.

          Annual audiometric screening is conducted by A.B.C. Corporation as
          part of it's overall health and safety program, in keeping with
          the specified guidelines of the Occupational Safety & Health
          Administration.  If you have further questions concerning your
          hearing test, you may seek consultation from my office.

          Hearing is a valued asset, not to be taken for granted by anyone.
          For this reason, you are urged to wear hearing protection if you
          work in an area designated as having high noise levels or if you
          engage in off-the-job activities where there is noise exposure.

                              Sincerely,



                              Jack Frost
                              Safety Director
```

Figure 9.4.   Employee notification letter for audiometric review category 2A.

reexamination may resolve the problem. However, some employees may persist in providing unsatisfactory hearing test results or may have symptoms or signs of ear disease and these individuals will merit referral.

Referral of all employees with minor hearing losses to an otologist or audiologist will result in added cost to both the employee and employer, and may be counter productive to the HCP. However, serious medical disorders and/or useful rehabilitation measures may be neglected if referrals are not made at all or are only made according to rigid, overly conservative criteria.

Referral procedures will vary considerably depending upon the personnel involved in the hearing conservation program in any particular industrial setting. If a physician is one of the team, then few referrals will be made for otitis externa or impacted cerumen. If an audiologist is present, then few referrals will be made

for audiometric evaluations. If referral is indicated, it will probably be less costly in professional fees and time off the job if referral is made to an otologist-audiologist team in the same office setting. The OSHA noise standard does not require that everyone with a standard threshold shift be referred for evaluation. The reviewing professional may make the judgment that additional evaluation is not necessary. It has been estimated that in a good, ongoing industrial hearing conservation program in an average industrial setting, no more than 1–2% of the personnel will require referral after periodic testing (4).

Referrals, in addition to obtaining an accurate appraisal of hearing sensitivity and a medical diagnosis, may have additional benefits. Counseling by a professional outside the industry may lead to better adherence to the advice given by the employer regarding hearing protection. Also, some employees with hearing losses about which nothing medical or surgical can be done, may benefit from hearing aids or other appropriate rehabilitation measures.

Referrals to an otologist or other physician who is not familiar with industrial hearing conservation programs may result in information which is quite adequate for medical purposes but which fails to provide information desired by the hearing conservation program director. Knowing whether a sensorineural hearing loss is possibly or probably due to noise on or off the job is helpful. Also, dizziness or balance problems that might be hazardous on the job should be noted. The employee may have been given medications which sometimes cause sedation. An otitis externa might preclude the use of HPDs of certain types. It is best to have an established referral source so that communication is easy and satisfactory between the referring individual and the consultant. Such an established referral pattern will save both time and money and will result in a better HCP. Some companies elect to pay referral fees for audiometric failures but not for ear pain or drainage or dizziness. The OSHA regulations require that the employer be responsible for work-related examinations. The determination of "work related" is not always clear cut. It is frequently a judgment call on the part of the reviewing professional or the company's medical consultant.

Under-Referral

It is easy to state that referrals should be kept to a minimum. It is difficult to define that minimum. A family physician sometimes has a difficult time deciding whether to refer a patient to a specialist. Certainly an OHC or technician should not be responsible for making referral decisions. The OHCs responsibility is to document the findings. The program director's action will vary depending upon his or her qualifications (physician, audiologist, safety engineer, nurse, etc.).

The referrals are of two types: audiological or medical. The OSHA regulations are quite clear as to which individuals must be identified on the basis of audiometric deficiencies. This is based on the definition of a standard threshold shift (STS) as an average change of 10 dB or greater in either ear at 2000, 3000 and 4000 Hz. The decision to refer for further evaluation, however, is at the discretion of the reviewing professional. Other more stringent or more liberal criteria will usually influence this decision (5).

We have already alluded to medical referrals. It is helpful to review the guidelines of the American Council of Otolaryngology (6) regarding medical referral. These are shown in Table 9.3.

Under-referral may result in savings in fees and hours off the job initially but can be costly in the long run. A hearing loss

Table 9.3.
Otologic referral criteria for occupational hearing conservation programs

1. History of ear drainage or vertigo (sensation of rotary movement) within past 12 months
2. Average hearing loss at 0.5, 1, 2 and 3 kHz greater than 25 dB.
3. Average hearing asymmetry of:
   More than 15 dB at 0.5, 1 and 2 kHz
   More than 30 dB at 3, 4 and 6 kHz
4. Average change from baseline audiograms of:
   More than 15 dB at 0.5, 1 and 2 kHz
   More than 20 dB at 3, 4 and 6 kHz
5. If a person has received otologic evaluation previously on the basis of failing the above screening criteria, he should be reevaluated if he has developed ear drainage or vertigo, or if he shows a significant change (as defined above) from the hearing level obtained at his previous otologic evaluation.

or ear disease may progress undetected and result in greater expense and lost time in the months ahead. It is better to refer than possibly overlook a potentially serious medical problem. But, when the professional who reviews the audiometric data and history does not believe either medical or audiological advantage would accrue from additional evaluation then such a recommendation should be deferred. This judgment may only be made by qualified professionals and clearly carries liability implications. If either a hearing loss or other signs of a medical disorder exist, these should be made known to the employee when referral is not recommended so that, if concerned about the findings, the employee can seek additional consultation independently.

Over-Referral

Over-referral lacks the inherent potential dangers of under-referral but it is costly in time and money. This is particularly true in the initial or start-up phases of an HCP. At the beginning, many of the employees will have had enough noise exposure in the past to demonstrate significant hearing loss. At the same time, very careful efforts are needed to introduce the HCP as a useful, essential aspect of the overall health and safety program. Referral of 70–80% of the employees on the basis of the baseline audiogram is likely to create suspicion and hostility toward the HCP among both labor and management. Production supervisors, whose cooperation is critical in the success of a HCP, will likely resent the loss of substantial production time or large scale scheduling problems that evolve from employees being absent for medical and/or audiological appointments.

The review and referral criteria in this chapter are offered only as one type of model. The variations are almost infinite. The primary point to be made is that a great deal of organizational effort must go into the development of systems for handling information if the HCP is to function efficiently. If such systems are in place, over-referral should not be a significant problem. In-house retesting and careful audiometric evaluations by qualified professionals should minimize audiometric referrals. It should again be stressed that good communication between the referring individual and the otolaryngologist and/or audiologist providing the professional consultation is essential. An ideal relationship would be one in which the HCP has been described in detail to the outside professional and the need for reinforcement of hearing conservation principles is recognized by the consultant.

Legal Manifestations

Whenever one deals in any manner with the health and/or well being of another individual, one immediately accepts a great responsibility and a tendency to be either praised or criticized. The latter, in our present litigation-minded society can be most costly. Good rapport between the employees and the hearing conservation team can minimize legal involvement. However, good audiometric technique may not be enough protection. Care of equipment, audiometric calibration, record keeping, referral policy, fitting of hearing protectors, and all aspects of an HCP may fall prey to legal action. In the opinion of one attorney, you should be able to show that you *know* about hearing conservation, that you *do* everything reasonable to enhance hearing conservation, and that you *care* about hearing conservation (7). It is also wise to be covered by good liability insurance.

Many aspects of professional and personal liability are discussed in Chapter 12.

SUMMARY

In this chapter we have discussed many of the day-to-day aspects that make the management of HCPs both a joy and a dilemma. Control of background noise and equipment calibration is challenging in the industrial environment. These components of the testing program must be constantly attended to in order to insure the validity of the tests. The administration of pure-tone, air-conduction audiometry is a rather simple, routine task. Regardless of the type of equipment used, the OHC must make accurate decisions about the reliability and validity of the results and the worker's history must be carefully recorded.

The program professionals also have their work cut out for them. In addition to the organization and supervision of the testing component, procedures and guidelines for review of the audiograms and referral for follow-up must be implemented and monitored. Managing the large volumes of paper associated with a HCP is no mean task. We have recommended the use of computerized systems for data management and provided an example of one such system. The need for careful consideration of referral guidelines cannot be over emphasized. Neither over-referral nor under-referral is desirable and both have a substantial influence on the overall success of the HCP. Striking a balance between an industrial identification and monitoring program on the one hand and a clinical program on the other is an ongoing dilemma that requires all of the ethical, intellectual and moral resources that can be brought to bear.

References

1. Criteria for Permissible Ambient Noise During Audiometric Testing. ANSI S3.6 1977: New York, American National Standards Institute, 1977.
2. Specifications for Audiometers. ANSI S3.6 1969: New York, American National Standards Institute, 1969.
3. Dobie RA, Archer RJ: Results of otologic referral in an industrial hearing conservation program. *Otolaryngol Head Neck Surg* 89:294, 1981.
4. Feldman AS, Grimes CT: Review and referral of industrial audiograms: a professional dilemma, *ASHA* 19:231, 1977.
5. Feldman AS: Industrial audiogram review, *Hearing Aid J*, 35:18–20, 1982.
6. American Academy of Otolaryngology-Head and Neck Surgery: *Otologic Referral Criteria for Occupational Hearing Conservation Programs.* American Academy of Otolaryngology-Head and Neck Surgery, 1983.
7. Radcliffe D: Current Issues in Hearing Conservation, *Hearing Aid J* July/August, 1982.

CHAPTER 10

Judging Effectiveness of Hearing Conservation Programs

WILLIAM G. THOMAS

INTRODUCTION

The primary goal of any hearing conservation program is the elimination of noise induced permanent threshold shift (NIPTS) resulting from on-the-job noise exposure. Attaining this goal, however, is difficult, if not impossible, without a systematic method of judging the effectiveness of the hearing conservation program (HCP). Adequate measures of effectiveness are not as straight forward as might be assumed because of numerous factors which interact and affect the outcome of these measures. These factors include such items as: (a) improved auditory thresholds for some employees resulting from "learning effects" as multiple thresholds are obtained; (b) aging effects (AE) during the course of the HCP, especially programs that have been in operation for many years; (c) the standard threshold shift (STS) criteria used; (d) the choice of an appropriate sample of nonexposed subjects with whom to compare the noise-exposed population; (e) the differences that exist in both non-noise and noise-exposed groups as a function of race and sex; (f) the accuracy of testing and absence of temporary pathology in the original baseline audiograms; (g) the age of the HCP; and (h) the adequacy of personal hearing protection used and the effectiveness with which this protection is used by the employees, especially as it relates to prevention of temporary threshold shifts (TTS).

The concept of establishing an "Effective Hearing Conservation Program" has been an intergral part of the noise standard since its first inclusion (1969) in the Walsh-Healy Public Contracts Act. This concept has been included in all modifications of the noise standard, both promulgated and proposed, up to and including the standard promulgated in March, 1983 (1). However, a gradual change seems to have taken place in the definition of "effective" over the past decade. Initially, the focus of effective hearing conservation was more programmatic. That is, the program was defined by the components making up the program with little attention toward evaluating its effectiveness. In its initial Guidelines, the U. S. Department of Labor (1971) described five components necessary to establish an effective hearing conservation program: (a) noise surveys, (b) engineering and/or administrative controls, (c) employee education, (d) audiometric testing, and (e) personal hearing protection (2). This programmatic approach to the development of effective hearing conservation in industry was reiterated by numerous authors (3–13). The approaches suggested by these authors are similar, with particular emphasis put on various aspects of the program by individual authors.

While an adequate initial concept, the programmatic approach to effective hearing conservation does not guarantee that additional hearing loss due to on-the-job noise exposure will not be present nor does it offer any specific, systematic way of judging program effectiveness. For this reason, several authors have suggested various ways of analyzing the audiometric data base (14–23). Several of the aforementioned studies have been retrospective. One of the first serial studies reported hearing threshold levels for various noise exposures over a 3-yr period, with appropriate control populations (14). Although not designed to evaluate the effectiveness of the various hearing conservation programs, the methodology lends itself to this type analysis. In this study, the mean audiometric thresholds from various work locations were plotted in audiogram form over a 3-yr period, showing mean hearing threshold level (HTL) changes. Pell (18) reports the results of a 5-yr longitudinal study on approximately 2800 employees exposed to different noise levels divided into three categories. The analysis technique showed the distribution of change in HTL over the 5-yr period at various audiometric frequencies for three noise categories. Pell used this data to suggest that the higher levels of exposure caused no greater hearing loss after 5 yr than lower, safer levels when the employees were adequately protected with personal hearing protection devices (HPDs). Several problems exist in this population, however. First, the population was all male. Subsequent studies have indicated more hearing loss and a more rapid rate of change occurs in males, particularly white males (20, 21). Therefore, the possibility exists that many of the employees used in this study were at, or near, asymptotic hearing loss prior to the longitudinal study. Second, Pell indicates a higher proportion of young employees in areas of higher noise exposure. Subsequent data have indicated a "learning effect" on serial audiograms during the first four or five hearing tests (19, 21–24). This raises the possibility that the amount of hearing loss over the 5-yr

period might be underestimated because of improvements in threshold caused by "learning" over the testing period for audiometric naive subjects.

The methodology of using test-retest results from audiometric data bases was extended by Berger (20) to include an analysis of the employees that exceed various criteria for STS. Nine different STS criteria were used in the analysis. This type of analysis has been expanded further to include smoothed rate of change at various frequencies, control and industrial data for various populations subdivided by race and sex, maximum percentage of employees that improve their HTLs over those that decrease their HTLs, and single number ratings of HCPs (19, 21–23). It appears obvious from the aforementioned studies that analysis of audiometric data bases are essential in developing criteria for judging HCP effectiveness and that programmatic approaches do not necessarily guarantee adequate protection of workers in a particular program.

In this chapter, analysis of population data, as well as analysis of individual audiograms, will be discussed. Although information used in population analysis derives from individual data, the analysis techniques are quite different. Since large-number statistics can usually be used in population data, small changes in mean HTL for a particular group may be extremely significant, while a ±10-dB change in an individual audiogram may be considered within normal limits.

JUDGING EFFECTIVENESS FROM POPULATION DATA

Background

In order to judge the effectiveness of a particular HCP in reducing on-the-job noise exposure and subsequent hearing loss resulting from such exposure, some quantifiable measure must be available. The obvious choice appears to be the results of periodic hearing tests. The only other aspect of an HCP that can be quantified with any degree of accuracy is the noise survey; however, a direct relationship between noise levels and hearing loss presently does not exist. This relationship is complex and depends on such factors as total noise dose, noise spectrum and "individual susceptibility." The choice of the audiogram as the most likely measure of effectiveness is not meant to imply that audiometric tests are free from errors or artifacts. It is simply to suggest that results of hearing tests are more directly related to the effectiveness of the over-all HCP than other parts of the program and, in fact, reflect the effects of such aspects as engineering controls, education and the use of personal HPDs. In addition, audiometric results lend themselves favorably to data reduction and statistical analysis.

Results of audiometric tests can contain numerous errors and artifacts, a topic discussed in more detail in the next section. Errors and artifacts become more of a problem in evaluating individual audiograms, however, than does the evaluation of population data. Many errors in measurement will be random and statistical procedures on large data bases will tend to cancel these random fluctuations. It is common for individual audiograms to fluctuate by ±10 dB on successive tests without apparent cause, while a 1- or 2-dB change might be highly significant in total population data. Partly because of large fluctuations in individual audiograms, the majority of work thus far in evaluating effectiveness of HCPs has used population data.

The evaluation of audiometric data bases offers additional advantages. Data can be subdivided in numerous ways to point out potential trouble areas by shift, department, etc., especially in the use of HPDs and the effects of educational programs. While not directly related to individual employees and the additional hearing loss an individual employee may acquire, data base analyses can become an important management tool in evaluating the over-all effectiveness of the program.

Factors Affecting Population Analysis

Baseline Data

In the early 1970s, many industries initiated audiometric testing of their employees as a direct result of changes to the Walsh-Healy Public Contracts Act and passage of the Occupational Safety and Health Act of 1970. The testing frequently was accomplished without adequate preparation, and utilized technicians with limited experience. Hearing testing was a unique experience to many employees, as well. This combination produced many erroneous thresholds which were considered baseline data. These were compared to subsequent audiograms to determine the presence or absence of STS. Even in the absence of erroneous threshold data, some baselines are contaminated by physiologic changes to the auditory system which may improve over time. Fluctuations in auditory thresholds resulting from inaccurate audiograms or from resolving ear pathology create problems for data analysis, particularly if a significant number of employees are involved. It is obvious that care should be taken in establishing baseline audiograms and that inaccurate or questionable data should not be entered into the record for later comparison. These judgments, however, require experience and some amount of insight on the part of the hearing conservationists. This is particularly true when ear differences exist which might exceed interaural attenuation values, inconsistencies are noted in the employee's responses, inadequate instructions are given, unacceptable testing techniques are used, or excessive noise is present in the testing environment.

Although some improvement in auditory threshold might be expected because of learning effects for two or three tests following the initial audiogram (23, 24), excessive improvements resulting from errors in baseline audiograms or resolving ear pathologies can influence the data analysis and overestimate the effectiveness of the HCP. Therefore, great care should be exercised in the establishment of baseline auditory thresholds. Of course, the same care should be incorporated in all hearing tests, but the importance of the baseline in future comparisons enhances the need for accuracy on that particular test. The significance of baseline audiograms in test-retest comparisons emphasizes the desirability of upgrading baseline data as the need arises, an option permitted by the Noise Standard promulgated in 1983 (1). The concept of baseline adjustment will be discussed in a later portion of this chapter.

Temporary Threshold Shift (TTS)

Although numerical estimates are unavailable, the presence of TTS in baseline and subsequent audiograms in industrial populations is probably considerable. The presence of TTS in annual tests may reflect the actual state of the employee's auditory threshold and indicate a need to counsel or educate the employee to the dangers of excessive noise exposure (on and off the job) and to fit, or refit, personal HPDs. The general purpose of the HCP is to detect potential hearing loss early and to institute effective measures to eliminate or slow its progress. The presence of TTS in the baseline audiograms, however, can lead to misinterpretation of HCP effectiveness. While errors in the establishment of baseline data may tend to be randomly distributed with respect to HTL over the population, TTS constantly displaces threshold toward worse hearing. The decay or complete remission of TTS on subsequent audiograms, particularly if a large number of employees are involved, may contribute to an overestimation of effectiveness for a particular HCP.

The presence of TTS in the baseline audiogram may be more difficult for the conservationist, audiologist or physician to detect since it represents an actual change in threshold and may not be associated with employee inconsistency. Safeguards should be established to reduce the effect of TTS. These might include testing employees after a period of time away from noise exposure, when feasible; documented use of HPDs prior to audiometric testing; or accurate information regarding second jobs or hobbies. The possibility of TTS in the baseline audiogram also supports the need for baseline revision.

Audiometric Calibration

Everyone accepts the need for accurate calibration of instrumentation used to establish auditory thresholds. Standards are available describing performance criteria for this instrumentation (25). Although considerable inconvenience and time waste are associated with retesting employees when an audiometer is found out of calibration, this fact is not in question. A more subtle problem arises, however, when minor adjustments are made in the output of the audiometer during annual calibrations. The accepted tolerance in calibration standards range from ±3–5 dB, depending on frequency. At 4 kHz, for example, the accepted tolerance is ±4 dB. Therefore, it is possible for an 8-dB swing to occur and the audiometer still remain within calibration specifications. It is common for minor adjustments to be made in SPL output during annual calibration. For example, if the audiometer at 4 kHz is 4 dB below the ANSI value, it may be adjusted to the actual level, although it is within calibration limits at −4 dB. Annual tests performed with an audiometer that is 4 dB higher in output than the previous year will cause many employees to exhibit better thresholds by 5 dB. Minor adjustments of SPL output levels cause little concern in individual audiograms, since a ±5 dB threshold variation might be expected. A 4- or 5-dB change in the population mean HTL, however, would be extremely significant. Data is available on calibration changes affecting population means and possibly causing misinterpretation of HCP effectiveness (23). Minor adjustments made during annual calibration should be noted, if made. It is important that the individual or company performing the calibration supply data on the SPL levels before, as well as after, adjustments are made. If the audiometer is within specifications for SPL output it should not be altered, adhering to the old saying, "if it ain't broke, don't fix it."

Age Effects

Decreasing hearing as a function of age has been documented by numerous authors over many years (26–44). This loss of sensitivity resulting from physiologic aging is thought to involve most levels of the auditory system, although cochlear devascularization and loss of hair cells may be the prime factors (32). In general, hearing loss with age, or presbycusis, shows a gradual loss of sensitivity as a function of frequency. Unfortunately, sensitivity changes in the auditory system due to aging alone are difficult to ascertain because of other environmental factors which may affect the auditory system, including: noise, various disease processes, stress, diet, etc. Since it is generally impossible to differentiate hearing loss resulting from presbycusis and other environmental factors in our society, a more general description termed "age effects" has been used to describe decreased auditory sensitivity as a function of age (43). This term includes hearing loss from environmental variables, as well as physiological aging. Age effects (AE) play an important part in evaluating HCP effectiveness. As the age of a particular industrial population becomes greater, additional hearing loss is to be expected which is not necessarily associated with noise exposure, at least industrial noise exposure. Any measure of HCP effectiveness will have to take into account age effects. Otherwise, all HCPs will appear ineffective after a few years. For this reason, age corrections are included as an option in the current noise standard (1).

Reference Population

The importance of good AE data with which to compare industrial populations cannot be overemphasized. These curves become reference curves for direct comparison to industrial populations at various ages. Ideally, reference populations should include data from the same general geographic area and the same general socioeconomic levels. This helps to insure that the reference population is exposed to the same environmental factors and probably engage in the same hobbies and extra-work activities as the industrial population. This will help increase the probability that the only remaining variable between the two populations is on-the-job noise exposure. Data on reference populations and AEs are available in the literature (26, 30–33, 35, 40–42, 44, 45, 46). However, industries are encouraged to develop their own reference populations, when feasible. In larger industries, this can be accomplished with employees not working in noise areas. When this is not feasible, data can be used from other sources. Differences may exist, however, between published data and particular industrial populations, depending on subject selection criteria, socioeconomic levels and geographic areas represented in the reference population. This is particularly true in urban vs rural populations, since extra-work activities are likely to be quite different.

Sex and Race Differences

As previously stated, accurate non-noise-exposed AE data are important for comparison with industrial populations in judging the effectiveness of a particular HCP. Previous research has indicated differences in auditory sensitivity between male and female populations and between black and white populations, particularly above 30 yr of age (26, 29, 31, 35, 36, 40). More recent studies have further defined these AE differences (42, 44). Figures 10.1–10.4 show the smoothed, non-normalized mean hearing levels for male,

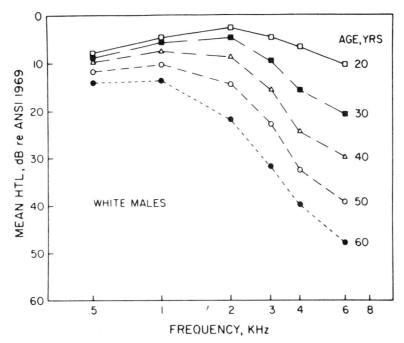

Figure 10.1. Smoothed, non-normalized hearing threshold levels (*HTL*) of white male nonindustrial noise-exposed subjects as a function of decade age. (From Royster LH, Thomas WG: *American Industrial Hygiene Association Journal* 40:504–511, 1979, (42).)

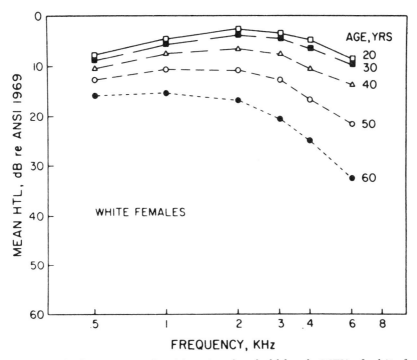

Figure 10.2. Smoothed, non-normalized hearing threshold levels (*HTL*) of white female nonindustrial noise-exposed subjects as a function of age. (From Royster LH, Thomas WG: *American Industrial Hygiene Association Journal* 40:504–511, 1979, (42).)

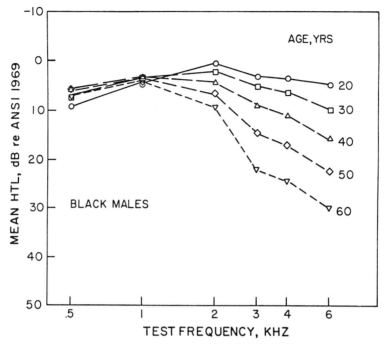

Figure 10.3. Smoothed, non-normalized hearing threshold levels (*HTL*) of black male nonindustrial noise-exposed subjects as a function of decade age. (From Royster LH, Driscoll DP, Thomas WG, Royster JD: *American Industrial Hygiene Association Journal* 41:113–119, 1980 (44).)

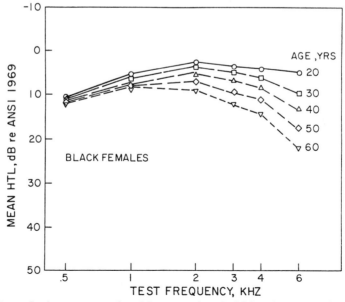

Figure 10.4. Smoothed, non-normalized hearing threshold levels (*HTL*) of black female nonindustrial noise-exposed subjects as a function of age. (From Royster LH, Driscoll DP, Thomas WG, and Royster JD: *American Industrial Hygiene Association Journal* 41:113–119, 1980 (44).)

female, black, and white populations as a function of age. These data are also included in Tables 10.1 and 10.2.

Figure 10.5 shows a comparison between male, female, black, and white groups. It can be noted from this figure that black females maintain the best hearing thresholds as a function of age, followed by white females and black males. The AE data for white females and black males are very similar. The AE data for white males, however, show a drastic departure from the other groups. This difference tends to accelerate in the older age groups. Race and sex differences in nonindustrial noise-exposed populations extend to the rate of change in decibels per year, as well as absolute threshold. Black females continue to show the smallest change over time, while white females show the most accelerated change above age 50 (42, 44).

Not only are differences noted in nonindustrial noise-exposed populations as a function of race and sex, these differences extend to industrial noise-exposed populations as well (47). The patterns for industrial noise-exposed populations are similar to the nonindustrial noise-exposed groups. That is, black females tend to show the least affects of noise exposure on auditory threshold, followed closely by white females and black males. White males continue to show the greatest hearing loss when exposed to industrial noise.

These data have significant implications on measures of HCP effectiveness. Industrial populations with a large percent of black female employees may tend to show less STS on annual retests and, thus, overestimate the effectiveness of the HCP because this population tends to show less hearing loss when exposed, or not exposed, to industrial noise. By the

Table 10.1.
Mean hearing threshold levels (HTL) and standard deviations (SD) for white male and female nonindustrial noise-exposed subjects as a function of age and frequency[a]

	White males															
Age group (yr): Age: No.:	5–14 11.2 39		15–19 17.6 42		20–29 25.6 74		30–39 35.1 47		40–49 43.1 55		50–59 55.0 24		60–69 64.6 14		70–79 72.5 6	
Frequency	HTL	SD	HTL	SD	HTL	SD	HTL	SD	HTL	SD	HTL	SD	HTL	SD	HTL	SD
Hz																
500	9.2	7.6	7.5	4.5	8.1	6.0	9.5	5.8	10.0	5.3	14.1	8.1	13.2	9.4	18.3	12.1
1000	6.8	8.1	3.7	4.8	5.2	6.6	7.1	5.0	8.1	7.2	12.9	10.0	11.4	11.0	23.9	13.1
2000	3.3	7.0	2.1	6.5	3.5	7.4	5.7	6.2	12.7	14.5	16.8	13.3	18.4	14.2	41.5	18.8
3000	3.9	6.9	4.7	6.1	5.7	9.1	11.3	11.2	20.3	16.8	26.4	17.1	31.3	17.6	50.4	20.8
4000	4.4	6.3	5.2	5.7	10.8	13.1	19.3	13.7	27.7	18.5	37.4	19.4	37.7	15.7	53.1	20.4
6000	11.4	10.3	8.0	7.5	17.0	20.0	21.8	15.3	33.0	21.9	49.2	18.5	44.8	15.7	59.6	11.9

	White females															
Age group: Age: No.:	5–14 12.1 46		15–19 17.6 60		20–29 24.5 81		30–39 33.4 60		40–49 44.6 47		50–59 53.3 49		60–69 63.5 25		70–79 73.7 15	
Frequency	HTL	SD	HTL	SD	HTL	SD	HTL	SD	HTL	SD	HTL	SD	HTL	SD	HTL	SD
Hz																
500	8.0	4.9	7.4	4.5	8.0	5.0	10.2	6.2	10.7	7.2	12.4	6.4	20.2	13.9	17.4	10.5
1000	5.0	5.2	4.2	3.9	4.9	4.5	7.2	6.1	8.5	8.1	9.8	5.9	20.2	14.0	21.1	9.9
2000	1.0	6.2	2.7	5.3	3.1	6.0	5.5	7.4	9.1	9.6	9.0	6.4	23.3	19.6	24.7	11.3
3000	3.9	8.0	3.2	7.2	3.2	5.9	6.1	8.3	9.4	7.9	13.0	8.2	26.1	22.8	31.8	11.7
4000	3.9	7.0	4.1	6.2	4.5	5.7	8.7	8.4	12.4	7.9	17.4	10.0	30.5	22.9	37.6	11.1
6000	7.6	9.0	7.9	6.8	8.2	7.8	12.8	8.5	17.3	9.7	21.3	12.1	39.6	22.3	51.2	13.6

[a] From Royster, LH, Thomas, WG: *American Industrial Hygiene Association Journal* 40:504–511, 1979 (42).

Table 10.2.
Mean hearing threshold levels (HTL) and standard deviations (SD) for black male and female nonindustrial noise-exposed subjects as a function of age and frequency[a]

	Black males											
Age group (yr):	15–19		20–29		30–39		40–49		50–59		60–69	
Age:	17.9		23.7		33.1		44.4		53.5		62.1	
No.:	28		68		40		24		22		8	
Frequency	HTL	SD	HTL	SD	HTL	SD	HTL	SD	HTL	SD	HTL	SD
Hz												
500	9.70	6.20	8.75	7.29	5.85	6.34	6.42	6.46	6.00	7.92	18.56	14.88
1000	4.36	5.43	4.02	6.14	3.91	4.81	3.08	6.02	4.70	9.99	15.38	16.30
2000	0.13	5.98	1.49	7.56	2.95	6.99	6.96	15.58	7.66	11.20	19.25	18.98
3000	2.13	6.51	4.09	8.36	5.36	7.99	12.00	16.21	15.36	12.86	27.06	19.53
4000	3.80	6.50	4.04	7.68	8.28	9.64	14.58	17.99	17.61	14.31	31.94	24.31
6000	4.04	6.91	6.74	7.79	10.95	12.31	17.88	15.45	22.98	14.29	37.94	25.92

	Black females											
Age group:	15–19		20–29		30–39		40–49		50–59		60–69	
Age:	17.5		23.5		34.0		44.5		53.9		62.5	
No.:	63		82		43		53		43		19	
Frequency	HTL	SD	HTL	SD	HTL	SD	HTL	SD	HTL	SD	HTL	SD
Hz												
500	10.75	8.36	10.22	5.85	12.34	7.75	10.88	6.94	11.52	7.74	14.45	9.49
1000	5.25	7.08	5.47	5.07	7.42	8.21	7.57	8.13	9.10	9.00	10.37	10.00
2000	2.82	6.19	2.19	6.60	5.92	10.90	5.46	12.12	8.05	9.48	11.37	10.78
3000	3.50	6.67	3.38	5.77	7.15	11.62	6.96	11.83	10.21	10.18	14.47	9.81
4000	4.33	7.96	3.80	5.24	8.42	11.37	8.57	11.84	12.66	10.41	13.18	7.51
6000	7.27	10.97	5.47	7.60	11.15	12.86	16.40	17.02	18.27	12.50	24.97	13.06

[a] From Royster LH, Driscoll DP, Thomas WG, Royster JD: *American Industrial Hygiene Association Journal* 41:113–119, 1980 (44).

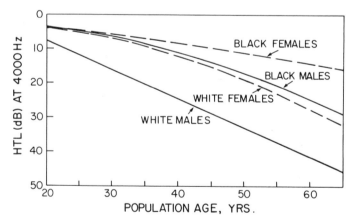

Figure 10.5. Comparison of smoothed hearing threshold level (*HTL*) curves at 4000 Hz for white males, white females, black males and black females as a function of age. (From Royster JD, Royster LH: Short course presented at annual meeting, American Speech, Language and Hearing Association, Toronto, Canada, November 20, 1982, (51).)

same token, industrial populations with large numbers of white male employees may show less effective programs because of the higher thresholds and greater rates of change found in this population, whether or not exposed to industrial noise. Figure 10.6 illustrates this point. When the total male industrial population (TM) is compared to the smoothed HTL curve for nonindustrial noise-exposed population (NINEP) white males, it appears that the industrial group has no

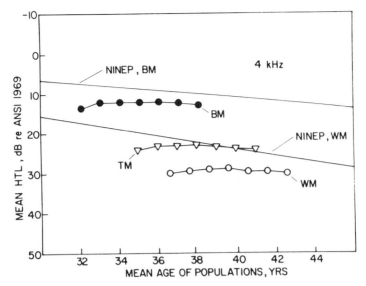

Figure 10.6. Mean hearing threshold level (*HTL*) variations for white male (*WM*), black male (*BM*) and total male (*TM*) industrial noise-exposed populations, compared to respective nonindustrial noise-exposed population (*NINEP*) curves at 4000 Hz. (Reproduced with permission, Royster LH, Royster JD, Thomas WG: *J Acoustical Society America* 68:551–566, 1980, (47).)

more hearing loss than the nonindustrial noise-exposed population. However, when black male and white male populations are separated and each compared to their respective NINEP curves, the additional hearing loss in the industrial population is apparent. It would seem reasonable, therefore, that measures of HCP effectiveness must take these factors into account and evaluate the various populations against their own AE and rate of change curves.

Learning Effect

Improvements in auditory threshold over the first three or four audiograms have been reported by several authors, with the learning effect (LE) generally having a range of 4–9 dB (24, 40, 45, 46, 48–50). In industrial populations, some of this effect might be due to a decrease in initial TTS. However, the same effect has been shown in non-noise exposed populations used as biological test subjects (19, 23). The fact that all improvements noted in auditory threshold over the first three or four tests cannot be explained by a decrease in TTS raises points for consideration in evaluating effectiveness of

HCPs. All studies found in the literature showing decreased hearing with normal aging or AEs, have used cross-sectional rather than longitudinal populations. That is, groups of subjects in various age decades are tested and mean values established. Each subject, however, is tested only once and the learning effect is not apparent in the AE curves. Therefore, a comparison between an industrial population and a reference, non-noise-exposed population tends to show improved mean thresholds for the industrial population over the first several tests, while the reference population shows a constant decrease in threshold over the same time period. This improvement in mean threshold for industrial populations has only been observed in effective HCPs. Figure 10.7, which shows an improvement in mean HTL for the industrial population to year 4 of the hearing conservation program at 4 kHz, illustrates this point.

Indicators of Effectiveness from Population Data

A number of population measures have been suggested as possible indicators of HCP effectiveness. All of these measures

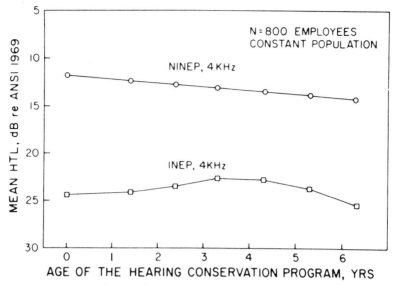

Figure 10.7. A comparison of mean hearing threshold levels (*HTL*) for nonindustrial exposed and industrial noise-exposed constant population (*NINEP, INEP*) at 4000 hz. (From Royster LH, Thomas WG: *American Industrial Hygiene Association Journal* 40:504–511, 1979, (42).)

involve test comparisons (14–23). Measures suggested in the literature include: (a) a comparison between a particular industrial population and an appropriate reference population matched for age, race, sex, and socioeconomic levels; (b) a comparison between baseline hearing tests and current hearing tests for a particular industrial population; and (c) a comparison between consecutive hearing tests within a particular industrial population to investigate trends in hearing loss. Suggested measurement techniques generally involve a comparison of mean HTLs, percent of employees exceeding some STS criteria on a particular test or comparing the rate of change in an industrial population and an appropriate reference population at a particular frequency, such as 4 kHz. It has also been suggested that indicators of HCP effectiveness have to take into account such factors as race and sex differences, learning effects and age (21–23, 40, 42, 44, 47). Thus far, most of the research has concentrated on the first 4–6 yr of a hearing conservation program, taking into account improvements in thresholds resulting from learning effects and resolving TTS.

Reference Populations

One of the best indicators of HCP effectiveness is a direct comparison of industrial data with an appropriate reference population. As previously indicated, reference data may be taken from available literature or, perhaps more appropriate, generated by an individual industry. Figure 10.6 demonstrates the need to separate populations by race and sex as a function of age in making this comparison. The current literature suggests significantly different mean HTLs and rate of change functions for male, female, black and white populations—both NINEP and industrial noise-exposed population (INEP) (40, 42, 44, 47).

A direct comparison between an INEP and an appropriate NINEP is illustrated in Figure 10.7. This figure also serves to illustrate the so called LE shown in industrial noise-exposed populations over the first three or four tests. An industrial population should demonstrate a gradually improving mean HTL when compared to an appropriate reference curve over this time period. Failure to show this improvement over the first several tests has been used to indicate a noneffective HCP (23).

The use of reference populations for comparison with several industrial data bases is also illustrated in Figure 10.8. Six different male industrial populations are separated by race and compared to their respective reference curves (population F contained only white male and female employees). Populations A and E show a steady improvement in mean HTL over the first four or five tests for both white males and black males. Populations C and G show initial improvement over three tests followed by a rather rapid decline, especially for white males in population G. Population B shows an interesting phenomenon with a large initial improvement on test 2, followed by a steady decline on tests 3 and 4. This particular type of pattern may represent calibration changes in the audiometric equipment (23, 51). Populations D and F fail to show a LE. Some variability is noted in population F; however, this group is represented by a small number of employees (N = 23) making the improvement noted

on test 3 difficult to evaluate. Evaluation of this type of data would suggest that populations A and E show effective programs, populations C and G show marginal programs and populations B, D and F show noneffective programs.

In addition to the use of mean HTL values, a comparison between industrial and reference populations in the rate of change at various frequencies has been suggested by several authors as a measure of HCP effectiveness (21, 23, 51). The smoothed rate-of-change levels for male, female, black and white reference populations at audiometric frequencies from 500–6000 Hz as a function of age can be found in Tables 10.3 and 10.4 (42, 44). These Tables indicate a difference between the various groups. For example, at 4 kHz, the white male population shows an initially high rate of change in decibels per year, with a gradual slowing of this trend for older age groups (i.e. 0.93 dB/yr at 20 yr of age vs 0.70 dB/yr at 65 yr). White females, black males and black females show a reversal in this trend. That is, the rate of change in decibels per year

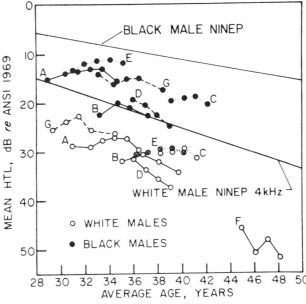

Figure 10.8.   Population mean hearing threshold levels (*HTL*) at 4000 Hz as a function of age for six white and black male populations, with respective *NINEP* curves. Population F contained only white male and female employees. (From Royster LH, Lilley DT, Thomas WG: *American Industrial Hygiene Association Journal* 41:40–48, 1980 (21).)

Table 10.3.
Smoothed rate of change in hearing threshold levels (HTL) for white male and female nonindustrial noise exposed subjects as a function of age and frequency[a]

Sex	Frequency	HTL in decibels per year: age in years									
		20	25	30	35	40	45	50	55	60	65
	Hz										
White male	500	0.05	0.07	0.10	0.13	0.16	0.18	0.21	0.24	0.26	0.29
	1000	0.05	0.09	0.14	0.18	0.23	0.27	0.32	0.36	0.41	0.45
	2000	0.13	0.22	0.30	0.39	0.47	0.56	0.64	0.73	0.81	0.90
	3000	0.43	0.50	0.56	0.62	0.68	0.74	0.80	0.87	0.93	0.99
	4000	0.93	0.91	0.88	0.85	0.83	0.80	0.78	0.75	0.72	0.70
	6000	1.00	1.00	0.99	0.96	0.94	0.91	0.89	0.86	0.84	0.81
White female	500	0.06	0.10	0.13	0.17	0.21	0.24	0.28	0.31	0.35	0.39
	1000	0.01	0.08	0.14	0.20	0.27	0.33	0.39	0.46	0.52	0.58
	2000	0.02	0.10	0.18	0.26	0.35	0.43	0.51	0.59	0.67	0.75
	3000	0.04	0.11	0.22	0.32	0.43	0.53	0.64	0.75	0.85	0.96
	4000	0.09	0.19	0.30	0.41	0.51	0.62	0.72	0.83	0.94	1.04
	6000	−0.06	0.11	0.27	0.44	0.60	0.77	0.93	1.10	1.26	1.43

[a] From Royster LH, Thomas WG: *American Industrial Hygiene Association Journal* 40:504–511, 1979 (42).

Table 10.4.
Smoothed rate of change in hearing threshold levels (HTL) for black male and female nonindustrial noise-exposed subjects as a function of age and frequency[a]

Sex	Frequency	HTL in decibels per year: age in years									
		20	25	30	35	40	45	50	55	60	65
	Hz										
Black males	500	−0.29	−0.23	−0.17	−0.11	−0.05	0.01	0.07	0.13	0.19	0.25
	1000	−0.07	−0.06	−0.04	−0.02	0.01	0.03	0.05	0.07	0.09	0.11
	2000	0.14	0.16	0.18	0.20	0.22	0.24	0.26	0.28	0.30	0.32
	3000	0.12	0.21	0.30	0.39	0.48	0.57	0.66	0.75	0.84	0.93
	4000	0.22	0.30	0.37	0.45	0.52	0.60	0.67	0.75	0.82	0.90
	6000	0.47	0.51	0.55	0.59	0.63	0.67	0.71	0.75	0.79	0.83
Black females	500	0.05	0.05	0.05	0.04	0.04	0.04	0.03	0.03	0.03	0.03
	1000	0.16	0.14	0.12	0.10	0.08	0.06	0.04	0.02	0.00	−0.02
	2000	0.12	0.13	0.14	0.15	0.16	0.17	0.18	0.19	0.20	0.21
	3000	0.12	0.15	0.17	0.20	0.22	0.25	0.27	0.30	0.32	0.35
	4000	0.18	0.20	0.21	0.23	0.24	0.26	0.27	0.29	0.30	0.32
	6000	0.31	0.34	0.36	0.39	0.41	0.44	0.46	0.49	0.51	0.54

[a] From Royster LH, Driscoll DP, Thomas WG, Royster JD: *American Industrial Hygiene Association Journal*, 41:113–119, 1980 (44).

becomes larger for older groups. The differences noted in rate of change in hearing levels as a function of age, like the absolute HTL differences, make it essential that industrial groups be compared to appropriate reference populations.

After the initial improvement in mean HTL noted in many programs, a direct comparison of rate of change in decibels per year between an industrial population and an age adjusted reference population at 4 kHz appears to be a good indicator of continuing HCP effectiveness. In order to make this judgement, the industrial populations should be compared to appropriate rate of change references separated by race and sex. Effective programs will show a rate of change no greater than the reference populations with increasing age. Although both populations will show increasing hearing loss with age, the two curves should remain parallel. Industries with noneffective HCPs will show a much greater change with age than the reference populations. Figures 10.6 and 10.7 illustrate this point. In Figure 10.6, both the black male (*BM*) and white male (*WM*) populations show an initial improvement in mean HTL, with the curves approaching a parallel function to the NINEP curve over six annual tests after baseline. Figure 10.7, however, shows an initial improvement in mean threshold over four tests, but the INEP slope turns downward more steeply than the NINEP curve after test 5. It is obvious that more years of data are needed to accurately identify this function and determine if the greater rate of change continues. This initial indication, however, might cause concern and initiate a reevaluation of the HCP, especially the use of HPDs. The characteristics of the population described in Figure 10.7 are obviously different from a population that fails to show any improvement and, in fact, continues to show a rapid, monotonic rate of change (i.e. population *D* in Fig. 10.8). The population in Figure 10.7 appears to have developed an effective HCP, but through lack of enforcement or loss of interest, the program has become less effective after several years. In contrast, population *D* in Figure 10.8 obviously has never developed an effective program.

Test-Retest Comparisons within Population Data

While a direct comparison of industrial data to appropriate reference data is probably the most accurate indicator of HCP effectiveness, valuable information can be obtained by test-retest comparisons within a particular industrial population. Several comparisons have been suggested in the literature (14, 15, 18–21, 23, 51). One of the earliest, and perhaps most fa-

miliar, involves a direct comparison between the mean HTL baseline audiogram and mean HTL audiograms for subsequent tests (14, 15, 18, 19). The direct comparison of two audiograms derived by taking the mean HTL values for baseline and a particular test year is relatively easy to accomplish. Unfortunately, it also gives very little useful information regarding the effectiveness of the program and is prone to misinterpretation. This type of data analysis gives no indication of the amount of change expected in a non-noise-exposed group over the same time period. In addition, to be meaningful, the data analysis would have to be corrected for age and separated by race and sex, since a predominance of one particular subgroup in the population could greatly influence the mean HTL values. Instead of plotting data in an audiometric configuration, more information can be gained by selecting a particular frequency for the test-retest comparisons and analyzing the results over time. For this purpose, 4 kHz has been used extensively in the literature.

Valuable information may also be gained in determining HCP effectiveness by evaluating the trend on subsequent tests. That is, measuring the differences that occur on tests 1 vs 2, 2 vs 3, 3 vs 4, etc., in addition to comparing baseline data to all subsequent tests (19–23). Mean population HTL values at 4 kHz or other frequencies of interest can be used for this analysis.

While most of the discussion thus far has dealt with mean HTL values, it is obvious that similar comparisons can be made on individuals exceeding a particular STS criteria. In this regard, it appears essential to include numbers of employees who exceed a given STS criterion in both a positive and negative direction. For example, if the current OSHA STS criterion is used (i.e equal to, or greater than, an average shift of 10 dB at 2, 3 and 4 kHz), employees who improve their auditory thresholds with regard to this criterion, "better" (B) would be evaluated, as well as those who show a decrease in excess of the criterion, "worse" (W). Individual auditory thresholds measured in industrial settings tend to show considerable fluctuation (52). When these fluctuations are added to decreasing TTS, learning and possible resolving pathologies, many employees would be expected to improve their auditory thresholds during a particular test year. The number of employees exceeding an STS criterion in a positive direction, compared to the number exceeding in a negative direction, has been used as a measure of HCP effectiveness (19–23, 51). These numbers are used to generate the percent of employees who improve (%B) and the percent of employees who get worse (%W). The ratio of these two numbers (% B : %W) appears to be a good indicator of effectiveness. Available data would suggest, at least for the first 4–6 test yr, that a ratio greater than 1.25 would be consistent with an acceptable program. Ratios between 0.75 and 1.25 would be considered marginal and those below 0.75 would be unacceptable. This concept is consistent with other data, at least in initial programs, since more employees might be expected to improve their auditory thresholds as a result of establishing an effective HCP than those that would decline. This particular type of analysis may not be appropriate in older programs where age effects are creating a greater decrease in auditory thresholds than improvements caused by learning, TTS and normal fluctuations. However, the evaluation of %B : %W may still be valid in older programs where age corrections are made and baselines are revised after STS has occurred. This concept will be discussed in more detail later in this chapter.

The use of two separate measures of effectiveness to increase predictability has been suggested by several authors (19, 21, 23, 51). Specifically, the rate of change in decibels per year is plotted against the %B :%W ratio. Values of these two mea-

sures judged to be acceptable, marginal and unacceptable for population subgroups can be found in Table 10.5. In this Table, particular values have been analyzed only for the first 4–6 yr of tests. This type of analysis may be displayed graphically, as shown in Figure 10.9 for the white male population. As indicated in Figure 10.9, a %B : %W ratio of 1.25 or greater and a rate of change in decibels per year of less than -0.18 would be considered acceptable, while a ratio of less than 0.75 and a rate of change of greater than 0.42 decibels per year would be considered unacceptable.

Age Corrections and Baseline Revisions

Two options are allowed in the 1983 version of the OSHA Hearing Conservation Amendment which will greatly affect the analyses of population data: correction for age and revision of baseline (1). Several of the effectiveness indicators described in the previous section cannot be used with corrected data. It is assumed, however, that correction for age and revision of baseline data will only be used to evaluate the presence of STS and that the raw audiometric data will still be available for analysis. Age correction and baseline revision should be used to evaluate the presence of STS. But, the uncorrected data would have to be compared to a reference population, for example, to determine the effectiveness of the program, using some of the analysis techniques described. Age-corrected data could be used in test-retest comparisons to determine %B : %W in relation to the STS criteria, however.

It is further recommended that baselines should be revised whenever an employee exceeds the STS criterion, in either a positive or negative direction. Of course, baselines should not be revised until the change in threshold is documented by retest of the employee. Baseline revisions would appear to be important for several reasons. First, initial baseline audiograms may be contaminated by excessive TTS,

Table 10.5.
Recommended rate of change values in decibels per year and %B : %W ratios for population subgroups[a]

Program classification	Population							
	White male		White female		Black male		Black female	
	ΔHL	%B : %W	ΔHL	%B : %W	ΔHL	%B : %W	ΔHL	%B : %W
Acceptable	<-0.18	>1.25	<-0.15	>1.25	<-0.16	>1.25	<-0.68	>1.25
Marginal	≥-0.18,≤0.42	≥1.25,≤0.75	≥-0.15,≤0.51	≤1.25,≥0.75	≥-0.16,≤0.84	≤1.25,≥0.75	≥-0.68,≤-0.32	≤1.25,≥0.75
Unacceptable	>0.42	<0.75	>0.51	<0.75	>0.84	<0.75	<-0.32	<0.75

[a] From Royster LH, Lilley DT, Thomas WG: *American Industrial Hygiene Journal* 41:40–48, 1980 (21).

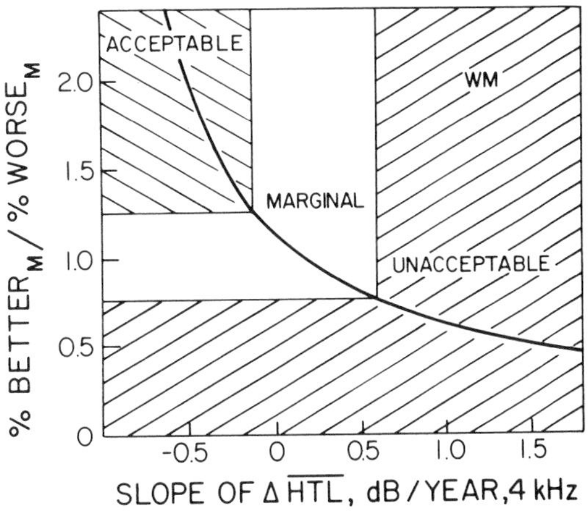

Figure 10.9. Ratio of %B : %W as a function of mean hearing level slope in decibels per year at 4000 Hz for white male populations. (From Royster JD, Royster LH: Short Course presented to annual meeting, American Speech, Language and Hearing Association, Toronto, Canada, November 20, 1982 (51).)

ear pathology or employee inconsistency. If subsequent audiograms show a significant improvement in auditory threshold, failure to revise the baseline to indicate better hearing may cause excessive STS to occur before it is detected. For example, if a particular employee showed a 40 dB hearing loss at a particular frequency or frequencies on the initial baseline caused by otitis media and subsequent tests showed normal hearing after resolving the otitis, the hearing threshold would have to show a drop of approximately 50 dB before meeting STS criterion when compared to the original baseline. Although this may be an extreme example, there is probably considerable ear pathology and TTS included in initial baseline audiograms. Second, employees showing decreased hearing which exceeds current STS criterion and is confirmed on retest should have their baselines revised to reflect these changes. In many cases, permanent changes in HTL may be gradual, finally reaching STS criterion. If subsequent audiograms are reviewed against original baselines, the employees will continue to show STS, although no additional change has taken place. It is probably detrimental to the integrity of the HCP to continue notifying employees of STS after the first notification when no additional change has occurred. Revising the baseline has an added advantage of helping to identify employees who show a second or third significant shift from baseline and, thus, may need extra counseling, a different type of HPD or removal from noise.

Revising the baseline in accordance with the new STS criterion raises several questions. When an employee exceeds STS criterion, should the entire audiogram be used as the new baseline or a revision of only those frequencies showing a shift? Since the new criterion uses an average of 2, 3 and 4 kHz, the entire audiogram should probably be replaced to reflect the new baseline. Another possibility is to store a single number reflecting the average of the three frequencies which can be compared to a single number reflecting the average of the three frequencies for subsequent years. However, using the single number method does not allow review and detection of additional hearing loss at 500 and 1000 Hz, frequencies extremely important in normal day-to-day communication. Since the new criterion effectively eliminates 0.5, 1 and 6 kHz from consideration in STS, some additional analysis may be needed to prevent significant amounts of hearing loss at frequencies essential for communication. This concept will be discussed further in the section concerning individual employee evaluations.

The use of a revised baseline may prove helpful in evaluating the effectiveness of a particular HCP. Individual audiometric thresholds in industry tend to be poorer and fluctuate more than those found in clinical studies (52). Since fluctuations of ±10 dB are not uncommon in industrial populations, revising baselines to account for previous STS, either positive or negative, may allow the use of %B : %W ratios as indicators of effectiveness in older programs. Table 10.6 gives an example of this

use. Data in Table 10.6 are taken from two departments in a large manufacturing company with base lines revised after STS. As indicated in this Table, 274 employees exceeded the current OSHA criterion in a positive direction and 325 in a negative direction during the current test year. The resulting %B : %W ratio was 1.20, indicating more improvement than decrement. This particular HCP is 12 yr old and analyses procedures used during the first 4–6 yr of the program may not be appropriate. The data from department 2 was also analyzed without baseline revision. This analysis indicated 10.8% of the employees with a positive STS and 2.5% with negative STS, or a %B : %W ratio of 0.23. Without baseline revision, this particular analysis procedure could not be used because age effects would eventually negate the negative threshold changes and produce very low %B : %W ratios. However, this procedure still appears valid if baselines are revised after STS.

Summary of Population Analysis

A number of analysis techniques have been suggested to evaluate the effectiveness of HCPs using population data. The majority of these techniques have concentrated on the first 4–6 yr of testing. Factors such as race and sex differences, learning effects, adequate reference populations for each subgroup and age effects have to be considered. Measurement techniques have included: (a) mean HTL values compared to reference curves; (b) slope of the rate of change function compared to age-appropriate populations separated by race and sex; (c) test-retest comparisons within a particular industrial population from baseline to subsequent tests and between subsequent tests; and (d) the ratio of employees showing improved thresholds to those showing decreased thresholds. Although these indicators appear to show a high correlation with effective HCPs, several problems are inherent in their use. First, a particular

Table 10.6.
Ratio of %B : %W in two departments of older HCP after revision of baseline

| Department | Total No. | Exceeds STS criterion | | | | %B : %W |
| | | Worse | | Better | | |
		No.	%	No.	%	
1	2198	138	6.3	167	7.6	1.21
2	2333	136	5.8	158	6.8	1.17
Total	4531	274	6.0	325	7.2	1.20

company would have to have audiometric records computerized and have access to relatively powerful computing facilities. In addition, either commercially available software or extensive software development would be required for many of the analysis techniques described. The time required to make many of the measurements without the availability of adequate hardware and software systems would be prohibitive. Second, the validity of many of the measures depends on the presence of a constant population (23). Most of the research thus far has used subpopulations which have remained constant over the testing periods reported. Creating subpopulations within an industrial setting for comparison purposes requires a considerable amount of additional work and would be difficult or impossible without adequate computer facilities. Even with adequate facilities, the constant subpopulation would tend to get smaller with each annual test as employees leave the work force and new employees are hired, eventually reaching a point where the subpopulation may not adequately represent the entire population. Of course, different subpopulations could be created with new employees. However, the number of analyses and the amount of record keeping will increase greatly.

Many of the techniques described in the literature are important from a research point of view and have added valuable information to the understanding of variables associated with HCP effectiveness. However, many of these techniques may be impractical for medium or small industries because of the data reduction and analysis required and because of the number of employees necessary to get adequate statistical samples.

Baseline audiograms used for comparison purposes should be revised after employees exceed STS criteria in either a positive or negative direction. A relatively easy method of measuring HCP effectiveness uses the ratio of employees exceeding some STS criteria in a negative direction compared to those exceeding in a positive direction for a particular test year. Even in older programs, this ratio should be close to unity with baseline revision. Another simple indicator is the percent of employees exceeding STS criterion in a positive direction only. For this measure, less than 6–8% of the employees should show additional hearing loss in effective programs (23). Because industrial populations are susceptible to the same auditory pathologies as nonindustrial populations, this percentage will never reach zero. In large populations, these analyses will be more accurate if separated by race and sex.

INDIVIDUAL EMPLOYEE EVALUATION

The evaluation of increased hearing loss in individual employees is more straight forward than population analysis and usually entails a direct comparison of current test with some baseline function, either original or revised. Since HTL values are measured against previous thresholds from the same individual, factors such as race and sex differences are not of consequence. In addition, learning effects are generally too small to significantly alter individual thresholds. A major problem in audiometric testing of individual employees is distinguishing true STS from normal fluctuations in threshold. Other problems involve the STS criteria used, revision of baseline and increased hearing loss at frequencies other than those used to determine STS.

Fluctuation in Individual Hearing Threshold Levels

Fluctuations in HTLs on test-retest have been reported by numerous authors (45, 46, 49, 50, 52, 53). Using well trained subjects under laboratory conditions, the standard deviations have ranged from 3–6 dB, with greater variability at higher frequencies. In "field" studies using naive subjects, standard deviations of the difference scores between test and retest have ranged from 6–10 dB, with variability tending to increase as time between test and retest is increased. These so-called "normal" fluctuations between two tests raises questions with regard to evaluation of individual audiograms in industry. Using available data from the literature, a decrease in HTL of 10 dB or more at one frequency might be expected to occur approximately 15% of the time, and still be considered a "normal fluctuation." With industrial audiograms secured approximately 1 yr apart, the variability would probably increase. This amount of variability is not restricted to audiometrically naive subjects. A study of eight employees used as biological calibration subjects over 74 tests showed fluctuation of 10 dB or more at one frequency occurred in 39% of the tests. These data revealed that one frequency might be expected to show a deviation of 10 dB or more 5% of the time, indicating that this amount of fluctuation is not restricted to the audiometrically naive.

Current OSHA criterion uses an average of three frequencies to establish STS. Previous data has indicated that normal fluctuations in thresholds are independent of frequency while noise-induced

hearing loss (NIHL) may be frequency dependent. Therefore, a three-frequency average will tend to reduce chance fluctuations. However, false-positive identifications may still reach a 15–20% level in industrial populations using an average of 10 dB or greater criterion (52).

Currently, there appears to be no satisfactory way to absolutely identify false positive changes in threshold. The most efficient method would be to increase the action level to 15 or 20 dB for STS identification, thus decreasing the probability of chance fluctuations reaching this level in a normal population. Of course, this procedure will reduce the efficiency of a hearing conservation program and allow more actual hearing loss prior to action. A compromise approach is to routinely retest individuals showing STS, either positive or negative. The probability of chance fluctuations occurring on two consecutive tests is considerably lower than on one test alone.

It is obvious that different criteria for STS will greatly affect the number of employees identified. Various criteria have been proposed, including: different action levels at each frequency; single frequency shifts; average shifts; and single frequency shifts occurring on two subsequent tests.

Evaluation of STS

While numerous criteria have been proposed to identify STS resulting from on-the-job noise exposure, the Hearing Conservation Amendment promulgated in March 1983, has established, at least for the present, STS criterion (1). This criterion utilizes an average shift of 10 dB or greater at 2, 3 and 4 kHz in either ear. The presence of STS on a particular audiogram triggers additional action that must be taken. This includes: (a) notification to the employee in writing within 21 days of STS determination; (b) fitting with protectors employees exposed to an 85 dB TWA that show a STS and are not currently wearing HPDs, training them in the use of the protectors and requiring the use of the protectors; (c) refitting employees showing a STS and currently wearing HPDs, retraining in their use and furnishing protectors with greater attenuation, if necessary; (d) referring employees for audiologic and/or otologic evaluations if additional tests are necessary or medical problems are caused or aggravated by the use of ear protectors; and (e) informing the employees of the need for otologic evaluation if pathology is suspected which is unrelated to the use of HPDs. As previously indicated, a retest within 30 days for employees showing STS is an option. If the retest fails to confirm the STS, it may be used as the annual audiogram.

According to the current Noise Rule (Appendix I), comparison between baseline and current audiograms may be made by a technician, with problem audiograms reviewed by a professional. Many industries, however, prefer to have all audiograms, not just those showing STS, reviewed by an audiologist, otologist or the plant physician. The written 21-day notice requirement appears to take effect after determination of STS, whether that determination is made by the technician, the plant physician, a consulting audiologist or otologist, or after a retest. Only audiograms which may be considered problems *must* be reviewed by an audiologist, otologist or other physician. In addition, age correction *may* be applied to the audiograms to determine STS.

Baseline Revision

As previously stated, baseline revision is permitted as an option in the current Noise Standard (1). Under this interpretation, baselines may be revised for either positive or negative STS. Revising the baseline of an employee whose hearing has improved or decreased above a particular criterion level would appear to be extremely important in evaluating the effectiveness of the HCP and as a comparison for possible future shifts in the employee's HTL. Many employees will show

at least one STS during a 10- to 15-yr work period resulting from continued noise exposure, chance fluctuations in HTL, aging, TTS or some other auditory pathology. An employee who shows two or three STSs, however, presents a much more serious problem in hearing conservation. Perhaps the most convenient way to identify an employee who continues to lose hearing, even with increased conservation efforts, is to revise the baseline each time a STS occurs.

Hearing Loss at Frequencies Other than 2000, 3000 and 4000 Hz

Hearing loss can occur at frequencies other than those used to determine the presence of STS under the current OSHA criterion. In an unpublished study involving the effects of STS criteria on the number of employees identified, threshold shifts were found to be a function of frequency (53). Figure 10.10 shows data from more than 900 employees using a 20-dB shift criterion at any frequency. As indicated in this figure, the largest number of shifts occurred at 6000 Hz, followed in succession by 4000, 3000, 2000, 1000 and 500 Hz. These data were collected on employees taking part in a hearing conservation program for the past 12 yr. This study also indicated that the great majority of shifts (72%) occurred at only one frequency. The involvement of two frequencies exceeding a 20-dB criterion dropped to 18%, while three frequencies dropped to 4% for this particular population. An important point, however, is that 46% of the shifts occurred at frequencies not included in the current STS criterion (i.e. 500, 1000 and 6000 Hz). Therefore, to adequately protect hearing, some evaluation should be made for frequencies other than 2000, 3000 and 4000 Hz. It is recommended that an average of 25 dB or greater at 500, 1000 and 2000 Hz be used as an additional criterion for review. Employees showing an average hearing loss of 25 dB or greater through the so-called "speech frequencies" may need rehabili-

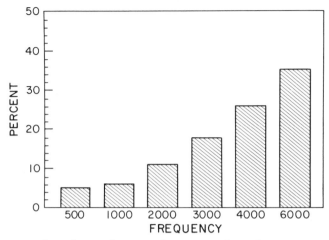

Figure 10.10.   Percent of employees from one large manufacturing company showing a STS of 20 dB as a function of frequency.

tation programs much different from those specified by OSHA. This is particularly true since low frequency hearing loss has a much higher probability of involving auditory pathology requiring otologic evaluation. In addition, those employees who cannot benefit from medical or surgical intervention may need help in the form of amplification to improve everyday communication skills.

Summary of Individual Evaluation

The evaluation of individual audiograms from employees exposed to on-the-job noise entails a comparison of the current annual audiogram to some baseline in order to determine if STS has occurred. In order to accomplish this task, it is recommended that individual audiograms should be age corrected and that baselines should be revised when a STS occurs. Published data have indicated that hearing threshold levels tend to fluctuate, especially in audiometrically naive subjects and when retests occur remote in time from the previous test. Because of the ramifications of identifying a STS, it is suggested that each employee showing STS be retested within 30 days to determine if the shift persists, ideally after the employee has been away from noise for

some period of time. This procedure should reduce the number of false-positive identifications and be cost effective in the long run. Age-corrected individual audiograms will further reduce the number of employees showing STS from age effect changes in threshold levels, although it is doubtful that these effects will be totally eliminated. Revised baselines, either in a positive or negative direction, will allow more accurate evaluation of HCP effectiveness and aid in the identification of individual employees who show a progressive decrease in hearing.

Since hearing loss can occur at frequencies other than those used for STS determination, further analysis and review should be accomplished on audiograms exceeding a given criterion. It is suggested that an average loss of 25 dB or greater at 500, 1000 and 2000 Hz be used for this criterion. In addition, "problem" audiograms should be reviewed carefully. These might include questionable threshold accuracy, the possibility of functional hearing loss, unusual audiometric configurations and ear differences which may exceed inter-aural attenuation values. The audiologist, otologist or plant physician is faced with certain ethical and legal questions when reviewing industrial audiograms. These questions go far beyond simple compliance with OSHA requirements and are compounded by the very restricted amount of information available.

OTHER CHARACTERISTICS OF AN EFFECTIVE HEARING CONSERVATION PROGRAM

Several methods have been described to judge the efectiveness of an industrial HCP. All of these methods involve some form of data analysis and many lend themselves to sophisticated statistical analysis. Other characteristics of an effective HCP have been described which are more subjective in nature (22). These characteristics include such elements as: management support; communication among various elements of the HCP and affected employees; enforcement programs for HPDs; the presence of a single key individual in the program; and the availability of effective HPDs. The general effectiveness and smoothness of operation will depend greatly on active support from management. This characteristic was described many years ago by Maas (5) and remains important to the present time. Communication among various elements of the HCP and effective communication with employees is also extremely important. In many industrial settings, responsibility for the HCP is divided between several departments, including: medical, personnel, safety, industrial relations, engineering, and supervisory personnel. It is essential that these areas communicate with each other, especially in regard to results of noise surveys, engineering and/or administrative control projects, audiometric data, education and the use of HPDs. For example, new equipment start-ups and changes in noise levels are important information to other departments responsible for portions of the HCP, particularly those individuals responsible for audiometric testing and ear protectors. By the same token, the results of annual audiometric testing may point out potentially hazardous areas or lack of HPD useage.

Numerous articles have mentioned the importance of an active enforcement program for HPD useage. Although education can improve the useage of HPDs, a clearly stated policy is very important. This policy usually includes verbal warnings, written warnings, suspension and termination for repeated violations for lack of HPD use in posted areas. To be effective, this program must have management support and apply to *all* employees and personnel of the company.

Although responsibility for various aspects of the HCP may be divided between several areas, the most effective programs appear to have one key individual who assumes responsibility for coordination of the entire program. This individual is usually someone with daily responsibility for a portion of the program and close connections with employees, such as the audiometric technician or plant nurse. This individual usually becomes the critical link in communication between management and hourly employees with regard to the HCP.

While data base analysis and individual audiogram analysis remains the focal point in juding HCP effectiveness, most effective programs also display the characteristics mentioned above. It is obvious that all of these areas are necessary and complement each other. Lack of management support or HPD enforcement will eventually show adverse effects in data base analysis. Conversely, HCP effectiveness, as evidenced by data base analysis, usually results from well planned programs with support and communication beween the various levels. Effective HCPs tend to be found in companies with good safety records, good employee relations and employee job satisfaction, raising the possibility that a major factor in HCP effectiveness may be a general concern for employee well-being.

References

1. Occupational Safety and Health Administration: Occupational noise exposure; hearing conservation amendment; final rule. *Federal Register* 46:9738–9785, March 8, 1983.
2. U.S. Department of Labor. *Guidelines to the Department of Labor's Occupational Noise Standards*, Bulletin 334, Washington, DC, US Department of Labor, 1971.
3. Bearce GR: Hearing conservation—a call for action. *Sound Vibration* 9:24–28, 1975.
4. Sataloff J, Michael P: *Hearing Conservation.* Springfield, Ill, Charles C Thomas, 1973.
5. Mass R: Industrial noise and hearing conservation. In Katz J (ed): *Handbook of Clinical Audiology*, Baltimore, Williams & Wilkins, 1972.
6. Feldman, A: Industrial hearing conservation programs. In Henderson, D, Hamernik, R, Dosanjh, D, Mills J (eds): *Effects of Noise on Hearing.* New York, Raven Press, 1976.
7. Spindler DE, Olson RA, Fishbeck WA: An effective hearing conservation program. *Am Ind Hyg Assoc J* 40:604–608, 1979.
8. Dear TA, Karrh BW: An effective hearing conservation program—federal regulation or practical achievement? *Sound Vibration*, 13:12–19, 1979.
9. Walker JL: A successful program of hearing conservation. *Ind Med* 41:11–14, 1972.
10. Michael P: Hearing conservation. *Mining Congress J* June:74–82, 1972.
11. Karrh BW: Effective hearing conservation programs. In *Noise-Con 73.* Washington DC, National Conference on Noise Control Engineering, 1973.
12. Glorig A: Industrial hearing conservation. In *Noise-Con 73.* Washington, DC, National Conference on Noise Control Engineering, 1973.
13. Mellard TJ, Doyle TJ, Miller MH: Employee education—the key to effective hearing conservation. *Sound Vibration* 12:24–28, 1978.
14. Hickish DE, Challen PJR: A serial study of noise exposure and hearing loss in a group of small- and medium-size factories. *Ann Occup Hyg* 9:113–133, 1966.
15. Summar TM: Industrial hearing conservation (a report on a longitudinal study). *Natl Safe News* 100:52–54, 1969.
16. Summar TM: An effective hearing conservation program in industry-today. In, *Inter-Noise 76.* Washington, DC, Proceedings of the International Conference on Noise Control Engineering, April, 1976.
17. Pell S: An evaluation of a hearing conservation program. *Am Ind Hyg Assoc J* 33:60–70, 1972.
18. Pell S: An evaluation of a hearing conservation program—a five-year longitudinal study. *Am Ind Hyg Assoc J* 34:82–91, 1973.
19. Lilly D: *Analysis Techniques for Evaluating the Effectiveness of Industrial Hearing Conservation Programs.* (Master's thesis presented to Graduate Faculty, NC, State University, Raleigh, NC, 1980.)
20. Berger EH: *Analysis of the Hearing Levels of an Industrial and Nonindustrial Noise-Exposed Population.* (Master's thesis presented to Graduate

Faculty of NC, State University, Raleigh, NC, 1976).
21. Royster LH, Lilly D, Thomas WG: Recommended criteria for evaluating the effectiveness of hearing conservation programs. *Am Ind Hyg Assoc J* 41:40–48, 1980.
22. Royster LH, Royster JD, Berger EH: Guidelines for developing an effective hearing conservation program. *Sound Vibration,* 16:22–25, 1982.
23. Royster LH, Royster JD: Methods of evaluating hearing conservation data bases. In Alberti, PW (ed): *Personal Hearing Protection in Industry.* New York, Raven Press, 1982.
24. Thomas WG, Royster LH, Scott III, CE: Practice effects in industrial hearing screening. *J Am Aud Soc* 1:126–130, 1975.
25. ANSI-S3.6-1969: *American National Standard Specifications for Audiometers,* New York, American National Standards Institute, 1970.
26. Bunch CC, Raiford TS: Race and sex variations in auditory acuity. *Arch Otolaryngol* 13:423–434, 1931.
27. Steinberg JC, Montgomery HC, Gardner MB: Results of world's fair hearing tests. *J Acoust Soc Am* 12:291–301, 1940.
28. Webster J, Himes H, Lichtenstein M: San Diego country fair hearing survey. *J Acoust Soc Am* 22:473–483, 1950.
29. Hinchcliffe R: Presbycusis in the presence of noise-induced hearing loss. In Robinson DW (ed): *Occupational Hearing Loss.* New York, Academic Press, 1971.
30. Glorig A, Nixon J: Distribution of hearing loss in various populations. *Ann Oto Rhino Laryngol* 69:497–516, 1960.
31. Post RH: Hearing acuity variation among negroes and whites. *Eugen Q,* 11:65–81, 1964.
32. Corso JF: Age and sex differences in pure tone thresholds. *Arch Otolaryngol* 77:53–73, 1963.
33. Shepard DC, Goldstein R: Race differences in auditory sensitivity. *J Speech Hear Res* 7:389–393, 1964.
34. Rosen S, Bergman M, Plester D, El-Mofty A, Satti MH: Presbycusis study of a relatively noise free population in the Sudan. *Ann Otol Rhinol Laryngol* 71:727–735, 1962.
35. Roberts J, Bayliss D: *Hearing Levels of Adults by Race, Region and Area of Residence, United States 1960-1962.* National Center for Health Statistics, Series II, No. 26. Washington, DC, U.S. Department of Health, Education and Welfare, Public Health Service, 1967.
36. Spoor, A: Presbycusis values in relation to noise-induced hearing loss. *Int Aud* 6:48–57, 1967.
37. Taylor W, Pearson J, Mair A: Hearing thresholds of a nonnoise-exposed population in Dundee. *Br J Ind Med* 38:114–122, 1967.
38. Kell RL, Pearson J, Taylor W: Hearing thresholds of an island population in north Scotland. *Int Aud* 9:334–349, 1970.
39. Townsend TH, Bess FH, Fishbeck WA: Hearing sensitivity in rural Michigan. *Ann Ind Hyg Assoc J* 36:63–68, 1975.
40. Berger EH, Royster LH, Thomas WG: Hearing levels of nonindustrial noise exposed subjects. *J Occup Med* 19:664–670, 1977.
41. Robinson DW, Sutton GJ: *A Comparative Anal-*

ysis of Data on the Relation of Pure Tone Audiometric Thresholds to Age. Teddington, Middlesex, UK, National Physical Laboratory Acoustical Report No. Ac84. 1978.

42. Royster LH, Thomas WG: Age effect hearing levels for a white nonindustrial noise-exposed population (NINEP) and their use in evaluating industrial hearing conservation programs. Am Ind Hyg Assoc J 40:504–511, 1979.

43. Glorig A, Davis H: Age, noise and hearing loss. Ann Otol, 17:556–571, 1961.

44. Royster LH, Driscoll DP, Thomas WG, Royster JD: Age effect hearing levels for a black nonindustrial noise-exposed population (NINEP). Am Ind Hyg Assoc J 41:113–119, 1980.

45. Robinson DW, Shipton MS, Whittle LS: Audiometry in industrial hearing conservation-I. NPL Acoustic Report No. Ac64. Teddington, Middlesex, UK, National Physical Laboratory, 1973.

46. Robinson DW, Shipton MS, Whittle LS: Audiometry in industrial hearing conservation-II. NPL Acoustic Report No. Ac71. Teddington, Middlesex, UK, National Physical Laboratory, 1975.

47. Royster LH, Royster JD, Thomas WG: Representative hearing levels by race and sex in North Carolina industry. J Acoust Soc Am 68:551–566, 1980.

48. Stephens SDG: Some individual factors influencing audiometric performance. In Robinson (ed): Occupational Hearing Loss. New York, Academic Press, 1971.

49. Delany ME: On the Stability of Auditory Thresholds. NPL Aero Report No. Ac44. Teddington, Middlesex, United Kingdom, National Physical Laboratory, 1970.

50. Robinson DW, Whittle LS: A comparison of self-recording and manual audiometry: some systematic effects shown by unpractical subjects. J Sound Vibration 26:412–62, 1973.

51. Royster JD, Royster LH: Evaluating the Effectiveness of Hearing Conservation Programs by Analyzing Group Audiometric Data. Short course presented at the annual meeting of the American Speech-Language-Hearing Assoc., Toronto, Ontario, 1982.

52. Dobie RA: Reliability and validity of industrial audiometry: implications for hearing conservation program designs. Laryngoscope, 93:906–927, 1983.

53. Thomas WG: Effects of STS criteria on the number of employees identified. (Unpublished data.)

CHAPTER 11

Hearing Handicap and Workers' Compensation

WILLIAM MELNICK

HISTORY OF COMPENSATION FOR HEARING LOSS

The practice of compensating an employee for industrial injury began in Europe during the industrialization period of the 19th century. Workmen's compensation started in Germany in 1884. The purpose of this compensation was to pay victims of industrial accidents for the time they were disabled and incapable of earning an income. Prior to the initiation of this compensation, the industrially disabled worker had to depend on charity for survival. The Germans believed that industrial accidents were inevitable. They introduced the idea that part of the cost of production should include compensation of those incapacitated by industrial accidents. The basis of this compensation was purely economic and was to be paid only when the worker was unable to earn. There was no concern were the worker injured as long as that injury did not prevent the person from continuing to work (1).

Britain incorporated the German philosophy of compensation in the British Workmen's Compensation Act of 1906. This Act not only provided for compensation for injury resulting from industrial accidents, but also included compensation for specific diseases attributable to certain occupational conditions. As was the case in Germany, compensation was only paid to those who were unable to earn an income. Since loss of wages seldom occurred as a result of industrial hearing loss, it was not included as one of the compensable diseases. In 1946, the British law was changed by the National Insurance Act which dropped the requirement for loss of wages as a condition for compensation. However, it was not until 1975 that legislation was introduced in the United Kingdom allowing claims for noise-induced hearing loss as an occupational disease (1).

Prior to passage of the Compensation Act, a worker could sue for damages under the tort system (civil action) of the British common law. A successful suit under common law for industrial hearing loss required proof, by the plaintiff, of exposure to a hazardous noise; a resulting hearing loss which constitutes a handicap; and negligence on the part of the defendant (2). In many cases this proof is difficult to establish. Successful suits under common law were relatively rare. There were some, however, and these cases resulted in sizable awards which created an economic hardship for the employer involved. Lengthy litigation was also costly, financially and in employee morale. Suits under the common law were unsatisfactory for everyone involved, and it was this dissatisfaction which lead to the introduction of worker's compensation, a type of no-fault insurance (3).

The first Employee's Compensation Act in the United States was introduced in 1908 as a federal statute (1). Workers' compensation laws were enacted by all except 6 states between 1911 and 1920 (3). Under these early compensation laws, traumatic hearing loss was included as a compensable injury but noise-induced hearing loss was not, and compensation was awarded only when there was loss of wages.

There are two landmark cases which had a major influence on compensating workers for occupationally noise-induced hearing loss: (a) Slawinski vs J. B. Williams & Co., New York, in 1948 (4); and (b) Wojcik vs Green Bay Drop Forge Company, Wisconsin, in 1953 (5). Mr. Slawinski, who worked as a drop-forger, filed a claim for compensation for occupational hearing loss as an industrial disease and not on the basis of accidental injury. His employer contested the claim contending that occupational hearing loss was not a disease covered by the act, and that there was no loss of wages. Mr. Slawinski was awarded the compensation. The decision was appealed by the defendants to the higher courts of New York. The appellate courts supported the original decision (1).

In Wisconsin, another drop-forger, Mr. Wojcik, successfully filed a claim for compensation for occupational hearing loss even though there was no loss of income. Based on an appeal by the employer, the decision by the Wisconsin Compensation Commission to make the award was reversed by a circuit court judge. In 1953, the Wisconsin Supreme Court supported the original judgement to compensate, ruling that loss of wages was not a requirement for justifying compensation for hearing loss induced by occupational noise. This ruling and subsequent actions in Wisconsin, affected compensation procedures in many of the other states in this country, and in many industrial countries of the world.

Noble (1) calls attention to an interesting relationship between compensation of veterans following World War II and changes in the philosophy and administration of industrial compensation for hearing loss. Before this war, claims had been made under both common law and statute law for acoustic and physical auditory trauma. The first claim for hearing loss induced by chronic exposure to hazardous industrial noise was not awarded until after World War II. Veterans, not only in the United States but in other countries as well, were compensated for hearing loss regardless of whether this loss was the result of a traumatic event or whether it resulted from repeated exposures to hazardous noise. This compensation provided precedent for industrial compensation for hearing loss which was not the result of a traumatic accident, but for the much more common occupationally noise-induced hearing loss.

Since the 1950s there has been a progressive increase in the number of states which include noise-induced hearing loss as compensable under their workmen's compensation laws. In 1963, 49 of the 50 states had provisions for deafness caused by accident, while 31 states covered industrially noise-induced hearing loss (6).

A report from a National Presidential Commission on State Workmen's Compensation Laws published in 1973 (7) called attention to the inequity and inadequacy of compensation rules, in general. Since that time, many states have passed laws which have extended eligibility and increased benefits. A survey conducted in 1977 showed that 41 states had statutes which would permit compensation for partial noise-induced hearing loss, while 9 states (some of the most industrialized) had requirements so restrictive that noise-induced hearing loss was essentially not compensable (8). Hearing loss compensation has paralleled these general trends with increasing benefits, a reduction in the statutes of limitation and a relaxing of other administrative restrictions.

DEFINITIONS OF IMPAIRMENT, HANDICAP AND DISABILITY

One source of confusion to people concerned with the relationship of impairment and handicap is the imprecise way these terms are used. Frequently these two terms are used interchangeably and are treated as if they were synonymous with still another term, disability. To reduce the confusion, the Committee on Hearing and Equilibrium of the American Academy of Otolaryngology-Head and Neck Surgery (AAO-HNS) has provided the following specific definitions for permanent impairment, handicap and disability (9).

Permanent Impairment

Permanent impairment is function outside the range of normal. Hearing impairment exists when any anatomic or functional abnormality reduces hearing sensitivity. This function should be evaluated after maximum rehabilitation has been achieved and when the impairment is nonprogressive. The determination of impairment is basic to the evaluation of permanent handicap and disability.

Permanent Handicap

Permanent handicap is the disadvantage imposed by an impairment sufficient to affect the individual's efficiency in the activities of daily living. Handicap implies a material impairment; conversely, the concept "material impairment" implies that there is a narrow range of hearing impairment beyond the statistical range of normal hearing, which does not produce hearing handicap.

Permanent Disability

An actual or presumed inability to remain employed at full wages is permanent disability. A person is permanently disabled or under permanent disability when the actual or presumed ability to engage in gainful activity is reduced because of handicap, and when no appreciable improvement can be expected.

These definitions represent a sequence. Impairment can exist without there being a handicap or a disability. For handicap to exist usually implies a greater degree of impairment, but it need not constitute an economic or legal disability. Disability requires a handicap specifically in the functional ability related to employment (10).

The preceding definitions as stated by the AAO-HNS have not received universal acceptance. To some, the term handicap has a much more personal connotation. Hardick et al. (11) define hearing handicap as alterations in an individual's life which result from hearing impairment and limitations of auditory performance imposed by this impairment. Handicap can only be determined by the involved individual or by observation of the individual in everyday life. This definition of handicap involves subjective, nonmedical factors such as age, sex, education, and socioeconomic factors. With this definition, even an impairment which produced a disability need not be a handicap. Although there is disagreement regarding the definitions proposed by the AAO-HNS, these definitions will apply throughout this chapter.

ESTIMATING AUDITORY FUNCTION

If compensation for hearing handicap is to be awarded, a method for estimating auditory function is absolutely necessary. Impairment may be structural or functional. Since the important sensory structures of the person seeking compensation for hearing dysfunction are not accessable for examination, methods devised for this compensation must depend on estimating the effects of auditory damage on the uses of hearing. Developing an exhaustive list of these uses to serve as a basis for estimating hearing handicap would be a difficult, if not impossible, task. The number of potential uses of the auditory sense is enormous.

Hearing function is inferred from the dimensions of the sounds which can be heard correctly. These dimensions include the intensity, frequency and spectral complexity of the acoustic signal. Auditory functions which have received the most attention for purposes of compensation are the ability to detect faint signals, and the discrimination of speech both in quiet and in a noisy background.

Understanding speech is an extremely important auditory function. Perhaps, it is the *most* important use of the auditory sense for human beings. Hearing loss compensation schemes, generally, assume that if there is no handicap in receiving and understanding speech, then a handicap is not likely to exist for hearing other sounds important for daily living. It is further assumed that the speech signal is complex enough in its acoustic and temporal properties that measures of hearing for speech provide an excellent estimate of overall hearing function.

Predictive indices which reliably and accurately estimate hearing handicap have many potential uses. The legal acceptance of the liability of employers for hearing handicap resulting from employment conditions, and the award of financial compensation for this handicap, have been major sources of impetus for development of hearing handicap scales. Equitable payment of compensation requires that an assessment method not only be able to demonstrate that hearing handicap exists but also be able to demonstrate the degree of this handicap. The size of the monetary award should bear a proportional relationship to the extent of the handicap.

For compensation purposes, the predictive method should be reliable and valid. Ideally, scales of hearing handicap should assess and relate all of the factors which contribute to the handicap. Unfortunately, no such scale exists. Nevertheless, a number of methods have been developed and have been proposed for use in determining the amount of compensation.

Predictive methods might involve pure tone audiometry, speech audiometry, self-evaluation techniques or some combination of these three types of hearing assessment. Clinical measures of hearing, mainly, provide indications of hearing impairment. Of the three procedures, as currently practiced, pure tone audiometry is the most reliable, while the self-assessment scaling is the most valid estimator

of hearing handicap (at least face validity). If speech can be assumed to be the most important acoustic stimulus, then speech audiometry occupies a middle ground between the other two techniques. From the standpoint of test reliability, it is not as reliable as pure tone audiometry, but more reliable than the self-assessment scales. Because it directly measures performance with speech signals, speech audiometry has more face validity for predicting communicative handicap than pure tone measures, but is not as valid as the self-assessment scales for estimating the more global aspects of hearing handicap. Development of scales of hearing handicap is plagued with an inherent incompatability; the need for a purely objective, unidimensional measurement of a uniquely subjective, multidimensional construct.

Pure Tone Audiometry

Without question, the most frequently used method for describing auditory function is the pure tone audiogram. The pure tone audiogram is a set of measures that compare a person's ability to detect the presence of faint pure tones in a quiet environment to the same ability of a population with normal auditory systems. Therefore, the audiogram is ideal for identifying whether or not auditory impairment exists. Because of its simplicity, its perceived objectivity, and its worldwide application and standardization, pure tone audiometry also has become the most widely used basis for predicting auditory handicap, particularly for compensation purposes.

Most auditory professionals would agree that the task of detecting the presence of pure tones is a much simpler task than speech perception and understanding. Understanding of speech is so important to human society that there is almost universal agreement that estimates of auditory handicap should be based to a large extent, if not entirely, on the magnitude of the effect of auditory pathology on this ability. Over the past half-century, considerable research has been devoted to describing the relationship of threshold hearing levels for tones and speech communication. Schemes which have been devised using pure tone audiometry to award compensation for hearing handicap have relied to some extent on this research.

Several formulas have been proposed for calculating hearing handicap from pure tone hearing levels. Debate continues on the elements comprising these formulas, and the appropriate relationship of these elements. There are differing opinions on how hearing sensitivity is to be represented for a given ear. If threshold hearing levels are to be averaged for several frequencies, what are these frequencies to be? Are the chosen frequencies equally important for understanding speech, or should some frequencies be given more weight in calculating handicap?

There is general agreement that some amount of hearing loss can exist without creating a communicative handicap; not all people with normal hearing have threshold hearing levels at audiometric zero. How much hearing loss represents a significant departure from normal sensitivity or, more importantly, at what level does this hearing loss become handicapping? There is disagreement about what degree of impairment constitutes total hearing handicap. At what level should a hearing loss be considered total? Hearing sensitivity is not always the same for both ears. How should hearing sensitivity for the two ears be unified in the equation for calculating hearing handicap? How much more important is the better ear? There is no unanimity about the relationship of hearing handicap to hearing impairment. How does handicap increase as a function of increasing hearing impairment? With all of these potential sources of disagreement, the fact that there are differences in the formulas for calculating compensable hearing loss from pure tone

threshold information is not surprising. These differences shall be discussed in greater detail later in this chapter.

Speech Audiometry

Two measurement procedures which use speech stimuli as independent variables have achieved widespread clinical application for deriving indices of hearing impairment. One of the procedures provides an estimate of sensitivity for speech signals and the measure is called the speech reception threshold (SRT). The other procedure makes use of stimuli presented at suprathreshold intensities, and provides an estimate of acuity for speech. The results of this procedure is known as the speech discrimination score.

There are some audiologists who are dissatisfied with the use of pure tone thresholds to derive estimates of hearing handicap. Since SRT and speech discrimination tests are diagnostically useful, why not use these measures as descriptors for hearing handicap? If one assumes that hearing for speech is the most important function to be considered for predicting handicap, then it is logical to argue that assessment of handicap should be accomplished using speech audiometry, if not alone, certainly in addition to pure tone threshold information. In fact, the Veteran's Administration (VA) does use a combination of pure tone and speech audiometry to evaluate claims for compensation from those incurring hearing loss while serving in the military (11).

The application of speech measures by the VA is patterned after the procedure described by Davis (12) called the Social Adequacy Index (SAI). This index was developed in an attempt to estimate a person's ability to follow everyday conversational speech. The SAI is based on measures of speech intelligibility at three different intensities taken as representative of faint, average and loud speech conversation. The SAI is the mean of the discrimination scores obtained at these three levels. A table was devised which permitted the clinician to calculate the index using the SRT and the maximum intelligibility score, in a way similar to that followed by the VA in calculating handicap.

The SAI has not received wide use or acceptance. The reasons for this lack of success include lack of standardization of speech test material and methodology; insufficient information regarding the relationship of the speech measures and ability to function in everday speech situations (13). Noble (1) adds another important criticism of the index. Validation was established on patients who had hearing disorders which were either totally or partially conductive, hardly a representative sample of the hearing-impaired population. Giolas (14) reports that the SAI may overestimate difficulty with conversational speech. However, in a later publication, Giolas (15) notes a close correlation of the Index to self-reports of hearing handicap (16, 17) and speculates that the Social Adequacy Index may be a more valid estimate of hearing handicap than its limited use implies.

Despite the criticisms of using speech tests for determining hearing handicap and of the two dimensional estimate of this handicap as proposed by the SAI, the VA continues to use this approach. The VA method involves categorizing hearing impairment into one of six categories simply designated by the alphabetic letters A through F. These categories are determined by entering a two-dimensional table with the measures of the speech reception threshold and measures of speech discrimination for a given ear. Pure tone threshold averages for 500, 1000 and 2000 Hz can be used as a substitute for the speech reception threshold. The binaural-impairment percentage is determined by entering the monaural information into another table. The categories of monaural hearing impairment and the binaural percentages of impairment were determined by a group of consultants (11). The method used by the consultants to establish these values is obscure.

Suter (18) provides a summary of the criticisms of the inadequacies of speech audiometric measures for assessing handicap. Not only are the speech stimuli not standardized, but the conditions under which these stimuli should be presented have not achieved consensus. Should speech be presented in a noise background? What should be the character of the noise? What should the speech-to-noise ratio be? The SRT correlates well with the pure tone average for 500, 1000, and 2000 Hz but does not correlate quite so well with speech discrimination scores. The usual procedure for obtaining a speech discrimination score is not typical of the everyday speech environment. The speech stimuli are typically presented under optimum listening conditions, with speech intensity such that performance is maximized against a quiet environment. This could hardly be considered typical of the speech conditions ordinarily encountered. The most frequently employed speech material is usually recorded with special attention to clear speech articulation delivered at a carefully controlled pace. In ordinary daily speech communication, the speech signal is often spoken hurriedly, with sloppy articulation and frequently the speaker is turned away from the listener. No matter how attractive use of speech would be in determining hearing handicap, development of test materials and procedures have not reached the point where it is feasible.

Self-Assessment Handicap Scales

Both pure tone and speech audiometry are methods for measuring hearing impairment. Impairment can be assessed with relative objectivity and precision. Because of the personal nature of a handicap, it is not as easy to quantify. Clinicians working to minimize communicative and psychological problems imposed by auditory impairment need to have more detailed information regarding the effects of the impairment on the individual. This need motivated development of self-assessment scales of hearing handicap.

Despite several attempts to produce an acceptable scaling method for this assessment, none has thus far appeared which has achieved common acceptance. High et al. (16) developed the Hearing Handicap Scale in 1964. This scale has been criticized as being too narrow in scope, and because the items were more related to hearing sensitivity than to problems of speech discrimination (19). Items on this scale were limited to the ability to hear and carry on conversations. There are no items which are concerned with vocational and attitudinal problems.

In 1970, Noble and Atherley (20) published the Hearing Measurement Scale. This self-assessment procedure was designed for use particularly with people experiencing sensorineural hearing loss resulting from noise exposure. Although this scale was originally designed to be administered in an interview situation, Noble (21) has adapted it to a paper-pencil method of administration. The Hearing Measurement Scale consists of 42 items divided into seven sections: speech hearing; acuity for nonspeech sounds; localization; emotional response; speech distortion; tinnitus; and personal opinion. This procedure shows promise as a method for assessing hearing handicap. Although the scale was designed specifically for use with adults experiencing hearing loss from noise, there is some evidence that it might be useful with other types of hearing loss in other populations (22).

Another promising scale for hearing handicap is the Hearing Performance Inventory published in 1979 by Giolas et al. (23). The developers recognized some of the limitations of earlier scales. They attempted to rectify the perceived problems, particularly the scope and the consistency and reliability of the items contained in the instrument. The original version of the Inventory consisted of 158 items but was subsequently reduced to 90 (24). These items, as in the case of the Hearing Measurement Scale, are divided into sections which permit the generation of a hearing performance profile. These sections include understanding speech, intensity, response to auditory failure, social, personal, and occupational areas. Evaluative data regarding this scale are meager, and are now in the process of being accumulated. The Hearing Performance inventory appears to be more comprehensive than other scales and may prove to be the most useful procedure available today for estimating the handicapping effects of hearing impairment (25).

A comprehensive review of all the proposed self-assessment scales of hearing handicap is not appropriate here. More thorough discussions of these methods can be found elsewhere (1, 15, 25). These scales represent a procedure for describing the effects of hearing impairment on the daily function of the person experiencing the problem. With the exception of Noble (1), the originators of these self-assessment procedures do not recommend that they be used directly for purposes of awarding compensation. The validity and utility of these scales of handicap depend on the cooperation and truthfulness of the person providing the answers. Whenever there is a question of compensation, there is reason to suspect the motivation of the respondent. The value of these self-assessment procedures is more likely to be as methods for validating other techniques devised to decide if compensation should be awarded because of hearing handicap.

COMPENSATION SCHEMES

Without question, most of the schemes used to assess hearing handicap for purposes of awarding compensation are based on pure tone audiometric information. In this section, the makeup of these schemes, as well as their historical development, will be considered in some detail.

Historic Development

One of the earliest methods for relating pure tone hearing loss to hearing handicap was known as Fletcher's 0.8 rule. Fletcher, in a study relating pure tone threshold to speech threshold for spoken digits (recorded and live-voice) found that the average threshold for 500, 1000, and 2000 Hz correlated well with speech performance (26). The audible range for this average from 0–120 dB was converted, linearly, to a percentage scale with a slope of 0.83%/dB. The slope was later simplified to 0.8%/dB. This rule was not developed for the purposes of compensation (27). The beginning point for calculating hearing handicap was too low (0 dB), and the point taken to be total hearing handicap was too high (120 dB).

In 1941, Fowler (28) proposed a system which applied different weights to percentages assigned to the five frequencies 500, 1000, 2000, 3000, and 4000 Hz. These weights were 15, 25, 30, 25, and 5%, respectively. A little later, he revised this system eliminating 3000 Hz, and changing the weighting to 15% for 500 Hz, 30% for 1000 Hz, 40% for 2000 Hz, and 15% for 4000 Hz (29). Binaural percentage loss could be calculated from a table which Fowler prepared. The binaural weighting assigned to the better/poorer ears varied depending on the magnitude of the difference between the two ears.

At about the same time that Fowler proposed his method for determining hearing handicap, Sabine (30) developed another system. Although these two methods shared many common features, Sabine's procedure was based on the assumption that the auditory range was comprised of a finite number of discriminable units of pitch and loudness. He assumed that the perception of speech depended on the capacity to discriminate differences in pitch and loudness, and a loss of this capacity implied a proportional loss in the ability to handle speech communication. Sabine's system used Fletcher's coefficients of pitch and loudness as a function of frequency and intensity, particularly for the frequency range 500–2000 Hz. The underlying assumptions of Sabine's approach led to a differential weighting with increasing intensity requirements. Handicap was not a simple linear function of the magnitude of the hearing loss. Sabine also recognized that minor deviations from threshold hearing levels of 0 dB would not produce a noticeable handicap. Losses <10 dB did not enter into the calculation of percentage reduction in hearing capacity. Sabine assigned a better/poorer ear ratio of 8 to 1 for determining binaural handicap (1).

The Council on Physical Therapy of the American Medical Association in 1942 (31) proposed a method for quantifying hearing handicap which was influenced by both the Fowler and Sabine procedures (not surprising since they were both members of the Council). The proposed method assigned percentage values of hearing loss to octave intervals between the frequencies 256 and 4096 Hz at 10-dB increments from 10–90 dB (ASA 1951 audiometric zero). Percentage of hearing handicap could be determined by superimposing a person's audiogram on a chart, connecting the threshold hearing levels with a line, selecting the percentage values just above the connecting line, and summing these values. The binaural percentage was calculated using a weighting of 7 to 1 favoring the better ear.

The method proposed by the AMA in 1942 did not enjoy enthusiastic acceptance. It was found to be confusing and prone to error. The Council on Physical Medicine (formerly the Council on Physical Therapy) modified the proposed system and a revision was published in 1947 (32). The revision was known as the Fowler-Sabine method. The 1947 version was more like the system proposed by Fowler in 1942. The percentage values were placed at discrete frequencies rather than in octave intervals and the weights assigned to the various frequencies were the same as selected by Fowler. Furthermore, the weights did not change with increasing intensity. Hearing handicap increased nonlinearly with increasing hearing loss in both of these earlier systems proposed by the AMA. Handicap was assumed to be a sigmoidal function of intensity, similar in shape to the speech articulation curve.

Although the 1947 revision simplified the system over that offered in 1942 by the AMA, it apparently was still too complex for the medical community. In 1955, the AMA Council on Physical Medicine and Rehabilitation (33) indicated its dissatisfaction with the Fowler-Sabine procedure. This Council felt that the 1947 system was not appropriate for people with sensorineural hearing loss and emphasized the need to establish with more precision the relationship between the pure tone audiogram and the ability to hear speech. The Council also indicated that the statistical limit of normal for pure tone audiometry was 15 dB (ASA 1951), and therefore hearing handicap should not begin below that level.

AAOO Method

The Subcommittee on Noise of the American Academy of Ophthalmology and Otolaryngology (AAOO) proposed another method in 1959 (34) which was subsequently adopted by the AMA in 1961. The AAOO system used the average of the threshold levels for 500, 1000 and 2000 Hz. Handicap (although called "impairment" in the AAOO publication) was not considered to begin until this average exceeded 15 dB and reached 100% at 82 dB. Handicap was taken to be a linear function of intensity, increasing 1.5% for each decibel increase in the three-frequency average. The better ear was given 5 times the weight of the poorer ear in establishing binaural handicap. According to the Subcommittee, hearing impairment (handicap) should be evaluated in terms of ability to hear everyday speech under everyday conditions. Evidence of this ability could be demonstrated by

hearing and repeating sentences correctly in a quiet environment. However, because of limitations of speech audiometry, the members of the Subcommittee felt that hearing level for speech should be estimated from measurements of pure tone threshold hearing levels.

The AMA, in 1971 (35), changed the decibel values for beginning and total handicap in order to be consistent with a change in the American National Standard Institute's reference threshold hearing level (ANSI, 1969) (36). Handicap was taken to begin at 25 dB instead of 15 dB, and total (100%) handicap became 92 dB.

The AAOO method for calculating handicap has enjoyed more acceptance nationally and internationally than any other proposed system. The acceptance has not only been by the medical community but in the legal arena as well. By 1979, it had been incorporated by 18 states into their workers' compensation laws. The system has been adopted by other state and federal agencies with only minor revisions (37).

The AAOO procedure has not been without its critics. Public hearings on the proposed standard for occupational exposure to noise held by the Department of Labor in 1975 served as a forum for this criticism. Suter (18) provides an excellent review of this testimony. The use of the simple average of the three frequencies 500, 1000, and 2000 Hz received the most criticism. Use of this procedure penalizes people with noise-induced hearing loss by giving equal weight to these three frequencies while ignoring hearing loss for frequencies above 2000 Hz, despite the fact that most of the noise-induced hearing loss occurs at higher frquencies. The National Institute for Occupational Safety and Health (NIOSH) in its published criteria (38) for an occupational noise exposure standard, recommended that the three-frequency average be based on 1000, 2000 and 3000 Hz rather than 500, 1000 and 2000 Hz. The reason for this recommended change was the demonstrated importance of higher frequencies for understanding speech in background noise, which more closely approximates everyday listening conditions. For similar reasons, the British Standard for Assessment of Occupational Noise Exposure (39) changed to the three frequencies 1000, 2000 and 3000 Hz.

The so-called "low fence" of 25 dB for beginning handicap was also criticized as being too high (40, 41). Basing his calculations on the Articulation Index (42), Kryter (40, 41) predicted that a person with a 26-dB hearing loss would correctly repeat only 90% of sentences at a normal conversational level and 50% of monosyllabic words at a weak conversational level (in quiet at a distance of 1 m). Kryter (40, 41) recommended that 15 dB be taken as the level of beginning handicap if the three frequencies 500, 1000, and 2000 are used.

The assumption by the AAOO that hearing for everyday speech under everyday listening conditions is represented by the person's ability to hear and receive sentences in a quiet environment is questionable. Kryter (41) maintains that these conditions are not representative of the typical conditions of speech communication.

AAO-HNS, 1979 Method

As a consequence of these criticisms and the availability of new information, the AAOO formula was revised once more. The Committee on Hearing and Equilibrium of the American Academy of Otolaryngology-Head and Neck Surgery (AAO-HNS, formerly the AAOO) in 1979 (43) recognized the importance of hearing at frequencies above 2000 Hz for speech understanding particularly in realistic noisy environments. The frequency 3000 Hz was added and the three-frequency average became a simple four-frequency average. All other features of the AAOO system were retained.

ASHA Task Force Proposal

Dissatisfaction with the AAOO method of 1959 motivated other agencies to engage in the development of more acceptable systems. A task force was appointed by the American Speech-Language-Hearing Association for this purpose and, in a report published in 1981 (44), recommended another formula for determining the percentage of hearing handicap. Although recognizing the inadequacies of a single test for establishing auditory function, the task force found no alternative to be more acceptable than the use of pure tone audiometric measures. Using information available in the published literature as support, the ASHA task force recommended the use of a simple average of the four frequencies 1000, 2000, 3000, and 4000 Hz with beginning handicap occurring when the average loss exceeds 25 dB and total (100%) handicap at 75 dB. Noting the lack of published data supporting the effect of differing degrees of hearing loss for the two ears on overall hearing handicap, the report advocated the continued use of the weighting to 5 to 1 in favor of the better ear for determining binaural handicap until a solid basis for another ratio is established. Finally, for reasons of simplicity, the task force recommended that percent handicap increase linearly at the rate of 2%/dB from the lower limit of 25 dB to the upper limit of 75 dB. The task force specifically intended that this system for calculating handicap be applied for purposes of workers' compensation in adults, implying that it may not be appropriate for other purposes in other populations.

Ohio State Proposal

The Department of Labor's Office of Worker Compensation Programs (OWCP) uses the average hearing level for 1000, 2000 and 3000 Hz. The remainder of the formula is the same as that described for the AAOO method. The elimination of 500 Hz from the averaging process, and the liberal payment schedules, make the

OWCP the most generous source of compensation in the United States (18).

Because of this generosity, the OWCP compensation scheme was criticized by other Federal fiscal agencies. The Employment Standards Administration of the Department of Labor contracted with the Ohio State University to survey the literature and, on the basis of the survey, to recommend a compensation strategy which would equitably assess occupationally induced hearing loss (11). From the survey, it became apparent that the schemes used for determining handicap were, to a large degree, systems which measured impairment, and only indirectly and imprecisely estimated handicap. The principal recommendation of the investigators from Ohio State was for the OWCP to consider adopting an impairment criterion for its compensation; impairment as defined by the AAO-HNS (9) as "a shift for the worse, in either structure or function, outside the range of normal." Use of the impairment scheme requires a decision of what constitutes the range of normal. The Ohio State system turned to data available from large-scale hearing surveys, and defined (arbitrarily) the normal range as those people with threshold hearing levels which fell within ±2.5 SD of the mean of the large-sample distributions. An erroneous designation of abnormal for 1% of the population was considered acceptable. Based on the information from the hearing surveys and this definition of the normal range, beginning impairment was proposed to be 15 dB. Use of this starting point for impairment was contingent on the acceptance of the use of an age correction to account for the well documented decrease in hearing sensitivity with increasing age. The Ohio State procedure, therefore, would require a variable low fence for purposes of compensation because both the mean threshold hearing level and the variance of the general population has been demonstrated to be dependent on age.

The Ohio State method differed from other compensation schemes in several other aspects. It recommended the use of a five-frequency average in assessing impairment. The proposed frequencies were 500, 1000, 2000, 3000, and 4000 Hz. The upper limit of the functional auditory range was proposed as 70 dB. Impairment was to increase linearly as a function of the decibel value of the five-frequency average between the level of beginning impairment and the upper limit. Each ear was to be given equal weighting in calculating binaural impairment. The Ohio State system departs from most of the other compensation schemes not only in the details of the procedure but also, and perhaps more importantly, in the underlying philosophy. It has yet to be adopted by any state or federal agency.

Compensation Schemes in Other Countries

Industrial countries around the world are faced with the problem of occupationally noise-induced hearing loss and compensation for that hearing loss. The compensation schemes adopted by these countries have some aspects in common with the systems used in the United States and some features which vary considerably. The method for assessing auditory function is almost universally based on pure tone audiometry. The United Kingdom uses the simple average of hearing threshold levels for 1000, 2000 and 3000 Hz. Compensable hearing loss begins at 40.5 dB and increases at a rate of 2%/dB above this low fence. Binaural function is calculated using a ratio of 4:1 favoring the better ear (45).

The provinces of Canada, generally, have adopted the system proposed by the AAOO. However, since 1972, Ontario has used a formula based on the average of 500, 1000, 2000, and 3000 Hz. with a low fence of 35 dB. The better/worse ear ratio for assessing binaural handicap is 5:1. The growth rate of hearing handicap is nonlinear varying from 1–3%/dB as degree of impairment increases. The upper limit of hearing loss in this scheme is reached at 96.6 dB (45).

The Australian system (46) is modeled after the AMA procedures of 1942 and 1947. Percentage ratings are derived separately for the 6 frequencies 500, 1000, 1500, 2000, 3000, and 4000 Hz. Unlike the systems previously described, these percentages are added rather than averaged. Hearing loss is weighted differently for these 6 frequencies, with the greatest weighting assigned to 1000 Hz. Percentage hearing loss increases nonlinearly in this scheme, with the growth rate decreasing with increasing hearing impairment. Impairment begins at 20 dB for all of the test frequencies except 4000 Hz. At this frequency, the low fence is taken to be 25 dB. The better/worse ear ratio is complex and variable with magnitude of impairment, but on the average is about 6:1 (1).

Belgium uses a system similar to that applied in the United Kingdom. The procedure is based on the average of three frequencies, 1000, 2000 and 3000 Hz with a low fence of 55 dB (International Organization for Standards, ISO). The AAOO method is used in Denmark but beginning handicap is fixed at 60 dB (ISO). The method adopted in France is a modification of that of the AAOO. To establish the degree of hearing loss, the threshold hearing levels for 500 and 2000 Hz are added to twice the threshold level measured for 1000 Hz, and the sum is divided by 4. The low fence for the French system is 35 dB (ISO). West Germany does not use a specific system, but compensation is based on medical evaluation. The Netherlands makes no distinction between occupational and nonoccupational injury. Under its social security system, compensation is payable to victims of disease and injury regardless of the etiology, and no specific system is used for determining handicap from hearing loss. Japan uses a system patterned after that of the French but with a low fence of 60 dB (American Standards Association, ASA). The AAOO method is used in Brazil, Austria, Israel,

and Iran. Israel has adopted a 40 dB low fence. For purposes of compensation, Austria also requires a supportive medical evaluation and the demonstration of wage loss (1).

Although this review of compensation schemes from foreign countries is not exhaustive, it should be obvious that the schemes vary considerably from country to country. It also should be evident that the methods developed in the United States have exerted a strong influence, internationally.

COMPONENTS OF PURE TONE COMPENSATION FORMULAS

The preceding section clearly indicates that although there is variation in the several proposed methods for calculating compensable hearing loss, the pure tone schemes are essentially modifications of the same model. The major components of these systems are common. These components include the starting point for compensable hearing loss, or the low fence; the degree of hearing loss considered to be total, or the high fence; the pure tone frequencies to be considered in the calculation; weighting the hearing loss for the two ears for binaural function; a scaling method for relating the growth of hearing loss to the growth of handicap. The variation in the details of these common components reflects the inadequate definition of the correlation of pure tone sensitivity and speech function, the inherent imprecision of the relationship of hearing loss to hearing handicap, and differences in motivation of the developers of the compensation formulas.

Low Fence

As Suter points out, the low fence selected for estimating percentage hearing loss depends on the test frequencies used to represent auditory function (18). The most common low fence cited in this country is 25 dB as proposed by the AAOO (34) for the average of 500, 1000 and 2000 Hz and, more recently, by the AAO-HNS for the average of 500, 1000, 2000, and 3000 Hz (43). The 25 dB low fence had its origin in the proposal of the Subcommittee on Noise of the AAOO in 1959. At that time, the Subcommittee determined on limited clinical evidence that people began to have difficulty hearing sentences in quiet and sought medical advice when the average hearing loss for 500, 1000 and 2000 Hz exceeded 15 dB (ASA) (47). When the standard threshold hearing levels were changed to reflect more precise estimates of normal hearing sensitivity (American National Standards Institute, ANSI, 1969) the 15-dB low fence became 25 dB.

Davis (48) acknowledged that the 25 dB level may be more stringent than is warranted on the basis of beginning hearing dysfunction. This low fence, also, was selected to minimize the possible compensation of those people who did not experience compensable damage to their hearing but rather were born with hearing sensitivities which fell in the upper tail of the normal distribution of hearing sensitivity. This rational and justifiable economic objective was an important influence in the establishment of this conservative low fence for beginning hearing handicap.

Use of impairment as a basis for selecting a low fence requires a decision about what constitutes a significant deviation from normal function. Here too, there must be concern about the normal variation of hearing sensitivity among normal hearing people. Hardick et al. (11), as a result of an extensive review of studies of hearing sensitivity of young adults including those which served as the basis of the international standard for audiometric zero (ISO, 1964), concluded that the standard deviation for the distribution of normal hearing sensitivity fell between 5.5 and 6.5 dB. These investigators concluded that selection of a low fence of 15 dB would include 99.5% (mean +2.5 SD) of the normal distribution. Only 0.5% of the normal hearing adult population would

be classified impaired using this criterion. Hardick and his colleagues from Ohio State felt that this was a reasonable risk.

Suter (18) suggests that the low fence might be selected based on the hearing level at which hearing-impaired subjects began to perform differently than normal-hearing controls. Using the data of Acton (49) and from her own study (50), she reports that the appropriate low fence using her suggested criterion would be 9 dB for the average of the thresholds for 500, 1000 and 2000 Hz; 19 dB for 1000, 2000 and 3000 Hz; and 22 dB for the three frequencies 1000, 2000 and 4000 Hz.

The low fence could be based on estimates of handicap using self-assessment procedures. From a review of data from Merluzzi and Hinchcliffe (51), Schein et al. (52), and from the Health and Nutrition Examination Survey (1971–1975) (53), Hardick et al. (11) conclude that a 15 dB average for the frequencies 500, 1000, 2000, and 3000 Hz would be a reasonable low fence, not only from the standpoint of pure tone impairment, but also using the criterion of self-assessed handicap as well.

Selection of a low fence is not a simple matter. Several factors must be considered including the auditory frequency range, the normal variability of auditory function, the individual nature of handicap, and the economic impact of the level selected. To achieve medical, legal and public acceptance inevitably must involve judicious compromise.

High Fence

Selection of the high fence or hearing level at which hearing handicap is complete also has a significant effect on compensation computation but has not received as much attention as the low fence. The AAOO formula (34) set the upper limit for its three-frequency average at 92 dB. The stated rationale for establishing this level was that it approximated the point at which a person would be unable to hear shouted speech. Probably of equal importance is the fact that this level represents the upper limit or 100% hearing handicap for a simple linear scale which begins at 25 dB and increases at a rate of 1.5%/dB.

If impairment is to serve as the basis for the upper limit of hearing then one possible strategy would be to establish this level at the upper limits of the auditory range where acoustic stimulation produces the sensation of pain or extreme discomfort. Pain thresholds have been estimated to be about 140 dB; discomfort thresholds 120–130 dB (54); the upper limit of comfortable loudness is estimated to be in the 80–90 dB range. To establish the upper limit for hearing handicap at the extremes of the auditory range does not seem reasonable or practical, but it is a potential option.

Based on an extensive review of the information available in the literature, Hardick et al. (11) suggest several criteria for selecting the high fence: on the upper limit of normal comfortable loudness (70–85 dB hearing level, HL); predicted level at which a person cannot hear speech (80 dB average for 500, 1000 and 2000 Hz); predicted level for 10% discrimination of loud conversational speech (three-frequency average of 61 dB); lowest level for which a person is unable to hear shouted speech from across a room (57–72 dB three-frequency average); or the level at which a person cannot hear shouted speech close to the affected ear (67–76 dB average). From their investigation, the Ohio State group suggest that the high fence should be no higher than 80 dB HL and no less than 60 dB HL for the average of 500, 1000 and 2000 Hz, and offer as a reasonable compromise, 70 dB.

According to Suter (18), the trend is to lower the high fence from that proposed by the AAO-HNS and adopted by the AMA. She points out that the task force of the ASHA recommended a 75 dB limit for the average of hearing levels at 1000, 2000, 3000, and 4000 Hz, and that the formula adopted by Illinois sets the high fence at an average hearing level of 85 dB for the frequencies 1000, 2000 and 3000 Hz. However, Suter acknowledges this trend is not universal, and reports that New Jersey has established the high fence at 97 dB for the same three frequencies.

Test Tone Frequencies

The variability in the auditory frequency range to be used in estimating hearing handicap arises from the controversy regarding the relationship of pure tone threshold sensitivity to hearing for "everyday" speech. More accurately, the relationship of concern has been which frequency or combination of frequencies are more closely correlated to measures from clinical tests of speech sensitivity and acuity, assumed to be predictive of auditory function in "everyday" speech situations.

The three frequencies 500, 1000, and 2000 Hz have been considered important since the early work of Fletcher (26) at the laboratories of the Bell Telephone Company. He observed that much of the acoustic energy of speech was contained in the frequency range from 500–2000 Hz. Fletcher reported that tonal thresholds in this frequency region were closely related to speech detection thresholds. Subsequent studies demonstrated that this close relationship was maintained for measures of speech reception thresholds (SRT) (55–57).

Fletcher recognized the importance of another dimension of hearing for speech, auditory acuity or speech discrimination. The investigators from Bell Laboratories (58, 59) demonstrated that frequencies above 2000 Hz, specifically 4000 Hz, were correlated significantly with speech discrimination. Later studies continued to support the importance of frequencies in the 3000–4000 Hz range (49, 50, 60–63). From his review of the published data regarding the relationship of tonal thresholds to speech discrimination, Noble (1) concludes that if hearing handicap is validly represented by speech discrimination then the practice of using the three-frequency average 500, 1000 and 2000 Hz to represent this handicap is invalid. In fact, he questions the predictive accuracy of pure tone thresholds for auditory speech function in general.

Suter (18) argues that the strong correlation of 500, 1000 and 2000 Hz to the SRT is of little importance for assessment of hearing handicap. She reports that the SRT correlates poorly with the measures of speech discrimination. Suter is of the opinion that the discrimination of speech sounds is most important for everyday speech communication. Based on her interpretation of the unpublished information, most of the studies which have considered the relationship of pure tone thresholds to measures of speech discrimination support the inclusion of frequencies above 2000 Hz and excluding 500 Hz. Suter implies that the stated reason for inclusion of 500 Hz in the schemes proposed by the AAOO and AAO-HNS, i.e. the need for a scheme which could be applied to all types of hearing loss including those which are conductive, is irrelevant. She asserts that the principal use of the assessment scheme has been for medicolegal judgments involving compensation. The overwhelming majority of cases considered for this compensation are noise-related, sensorineural hearing losses.

Noble also indicates skepticism concerning the motivation of assessment systems which resist inclusion of frequencies above 2000 Hz and the continued use of 500 Hz in the averaging process. He believes the rationale for the frequencies used in the assessment is mainly economic. Noble (1, p. 134) states, "Management (aided by the medical profession) wants to minimize its losses in noise deafness claims. Labor wants to maximize its gains. In this instance, we see 'science' in the service of only one party to the dispute."

Some of the assessment schemes attempt to improve accuracy of predicting hearing for speech by weighting the thresholds obtained for the various test frequencies differently. Hardick et al. (11) conclude from their investigations that the amount of relevant research is limited but, from the the information that is available, differential weighting of the various frequencies would add little to estimates of speech processing ability. The chief effect, apparently, would be to reduce the calculated percent hearing loss without a significant increase in the precision for the estimates of speech function.

Scaling Compensable Hearing Loss

One generally accepted objective of the pure tone systems for assessing compensable hearing loss is that the amount of compensation should increase as the amount of hearing handicap increases. To accomplish this objective requires knowledge regarding the relationship of handicap to changes in pure tone hearing sensitivity. Because of the highly individual and variable nature of hearing handicap, precise information regarding this relationship is not available now, and is not likely to become available in the near future (if ever). Nevertheless, proposed compensation schemes have attempted to meet the objective by assuming a mathematical relationship between the degree of hearing loss and the magnitude of handicap.

Thus far, the most popular assumption has been that the compensable handicap should be directly proportional to the amount of hearing loss. The calculated percent of hearing handicap is taken to be linearly related to increasing hearing loss as measured in decibels. Although the decibel scale is logarithmic, in this particular application, it too is treated as if it were linear. Use of the linear relationship of hearing loss to hearing handicap is not based on firm scientific evidence, but rather on its mathematic simplicity and convenience.

Sabine (30) assumed that the prediction of hearing handicap should be based on the difference limen or differential sensitivity for changes in sound intensity. Since the decibel value of these intensity discriminations decrease with increasing intensity, handicap becomes an exponential function of hearing loss. The amount of hearing handicap per decibel of hearing loss increases in an accelerated fashion as the magnitude of hearing loss increases. The system used in Ontario, Canada has adopted this type of scaling (45).

Some of the proposed systems assume that handicap is a sigmoidal function of hearing loss. With this model, handicap grows slowly for mild losses, then increases rapidly through the moderate degrees of loss and finally tapers off as the loss becomes severe, resulting in the sigmoidal, or "S" shape. The proponents of this relationship base their assumption on measures of speech intelligibility as a function of intensity rather than on data obtained from people with hearing loss (18). The earlier AMA formulas (31, 32) and the Australian scheme (46) are examples of the application of the sigmoidal function.

The linear, exponential and sigmoidal scaling methods just described treat handicap as if it were, essentially, a continuous function of hearing loss. The scheme used by the Veterans Administration uses six discrete categories of handicap. This scheme does not recognize differences in the degree of hearing loss within these six categories. These minor differences only assume an importance in assessing handicap when they occur at the boundaries of the categories. If percentage of compensable hearing loss were graphed as a function of the pure tone average at 500, 1000 and 2000 Hz, it would have a "stair step" appearance characteristic of scales using discrete categories (11).

Better-Poorer Ear Weighting

Pure tone systems for assessing compensable hearing loss typically quantify the hearing loss for each ear separately and then combine these results in some fashion to produce an estimate of binaural handicap. The more sensitive ear is called the "better" ear and is usually accorded more weight than the less sensitive, "poorer" ear in deriving the composite binaural percentage of compensable hearing loss.

Most of the assessment methods assign a fixed weight to the better ear. The AMA methods of 1942 (31) and 1947 (32) propose a ratio of 7 to 1; the more recent methods of the AAOO (34), the AAO-HNS (43), and the procedure advocated by the task force of the ASHA (44) advocate a ratio of 5 to 1; while Macrae in Australia supports a ratio of 4 to 1 (64). Fowler (28) recommended that the better/poorer ear weighting vary as a function of extent and pattern of hearing loss.

The assignment of the weightings for most of the proposed pure tone schemes have been arbitrary with little or no experimental evidence available for support. The situation has not changed appreciably from that which existed in 1942 when Sabine (30) felt that the best one could do would be to make some general assumptions regarding binaural and monaural hearing, make a more-or-less arbitrary rule and wait for constructive criticism. The criticisms have come but for the most part have not been based on scientific investigation. The most popular better/poorer ear weighting ratios rely on the strength of clinical experience which, while respectable, does not provide the most solid foundation.

One notable exception to this lack of investigative support was the 4:1 ratio proposed by Macrae (64). His recommendation was based on a correlational study of the hearing levels for the better and the poorer ears with an estimate of handicap derived from a questionnaire. The 4:1 ratio was based on the results of a multiple correlation. Using this better/poorer ear weighting, Macrae obtained a correlation 0.91 between the binaural estimate and individual scores for the handicap questionnaire. It is interesting to note that in spite of the availability of Macrae's findings to the National Acoustic Laboratory in Australia, the method which they proposed and which was adopted, did not use this ratio. Because of some obscure "theoretical considerations," the Australian system uses a variable ratio which results in an average weighting of 6:1 (1).

The report from the Ohio State project recommends that the ears be given equal weighting, 1:1 (11). This recommendation was based on their decision that compensation be awarded based on impairment and not on supposed handicap. It also was based on the lack of evidence supporting any of the other proposed ear-weighting schemes.

The specific components of some of the better known pure tone compensations schemes are summarized in Table 11.1.

COMPENSATION STATUTES AND RULES

With the exception of federal employees and the military, compensation for occupational hearing loss is authorized and regulated by state law. Most often these rules and regulations are specified in the Worker's Compensation Laws of the individual states and are notoriously variable. The compensation situation for occupational hearing loss is not static but is subject to continual change. Social, economic, medical, and scientific forces demand this change. The interpretation and application of the rules and statutes also changes in time. This variability requires continual review and reappraisal to remain current and accurate. The most recently available comprehensive survey of the rules for compensating occupational hearing loss was made in 1978. Table 11.2 summarizes state compensation practices at that time. The contents of this Table are based on information published by Fox and Bunn (3) and Shampan and Ginnold (7) who have provided us with comprehensive and detailed reviews of that survey.

A striking feature of the state compensation programs for occupational hearing loss is that nine of the states, including a number of major industrial states, do not compensate for partial hearing loss. These states are Florida, Indiana, Louisiana, Massachusetts, Michigan, Nevada, New Mexico, Ohio, and Pennsylvania. In these states, if noise-related hearing loss is to be

Table 11.1.
Components of selected pure tone compensation schemes

Source	Averaged frequencies	Low fence	High fence	Better ear weighting	Scale
	Hz	dB	dB		
AMA[a] 1947	500, 1000, 2000, 4000 (weighted)	20	105	7:1	Nonlinear
AAOO 1959	500, 1000, 2000	25	92	5:1	1.5
AAO-HNS 1979	500, 1000, 2000, 3000	25	92	5:1	1.5
NIOSH	1000, 2000, 3000	25	92	5:1	1.5
ASHA (Task Force)	1000, 2000, 3000, 4000	25	75	5:1	2.0
Ohio State (recommended)	500, 1000, 2000, 3000, 4000	15 (adjusted for age)	55	1:1	2.5
Canada (Ontario)	500, 1000, 2000, 3000	35	96.6	5:1	Nonlinear
Britain	1000, 2000, 3000	40.5	90.5	4:1	2.0
Australia	500, 1000, 1500, 2000, 3000, 4000	Varies (~20 dB)	95	Varies (approx 6:1)	Nonlinear

[a] AMA, American Medical Association; AAOO, American Academy Ophthalmology and Otolaryngology; AAO-HNS, American Academy Otolaryngology-Head and Neck Surgery; NIOSH, National Institute of Occupational Safety and Health; and ASHA, American Speech-Language-Hearing Association.

Table 11.2.
State and federal hearing loss compensation programs[a]

	Occupational hearing loss compensable	Schedule in weeks for one ear	Schedule in weeks for both ears	Maximum compensation for one ear	Maximum compensation for two ears	Method/formula for assessing hearing loss	Waiting period	Time limit to file claim	Deduction made for presbycusis?	Loss adjusted for improvement with hearing aid?
Alabama	Yes	53	163	6,784	20,864	ME[b]	No	1 yr	—	No
Alaska	Yes	52	200	7,280	28,000	ME	No	D-2 yr	—	No
Arizona	Yes	25	60	15,625	41,220	AAOO[c] 1959	No	1 yr	No	No
Arkansas	Yes	40	150	3,500	13,125	ME	No	2 yr	No	P
California	Yes	—	—	—	—	AAO 1979	No	D-1 yr	—	Yes
Colorado	Yes	35	139	5,705	22,657	ME	No	3-5 yr	Yes	No
Connecticut	Yes	52	156	8,320	24,960	AAOO 1959	No	D-1 yr	No	No
Delaware	Yes	75	175	11,625	27,125	ME	No	D-1 yr	No	P
DC	Yes	52	200	20,632	79,356	AMA 47[d]	No	—	P	No
Florida	No-PPD	40	150	5,040	18,900	ME	No	D-2 yr	Yes	P
Georgia	Yes	—	150	—	16,500	AAOO 1959	6 mo	1 yr	No	No
Hawaii	Yes	140	200	26,460	37,800	AAOO 1959	No	D-1, 2 yr	Yes	No
Idaho	Yes	—	175	—	17,613	ME	No	1 yr	P	No
Illinois	Yes	100	200	24,116	48,232	NIOSH[d]	No	3 yr	No	—
Indiana	No-PPD	75	200	5,625	15,000	ME	No	2-3 yr	P	—
Iowa	Yes	50	175	12,200	42,700	AAO 1979	No	2 yr	P	No
Kansas	Yes	30	110	3,871	14,196	AMA 1947	No	1 yr	No	No
Kentucky	Yes	78	156	8,736	17,472	AAOO 1959	No	1-3 yr	No	Yes
Louisiana	No-PPD	—	—	—	—	ME	—	D-4 mo	—	—
Maine	Yes	50	200	11,586	46,344	AAOO 1959	30 dy	2 yr	Yes	No
Maryland	Yes	—	250	—	17,000	AAOO 1959	6 mo	2 yr	Yes	—

Table 11.2.—Continued

	Occupational hearing loss compensable	Schedule in weeks for one ear	Schedule in weeks for both ears	Maximum compensation for one ear	Maximum compensation for two ears	Method/formula for assessing hearing loss	Waiting period	Time limit to file claim	Deduction made for presbycusis?	Loss adjusted for improvement with hearing aid?
Massachusetts	No-PTI	150	400	4,500	12,000	ME	No	D-1 yr	P	No
Michigan	No-PPD	—	—	—	—	ME	—	D-4 mo	No	Yes
Minnesota	Yes	85	170	17,765	35,530	ME	No	D-3 yr	No	No
Mississippi	Yes	40	150	3,640	13,650	ME	No	D-2 yr	P	Yes
Missouri	Yes	40	148	3,800	14,060	AAOO 1959	6 mo	D-1 yr	Yes	Yes
Montana	Yes	40	200	3,760	18,800	AAOO 1959	6 mo	D-30 dy	Yes	No
Nebraska	Yes	50	100	7,750	15,500	AAOO 1959	No	D-6 mo	Yes	No
Nevada	No-PTD	—	—	—	—	AAO 1979	No	D-90 dy	No	No
New Hampshire	Yes	52	214	9,360	38,520	AAOO 1959	No	2 yr	No	No
New Jersey	Yes	60	200	2,400	8,000	NIOSH[d]	No	D-1, 2 yr	No	No
New Mexico	No-PTD	40	150	6,898	25,869	ME	No	1 yr	No	—
New York	Yes	60	150	6,300	15,750	NIOSH[d]	3 mo	D-90 dy/ 2 yr	No	No
N Carolina	Yes	70	150	12,460	26,700	AAOO 1959	6 mo	D-2 yr	No	No
N Dakota	Yes	50	200	2,000	8,000	ME	Yes	1 yr	No	Yes
Ohio	No-PTD	25	125	2,700	13,500	ME	—	6 mo	Yes	Yes
Oklahoma	Yes	100	300	6,000	18,000	ME	No	D-3, 18 mo	No	No
Oregon	Yes	60	192	5,100	16,320	0.5-6 kHz	Yes	D-6 mo	No	Yes
Pennsylvania	No-PTI	60	260	12,780	55,380	ME	No	120 dy	No	—
Rhode Island	Yes	17	100	765	4,500	AAOO 1959	6 mo	D-2 yr	No	No
S Carolina	Yes	80	165	13,760	28,380	ME	No	D-2 yr	Yes	No
S Dakota	Yes	50	150	7,750	23,250	ME	No	2 yr	No	Yes
Tennessee	Yes	75	150	7,500	15,000	ME	No	1-3 yr	No	Yes
Texas	Yes	—	150	—	13,650	AAOO 1959	No	6 mo	No	No

Table 11.2.—Continued

	Occupational hearing loss compensable	Schedule in weeks for one ear	Schedule in weeks for both ears	Maximum compensation for one ear	Maximum compensation for two ears	Method/formula for assessing hearing loss	Waiting period	Time limit to file claim	Deduction made for presbycusis?	Loss adjusted for improvement with hearing aid?
Utah	Yes	50	100	6,550	13,100	ME	6 mo	D–1 yr	Yes	No
Vermont	Yes	52	215	8,840	36,550	ME	No	1 yr	No	No
Virginia	Yes	50	100	9,350	18,700	AAOO 1959	No	D–2 yr	No	No
Washington	Yes	—	—	2,400	14,400	AAO 1979	No	D–1 yr	No	No
W Virginia	Yes	100	260	13,800	35,880	AAOO 1959	No	D–3 yr	P	No
Wisconsin	Yes	36	216	2,340	14,040	CHABA	2 mo	None	No	No
Wyoming	Yes	40	80	5,816	11,632	ME	No	D–1, 3 yr	Yes	—
U.S. Dept of Labor	Yes	52	200	35,625	137,020	NIOSH	No	D–3 yr	No	No

[a] Based on information published by Fox and Bunn (3) and Shampan and Ginnold (8).
[b] ME, medical evaluation; D, discovery; P, possible; PPD, permanent partial disability; PTD, permanent total disability; and PTI, permanent total impairment.
[c] AAOO, American Academy Ophthalmology and Otolaryngology; AAO, American Academy Otolaryngology; AMA, American Medical Association; NIOSH, National Institute for Occupational Safety and Health; and CHABA, National Research Council's Council on Hearing and Bioacoustics.
[d] Modification of indicated method; averaged for frequencies 0.5–6 kHz with 25 dB low fence.

compensable, the hearing loss must be judged to be total, in some instances using the criterion of impairment while in others, disability. Occupationally noise-induced hearing loss is rarely total. Consequently, this requirement virtually eliminates compensation for most of the employees whose hearing has been affected by industrial noise.

Ginnold (37) relates that in 1977, the distribution of paid compensation claims among the 50 states was remarkably uneven. In that year, only the nine states New Jersey, New York, West Virginia, Connecticut, Wisconsin, Minnesota, California, Oregon, and Washington paid more than a token number of claims. Of the 6095 paid claims for that year, 5780 are accounted for by these nine states, with New Jersey, alone, being involved in over half of the total number of cases. Although the details may have changed since the 1977 survey, the variability in the level of state compensation activity has not.

Ginnold (37) further reports that although workers compensation for occupational hearing loss had increased to 13 million dollars in 1977, this amount still only represented less than 0.1% of 14 billion dollars paid in workers compensation claims that year. The average dollar benefit per claim was small. In Wisconsin, the average claim in 1977 amounted to $2300. This low dollar benefit for hearing loss claims also was found in a more recent survey by Hefler (65), who projected the average award to be about $2000.

Table 11.2 underscores the considerable variation in maximum allowable benefits among the states. Shampan and Ginnold (7) calculated the average maximum benefit to be $21,700. They warn, however, that it is inappropriate to compare states on the basis of this maximum since there is little relationship between this figure and the number of awarded claims. New Jersey, for instance, has one of the lowest maximum benefits but has been involved with a high number of claims.

Federal Compensation Programs

Compensation for occupational hearing loss suffered by federal employees is authorized under the Federal Employees' Compensation Act (FECA) (66) and under the Longshoremen's and Harbor Workers' Program (LSHW) (67). Administration of these compensation programs is the responsibility of the Office of Workers' Compensation Programs (OWCP) in the Employment Standards Administration of the Department of Labor. The FECA covers all federal employees including blue collar workers at federal installations, while the LSHW covers civilians working in nonseafaring maritime occupations. The main groups of noise-exposed employees involved with the FECA are federal employees working in shipyards and airbases. This amounts to approximately 75,000 people. The LSHW covers about 50,000 workers (7).

The federal compensation program is more liberal than most of the state administered compensation systems. Shampan and Ginnold (7) list five factors responsible for the more generous compensation of the federal employees:

1. Use of the NIOSH compensation formula which is based on the average of 1000, 2000 and 3000 Hz with a low fence of 25 dB
2. To be eligible a worker need only be exposed to noise exceeding 85 dBA, with duration of exposure unspecified
3. Workers need not wait until retirement to file a claim
4. The FEC and LSHW have higher maximum benefits for total loss than any state ($135,000 for the FEC and $99,100 for the LSHW)
5. Employers do not have the authority to challenge rules and awards in individual cases.

In 1977, the OWCP compensated approximately 1800 workers under the provisions of the FECA, at a cost of about 14 million dollars. At the same time, approximately 500 employees were compensated in the LSHW program at a cost exceeding 3 million dollars. The combined total of over 17 million dollars exceeded the total of all state claims for that year (7).

Veterans Administration

The largest compensation program operated by the federal government is that operated by the Veterans Administration (VA). The estimated compensation for service-connected hearing impairments for 1980 exceeded 125 million dollars. In September of that year approximately 59,000 veterans claimed hearing impairment as their primary disability, while another 18,000 received payments for hearing loss as a secondary impairment (7). The cost of these compensation programs is enormous and, therefore, serves as a major incentive for aggressive hearing conservation programs by the Department of Defense.

OTHER FACTORS INFLUENCING COMPENSATION

The formula used for assessing compensable hearing loss is recognized as a major factor in determining the number of eligible claimants and the size of the monetary award. However, other factors can influence the level of compensatory activity and the amount of compensation paid to a claimant. These factors include definition of hazardous exposure, required waiting period between exposure and filing a claim, time limits on filing a claim, use of an adjustment for aging, choice of verifying physician, and level of union activity (7).

Hazardous Exposure

The definition of noise exposure which qualifies an employee as a potential recipient of compensation for occupational hearing loss could be a major factor in limiting the number of filed claims. More than half the states define hazardous noise either using the OSHA specification of 90 dBA for 8 hr, or the NIOSH recommendation of 85 dBA for the same dura-

tion. Utah requires that noise levels exceed 95 dBA. Some states recognize that the noise exposure is hazardous for certain occupations and simply accept a history of working in these occupations as sufficient documentation of potential noise-related hearing loss (7)

Waiting Period

The waiting period is the intervening time interval required between working in the hazardous noise environment and filing a claim for compensation. Ostensibly, this waiting period serves to minimize the influence of temporary hearing loss on threshold hearing levels measured for assessing compensable hearing loss. However, it has served as an administrative control of the filing of claims. The most common waiting period, adopted by 10 states, is 6 months. This period can hardly be justified on the basis of elimination of temporary hearing loss. More believably, the 6-month interval was chosen because of economic considerations (68). Because of this rule, most potential applicants cannot file a claim while working. Filing of a claim usually is delayed until an employee is eligible for retirement. As a consequence, many potential claimants die or do not feel that filing a claim is worth the trouble. In some states, where adjustments are made for aging, the waiting rule effectively is responsible for a reduction in dollar value of the award.

To underscore the economic effects of this waiting period, the federal compensation program (with its high level of claims activity) and the two states with the highest number of claims do not exercise such a restriction. Approximately one-third of the 32 states with few or no claims have a significant waiting period. Only two of the nine states with a high volume of claims have a required waiting interval, New York (3 months) and Wisconsin (1 month) (7). The New York waiting period simply requires the employee to use HPDs when exposed to occupational noise for a 3-month period following the date of discovery.

Filing Time Limits

Filing-time limits define the interval from time of injury or last exposure and the time when a filed claim could be accepted for processing. Some states have instituted a discovery rule. The discovery rule specifies that the time limits imposed on filing do not begin until employees have become aware of their disability. The nine states with a significant level of compensation activity all have discovery rules. In these states, the time limits following discovery range from 6 months to 3 yr. Of the states with few claims, 27 have filing time limits while only 4 of these states accept the "discovery" concept (7). In the states where the discovery rule does not apply, many of the workers retire before they are aware of the magnitude of their hearing problem, and without realizing their eligibility for a compensation claim. Frequently, this awareness does not come until after the filing time limit has expired, and the employees not only have lost some of their hearing, but also have lost the opportunity for remuneration for the hearing impairment.

Adjustment for Aging

Loss of hearing sensitivity as a function of age is a common finding of all large-scale surveys of hearing in the adult population of industrialized nations. Age-related hearing loss has been documented in these adults even when there is no history of hazardous exposure to occupational noise. In order that the employer not be burdened with the responsibility for hearing loss not resulting from the employee's work environment, eleven states have implemented compensation schemes which adjust the assessed compensable hearing loss for aging (7). An age adjustment can restrict the number of people eligible for compensation, as well as reduce the size of the financial award.

This adjustment would be particularly restrictive in states where lengthy required waiting periods dictate that claims would not be filed until the employee retires.

The adjustment for aging varies among the several states which have adopted its application. Wisconsin deducts 0.5% of the assessed percentage of compensable hearing loss for each year of age beyond 52. Missouri reduces the calculated hearing impairment by 0.5 dB for each year over 40. Since Missouri uses the compensation formula adopted by the AAOO in 1959, this adjustment decreases the percentage by 0.75%/yr after 40 yr of age. Other states, such as Connecticut and West Virginia, permit physicians to consider adjustments for aging in their assessment (7).

The concept of an age adjustment of hearing loss compensation has its opponents. There are those who feel that the deduction should not be made because the handicapping effect of a hearing loss is the same regardless of the cause and the age of person experiencing the loss. These critics contend that if the employee was exposed to hazardous noise conditions, then the noise exposure either caused or contributed to the hearing problem. The employer might not be responsible for the total hearing loss, but would be responsible for aggravation of an existing hearing loss because of hazardous working conditions (18).

The age adjustment also might be considered unwarranted and unfair because of the use of a conservative low fence. In Missouri, the low fence is 25 dB for the average of 500, 1000 and 2000 Hz, while in Wisconsin the fence is set at 35 dB for the three-frequency average using 1000, 2000 and 3000 Hz. Davis (48) reports that the low fence adopted by the AAOO in 1959 was deliberately set high enough to account for this aging effect.

Union Activity

The degree of labor union involvement in providing information and assistance to its members in filing claims exerts a significant effect on state compensation activity. In Wisconsin, claims increased from 80 in 1974 to 150 in 1975. This followed a 2-day workshop on compensation claims for occupational hearing loss which was conducted for a group of union leaders in 1974. Of the claims filed in Wisconsin in 1975, 75% were from nine unionized metalworking firms. The United Steelworkers of America in Milwaukee established a revolving fund to pay for a hearing test for any of its members. In 1979, this fund paid for over 100 hearing evaluations (37).

Five thousand claims were filed by employees of the Long Beach Naval Shipyard. The boilermakers union filed claims after management ignored union requests to correct the noise problem. The union held educational seminars on claims filing for its members. It hired highly qualified lawyers and hearing specialists. A large number of the claims were paid by the Federal Employee Compensation program (37).

In Chicago, the United Auto Workers sponsored hearing tests for its members and, in one of its employee newsletters, recognized the importance of compensation as a method to motivate management to improve the working environment. The United Auto Workers in one local in New Jersey handled 250 claims by its membership as a consequence of the activity of its president, who developed a hearing loss, himself (37).

Choice of Physician

Ginnold (37) reports that the choice of physician can be a major influence in claims for hearing loss compensation. This is particularly true in those states which use medical evaluation as the basis for assessing compensable hearing loss. Physicians hired by the employer or paid by the insurance carrier could be faced with a conflict of interest. On the other hand, a physician chosen by the employee is more likely to defend his evaluation of

the employee's hearing status and to testify on behalf of the claimant when the claim is contested by the insurer. Of the nine states with an appreciable level of compensation claims listed by Ginnold (37), seven permit the employee to choose the verifying physician.

PROFESSIONAL RESPONSIBILITY

Hearing health professionals provide important services in programs for compensating occupational hearing loss. As a consequence of their educational background, their clinical experience and their professional affiliations, audiologists and otolaryngologists can provide consulting services to state compensation boards regarding hearing loss provisions. When claims are being disputed, these professionals may serve as expert witnesses in legal proceedings which may arise. In states where the criteria for compensable hearing loss is not specified and medical evaluation is the basis for compensation, audiologic and otologic recommendations may be the primary consideration in making the award.

Hearing health professionals may serve as consultants to the affected employees and their unions. They can supply information and guidance to people seeking compensation for occupational hearing loss. They should be able to counsel the employee regarding the amount of hearing loss which exists, the expected effects of this hearing loss on the person's ability to function, the probability that the measured hearing loss is related to the worker's occupation, and the evidence required to substantiate a compensation claim.

Medical and Audiological Diagnosis

The diagnosis of noise-induced hearing loss is difficult to establish. It is even more difficult to attribute a given noise-induced hearing loss to a specific noise source.

Hazardous noise exposures damage the delicate sensory cells in the cochlea. The audiometric findings are those which would be identified as a cochlear, sensorineural hearing loss. There is nothing particularly unique about the cochlear hearing loss produced by excessive noise exposure and that produced by other agents. A noise-induced hearing loss usually is slow to develop. Therefore, a significant period of time passes before such a hearing loss becomes noticable. Change in hearing sensitivity over a period of time can result from a complex accumulation of effects from several sources. The aging process, itself, can produce a sensorineural hearing loss, presbycusis. The longer a person lives, the more probable it becomes that the person would be affected by a systemic viral or bacterial disease which produce cochlear damage, and a consequent senorineural hearing loss. Hearing loss arising from disease processes is called nosoacusis. Noise-induced hearing loss can be produced not only by occupational noise, but also by noises encountered in other everyday activities in an industrialized society, such as traffic noises, gunfire and lawn mowers, among countless others. The hearing loss resulting from this daily noise exposure is called sociocusis.

It is impossible to specify, precisely, what proportion of a complex, age-related hearing loss is due to a particular etiologic agent. The health professional must be satisfied with being able to state with some degree of probability that a given hearing loss was the result of a specific occupational noise exposure. The audiologist and otolaryngologist must make this statement of probability acceptable to those responsible for making a legal judgment. A preemployment assessment of an employee's hearing status reduces the uncertainty. If a hearing loss can be documented prior to employment, at least that portion of loss need not be attributed to subsequent occupational noise exposure.

As is frequently the case in medical diagnosis, a careful personal, occupational and medical history is of paramount importance. Reports of familial hearing loss might point to a progressive hereditary sensorineural hearing loss. Active participation in hobbies such as hunting and automobile racing might indicate exposure to hazardous noises outside the workplace. A documented history of systemic disease and drug therapy could indicate another source for the measured hearing loss.

The health professional must have an understanding of the relationship of noise exposure to hearing loss and be able to apply this understanding in interpreting information available for a specific compensation claimant. What was the noise level in the occupational environment? What is the typical daily duration of the noise exposure? What was the length of employment in the noisy job? Valid measurements of noise levels that exist today are unlikely to represent the levels that existed 10 or 20 yr ago. Exposure to noise levels below 80 dBA are not likely to produce significant hearing losses. Exposure to noise levels of 105 dBA for 8 hr/day, for a period of several years, without the benefit of hearing protection, almost certainly will produce measurable high frequency hearing loss. If the sensorineural hearing loss is unilateral, it is not likely that the hearing loss was produced by chronic industrial noise exposure.

Compensation and the prospect of financial gain have motivated claimants to exaggerate or feign hearing loss. The professionals responsible for assessment of hearing must be alert to the possibility that a hearing loss measured audiometrically could be nonorganic. Audiologic evaluation using tests designed to reflect on the validity of a measured hearing loss is indispensable for clinical programs involved with documenting the existence of a hearing loss for purposes of compensation.

SUMMARY

Exposure to hazardous noise in the workplace continues to be a major source of hearing loss in the United States and other industrial countries. Compensation by the employer for the social and financial consequences of this hearing loss has become a practice accepted by the legal community and by society as a whole. In the United States, this compensation is usually awarded under the authority of the Worker's Compensation Laws and is administered primarily by each individual state. People working for the federal government, either as civilians or as military personnel, are covered by federal compensation laws and fall under the jurisdiction of federal agencies. Over the past 2 decades, the trend has been for the responsible state and federal agencies to recognize the legitimacy of occupational hearing loss claims, to provide more coverage, and to increase the size of the award. More recently, perhaps because of problems arising in the economy of our country, this trend shows signs of slowing and even reversal.

Because the states are responsible for the statutes covering compensation for occupational hearing loss, there is significant variability in worker eligibility and the amount of money paid for a given hearing loss. The compensation systems have based the assessment of compensable hearing loss on audiometric measures of pure tone hearing sensitivity. These measures of hearing impairment are converted by some formula into presumed measures of hearing handicap. These formula are based, to some extent, on information regarding the relationship of pure tone threshold hearing levels to the ability to communicate in "everyday" speech situations. However, the equations developed for calculating hearing handicap rely on clinical observation and arbitrary decisions more often than solid scientific support.

The data which have been used to develop formulas were derived from groups of people and reflect average performance rather the performance of an individual. Compensation systems which use these hearing loss formulas can never be precise indicators of individual hearing handicap. The best that these systems can hope to offer is a reasonable estimate of handicap. This estimate can be improved by replacing the arbitrary elements of the hearing loss formulas with elements that have the scientific strength of investigative evidence which demonstrates their relationship to auditory communicative function. The hearing heatlh professional must accept the responsibility for conducting the necessary research which would establish the social impact of hearing loss. The results of this research should provide methods for calculating compensation which would reflect, more adequately, the handicap which this loss imposes.

References

1. Noble WG: *Assessment of Impaired Hearing*, New York, Academic Press, 1978.
2. Coles RRA: Medico-legal aspects of noise hazards to hearing. Med Leg J 43:3–19, 1975.
3. Fox MS, Bunn JH, Jr: Workers' compensation aspects of noise-induced hearing loss. In *Symposium on Noise—Its Effects and Control. Otolaryngol Clin N Am* 12:705–724, 1979.
4. *Slawinski v Williams & Co.*, 298 N.Y. 546, 81 N.E. 2d 93, aff'g 273 App. Div. 826, 76 N.Y.S. 2d 888, 1948.
5. *Wojcik v Green Bay Drop Forge*, 265 Wis. 38, 60 N.W. 2d 409, rehearing denied, 61 N.W. 2d 847, 1953.
6. Fox MS: Comparative provisions for occupational hearing loss. Arch Otolaryngol 81:257–260, 1965.
7. National Commission on State Workmen's Compensation Laws: *Compendium on Workmen's Compensation*. Washington, DC, Government Printing Office, 1973.
8. Shampan J, Ginnold R: The status of workers' compensation programs for occupational hearing impairment. In Kramer MB, Armbruster JM (eds): *Forensic Audiology*. Baltimore, University Park Press, 1982, ch 14, pp 283–323.
9. AAO-HNS: *Guide For The Evaluation of Hearing Handicap*. Rochester, Minn American Academy of Otolaryngology-Head and Neck Surgery, 1981.
10. Eldredge DH: The problems of criteria for noise exposure. In Henderson D, Hamernik RP, Dosanjh DS, Mills JH (eds): *Effects of Noise on Hearing*. New York, Raven Press, 1976, pp 3–20.
11. Hardick EJ, Melnick W, Hawes NA, Pillion JP, Stephens RG, Perlmutter DJ: *Compensation for Hearing Loss for Employees Under the Jurisdiction of the U.S. Department of Labor: Benefit Formula and Assessment Procedures*. Final report for contract no. J-9-E-90205. Washington, DC, U.S. Department of Labor, 1980.
12. Davis H: The articulation area and the social adequacy index for hearing. *Laryngoscope* 58:761–778, 1948.

13. Davis H, Silverman SR: *Hearing and Deafness*, ed 4. New York, Holt, Rinehart & Winston, 1978.

14. Giolas TG: Comparative intelligibility scores of sentence lists and connected discourse, *J Aud Res* 7:31–38, 1966.

15. Giolas TG: *Hearing-Handicapped Adults*. Englewood Cliffs, NJ, Prentice-Hall, 1982.

16. High WS, Fairbanks G, Glorig A: Scale of self-assessment of hearing handicap. *J Speech Hear Dis* 29:215–230, 1964.

17. Nett EM, Doerfler LG, Matthews J: *The Relationships Between Audiological Measures and Handicap*. (Unpublished Report, Vocational Rehabilitation Administration, Project no. 167, 1960.)

18. Suter AH: Calculation of impairment or handicap. In Kramer MB, Armbruster JM (eds): *Forensic Audiology*. Baltimore, University Park Press, 1982, ch 13, p 259–281.

19. Giolas TG: The measurement of hearing handicap: a point of view. *Maico Aud Libr Ser* 8:20–23, 1970.

20. Noble WG, Atherley GRC: The hearing measurement scale: a questionnaire for the assessment of auditory disability. *J Aud Res* 10:229–250, 1970.

21. Noble WG: The Hearing Measurement Scale as a paper-pencil form: preliminary results. *J Am Aud Soc* 5:95–106, 1979.

22. McCartney JH, Maurer JF, Sorenson FD: A comparison of the Handicap Scale and the Hearing Measurement Scale with standard audiometric measures on a geriatric population. *J Aud Res* 16:51–58, 1976.

23. Giolas TG, Owens E, Lamb SH, Schubert ED: Hearing Performance Inventory. *J Speech Hear Dis* 44:169–195, 1979.

24. Lamb SH, Owens E, Schubert ED, Giolas TG: Hearing Performance Inventory, revised form. Appendix G. In Giolas TG (ed): *Hearing Handicapped Adults*. Englewood Cliffs, NJ, Prentice-Hall, 1982, pp 189–199.

25. Davis JM, Hardick EJ: *Rehabilitative Audiology for Children and Adults*. New York, Wiley 1981.

26. Fletcher H: *Speech and Hearing*. New York, Van Nostrand Reinhold 1929.

27. Davis, H: Hearing handicap, standards for hearing, and medicolegal rules. In Davis H, Silverman SR (eds): *Hearing and Deafness*, ed 3. New York, Holt, Rinehart & Winston, 1970, pp 253–279.

28. Fowler EP: Hearing standards for acceptance, disability rating and discharge in the military services and in industry. *Laryngoscope*, 51:937–956, 1941.

29. Fowler EP: A method for measuring the percentage of capacity for hearing speech. *J Acoust Soc Am* 13:373–382, 1942.

30. Sabine PE: On estimating the percentage loss of loss of useful hearing. *Trans Am Acad Opthalmol Otolaryngol* 46:179–196, 1942.

31. American Medical Association, Council on Physical Therapy: Tentative standard procedure for evaluating the percentage of useful hearing loss in medicolegal cases. *JAMA* 119:1108–1109, 1942.

32. American Medical Association, Council on Physical Medicine: Tentative standard procedure for evaluating the percentage loss of hearing in medicolegal cases. *JAMA* 133:396–397, 1947.

33. American Medical Association, Council on Physical Medicine and Rehabilitation: Principles for evaluating hearing loss. *JAMA* 157:1408–1409, 1955.

34. American Academy of Ophthalmology and Otolaryngology, Committee on Conservation of Hearing: Guide for evaluation of hearing impairment. *Trans Am Acad Opthalmol Otolaryngol* 63:236–238, 1959.

35. AMA, Committee on Rating of Mental and Physical Impairment: Ear, nose, throat and related structures. In *Guides to the Evaluation of Permanent Impairment*. Chicago, American Medical Association, 1971, ch 8, pp 103–111.

36. ANSI S3.6-1969: *American National Standard Specifications for Audiometers*. New York, American National Standards Institute, 1969.

37. Ginnold RE: *Occupational Hearing Loss: Workers Compensation Under State and Federal Programs*. Washington, DC, U.S. Environmental Protection Agency Report EPA 550/9-79-101, 1979.

38. National Institute for Occupational Safety and Health: *Criteria for a Recommended Standard Occupational Exposure to Noise*. Report HSM 7311001, Washington, DC, U.S. Department Health, Education and Welfare, 1972.

39. BS 5330:1976: *Estimating Risk of Hearing Handicap Due to Noise Exposure*. London, British Standards Institution, 1976.

40. Kryter KD: Hearing impairment for speech. *Arch Otolaryngol* 77:598–602, 1963.

41. Kryter KD: Impairment to hearing from exposure to noise. *J Acoust Soc Am* 53:1211–1234, 1973.

42. French NR, Steinberg JC: Factors governing the intelligibility of speech sounds. *J Acoust Soc AM* 19:90–119, 1947.

43. American Academy of Otolaryngology-Head and Neck Surgery, Committee on Hearing and Equilibrium and the American Council of Otolaryngology, Committee on the Medical Aspects of Noise: Guide for the evaluation of hearing handicap. *JAMA* 133:396–397, 1979.

44. American Speech-Language-Hearing Association: Report of the task force on the definition of hearing handicap. *Asha* 23:293–297, 1981.

45. Alberti PW, Morgan PP, Fria TJ, LeBlanc JC: Percentage hearing loss: various schema applied to large population with noise-induced hearing loss. In Henderson D, Hamernik RP, Dosanjh DS, Mills JH (eds): *Effects of Noise on Hearing*. New York, Raven Press, 1976.

46. NAL: *Procedure for Determining Percentage Loss of Hearing*. Sydney, Austr, National Acoustics Laboratories, 1974.

47. Davis H: Some comments on "Impairment to hearing from exposure to noise" by KD Kryter. *J Acoust Soc Am* 53:1237–1239, 1973.

48. Davis H: A historical introduction. In Robinson DW (ed): *Occupational Hearing Loss*. New York, Academic Press, 1971.

49. Acton WI: Speech intelligibility in a background

noise and noise-induced hearing loss. *Ergonomics* 13:546–554, 1979.

50. Suter AH: *The Ability of Mildly Hearing-Impaired Individuals to Discriminate Speech in Noise.* Washington, DC, U.S. Environmental Protection Agency and U.S. Air Force Reports EPA 550/9-78-100 and AMRL-TR-78-4, 1978.

51. Merluzzi F, Hinchcliffe R: Threshold of subjective auditory handicap. *Internat Aud* 12:65–69, 1973.

52. Schein JD, Gentile A, Haase K: Development and evaluation of an expanded hearing loss scale questionnaire. *Vital Health Stat* 2:1–42, 1970.

53. Roberts J: Hearing levels of youths 12–17 years. *U.S. National Center for Health Statistics. Series 11. No. 145.* Washington, DC, U.S. Dept. of Health, Education and Welfare, 1975.

54. Silverman SR: Tolerance for pure tones and speech in normal and defective hearing. *Ann Otol Rhinol Laryngol* 56:658–677, 1947.

55. Harris JD: Free voice and pure tone audiometer for routine testing of auditory acuity. *Arch Otolaryngol* 44:452–467, 1946.

56. Carhart R: Speech reception in relation to pattern of pure tone loss. *J Speech Dis* 11:97–108, 1946.

57. Quiggle RR, Glorig A, Delk JH, Summerfield AB: Predicting hearing loss for speech from pure tone audiograms. *Laryngoscope* 67:1–15, 1957.

58. Fletcher H, Steinberg JC: Articulation testing methods. *Bell Syst Tech J* 8:806–854, 1929.

59. Steinberg JC, Gardner MB: On the auditory significance of the term hearing loss. *J Acoust Soc Am* 11:270–277, 1940.

60. Young MA, Gibbons EW: Speech discrimination scores and threshold measurements in a non-normal hearing population. *J Aud Res* 2:21–33, 1962.

61. Kryter KD, Williams C, Green DM: Auditory acuity and perception of speech. *J Acoust Soc Am* 34:1217–1223, 1962.

62. Ross M, Huntington DA, Newby HA, Dixon RF: Speech discrimination of hearing-impaired individuals in noise. *J Aud Res* 5:47–72, 1965.

63. Niemeyer W: Speech discrimination in noise-induced deafness. *Internat Aud* 6:42–47, 1967.

64. Macrae JH: *Notes on the Procedure for Determining Percentage Loss of Hearing (March 11, 1974).* Sidney, Austr, Commonwealth Department of Health, 1974.

65. Hefler AJ: Distribution of compensable impairment in industry. *Sound Vibr* 14:18–20, 1980.

66. Federal Employees' Compensation Act, U.S. Code 1976, Title 5, as Amended, 1977.

67. Longshoremen's and Harbor Workers' Compensation Act, U.S. Code 1976, Title 33, as Amended, 1972.

68. Sataloff J, Michael P: *Hearing Conservation.* Springfield, Ill, Charles C Thomas, 1973.

CHAPTER 12

Legal Issues: Licensure, Liability and Forensics

ANTHONY A. MURASKI

INTRODUCTION

The provision of professional services to industry involves many legal considerations for the audiologist. Among these are government statutes dealing with licensure and liability. In addition, the professional engaged in matters of public health and safety is likely to become involved in matters of forensics relating to worker compensation and other medicolegal questions. The audiologist, by tradition, has not been broadly involved in these issues which are commonly encountered in the private practice sector.

As audiologists have moved from institutional settings for the delivery of service these issues have become more relevant. The provision of service to industry in the area of occupational noise introduces a number of considerations that must be addressed by audiologists. The profession, being as it is, a newly licensed body, has yet to develop a so-called licensure mentality. Its practitioners are not involved with the possible restrictive impact of licensure as much as they are with its potential attributes.

This chapter will first explore the issue of licensure from an historical perspective. It will also examine the matter of professional lability and its impact on the provider of professional services. Finally, we will look at general considerations of forensics, including the application of audiological data to the law and testimony in medicolegal matters.

PROFESSIONAL LICENSURE AND THE PRIVATE PRACTITIONER

Governments have a constitutional mandate to protect the public health, welfare and safety of their citizens. Thus, the general purpose of licensing laws is to regulate professions in order to satisfy this mandate. A profession is a "vocation or occupation requiring advanced education and training, and involving intellectual skills" (1). Only those professions which provide services to the public have come under the scrutiny of the legislature to be possible candidates for licensure. Legislatures began enacting licensure statutes to regulate the health professions at the turn of the century (2).

There are both advantages and disadvantages of licensing professions. These are relative, depending upon ones perspective, either as a consumer of the services or as a member of the licensed profession. The main consumer advantage of licensure is the assurance that the services provided must meet basic standards of professional performance, and that a failure to meet such standards exposes the licensed individual to penalties. The often stated consumer disadvantage of licensure is that the profession occupies a monopoly for the licensee's own economic benefit. Arguably, the licensee does incur an economic benefit from licensure, not from aggregating monopolistic power, but from the fact that the marketplace will pay a higher premium for a statutory guaranty of performance standards. Thus, there is a prestige factor, as a result of licensure, which is derived from the fact that the public perceives that the licensed profession must have a greater value to society than the unlicensed profession if the legislature so deems to pronounce that it is worthy of licensure.

Then licensure has a profound effect on the future of a profession because it alone establishes a recognizable public and legal identity, which may result in financial independence and professional autonomy for the licensee. The primary disadvantage of licensure, from the licensee's perspective, is the continual need to update any changes in the licensing and related laws. Such update is the licensee's legal obligation in order to maintain his or her license. Also, the extra step of licensure may discourage individuals from entering certain professions.

Because of both economic and political reasons, legislatures are currently questioning the need to create more licensed professions. Certain economists have identified licensure as a factor in the rise of inflation (3). State legislatures have enacted so-called "sunset" legislation which has the sole purpose of automatically, at some prescribed date, deregulating the profession. Further, at a White House Conference on State and Local Regulatory Reform, President Carter stated:

> Regulations are quite often counterproductive. Many regulatory agencies at the local and the state government level, which I know from bitter experiences as a local and state official, and from the federal government level, protect monopolies (4).

Audiology as a Provider Discipline

Audiology, as a separate discipline, was created out of a social need to rehabilitate the thousands of injured servicemen returning from World War II who suffered hearing losses. Audiology, at that time, did not have a separate identity from the discipline of speech pathology (5). However, in the last 40 yr audiology has established its own identity, within the American Speech-Language-Hearing Association (ASHA), through its distinctive training programs and scholarship. Thus, the discipline of audiology has modeled other learned professions in its development, for its clinical training programs are sup-

ported by scholarly research, and most audiologists are members of a professional association which has established certification standards and a code of ethics.

STATE LICENSURE
The Florida Act and its Progeny

Prior to 1969, there were no licensure acts regulating the professional practices of speech-language pathologists and audiologists. The various state Speech-Language and Hearing Associations relied upon their professional code of ethics and self-regulation. However, many members of these associations were becoming alarmed by the persistent encroachment of related fields which advertized similar speech and hearing services, but without similar or any formal training and education. Also, it became clear that since professional codes of ethics had no legally binding effect, they were not as effective as licensure in promoting regulation.

On July 10, 1969, the nation's first licensure of speech pathologists and audiologists, as strongly supported by the Florida Speech and Hearing Association (FLASHA), became effective and, as seen in Table 12.1, by 1984 35 states had licensure statutes.

Licensure Provisions

The licensure acts are somewhat diverse in their rules and procedures. However, each licensure act has similar provisions such as a declaration of purpose; definitions of key words and phrases; persons exempted; a "grandfather" clause; qualifications for, and the examination of, applicants, including a provision for supportive personnel; a provision for a licensing board, and their duties and powers; a provision for the issuance of the license, and temporary license; a provision for licensure fees; the bases for expiration and renewal; a provision for reciprocal licensing; conditions for suspension and revocation; hearings and appeals; and penalties. The essential variations between state licensure acts involve the provisions

Table 12.1.
Licensed and unlicensed states

Licensed states	Unlicensed states
Alabama, Arkansas, California, Connecticut, Delaware, Florida[a], Georgia, Hawaii, Indiana, Iowa, Kentucky, Louisiana, Maine, Maryland, Massachusetts, Mississippi, Missouri, Montana, Nebraska, Nevada, New Jersey, New Mexico, New York, N Carolina, N Dakota, Ohio, Oklahoma, Oregon, Rhode Island, S Carolina, Tennessee, Texas, Utah, Virginia, Wyoming	Alaska, Arizona, Colorado, Idaho, Illinois, Kansas, Michigan, Minnesota, New Hampshire, Pennsylvania, S Dakota, Vermont, Washington, Wisconsin, W Virginia

[a] First state licensed

regulating exemptions and residency requirements, the temporary license or interim practice, reciprocity, and supportive personnel. These considerations must be addressed by audiologists providing services to industry and who move from one state to another and/or who use supportive personnel (6).

Status Exemptions

As shown in Table 12.2, all of the 35 states with licensure acts, have a provision for exempting persons based upon their status. As stated earlier, in order to receive the political and professional support from other groups, it was necessary to make certain status exemptions from licensure. Thus, physicians, and individuals who are physician supervised to perform hearing tests, such as nurses, are exempted.

The use of supportive personnel in the profession has been debated for almost 2 decades. Most hearing tests performed in

industrial hearing conservation programs (HCPs) are by audiometric technicians, a form of supportive personnel. ASHA's Committee on Supportive Personnel recently published guidelines for the employment and utilization of supportive personnel (7). This Committee outlined the prospective duties of supportive personnel which included the screening of speech, language, and/or hearing.

As seen from Table 12.2, 20 states have a provision for supportive personnel in their audiology and speech pathology licensure acts. The licensure acts do not exactly specify the qualifications of supportive personnel, who are generally referred to as audiology and speech-language pathology aides, but leave the determination of their qualifications to the state licensure boards, and their supervision to licensed speech-language pathologists and audiologists. While supportive personnel may be used by the licensed audiologist in hearing conservation pro-

Table 12.2.
Status exemption

Status	Exemption provision
Physicians	All 35 states
Nurses	All 35 states
Industrial technicians	Delaware, Iowa, Massachusetts, Mississippi, N Carolina, S Carolina, Texas
Supportive personnel	Alabama, California, Delaware, Florida, Georgia, Indiana, Iowa, Kentucky, Maine, Mississippi, Missouri, Montana, Ohio, Oklahoma, Oregon, Rhode Island, Tennessee, Texas, Utah, Virginia

grams, only seven states, according to Table 12.2, specifically provide an exemption for supervised technicians performing industrial screening.

Even if a licensure act does not specifically include a provision for supportive personnel to provide hearing tests, or to provide for an exemption for industrial audiometric technicians, this does not foreclose the possibility that the act may be interpreted to allow this activity. The attorney general of a state is the individual who has the responsibility of interpreting the legal effect of the state's licensure acts. For instance, North Dakota's State Board of Examiners of Audiology and Speech Pathology raised the following question to North Dakota's Attorney General:

> Whether persons who are not licensed can legally conduct hearing screening tests in public schools without supervision by a licensed audiologist.

North Dakota's Attorney General gave his opinion that, according to the licensure act, unlicensed persons could not lawfully conduct a hearing screening program in public schools with or without the supervision of a licensed audiologist. However, the Attorney General reasoned that the licensure act should be "construed liberally" and ruled that a "lay person" would be allowed to "assist a licensed audiologist" only under conditions of "total supervision" (8). It follows that it would be incumbent upon the audiologist responsible for HCPs in any given state to determine whether licensure statutes and regulations prohibit or limit the use of audiometric technicians who are supervised by audiologists.

Residency Exemptions

According to Table 12.3, only 16 states have temporarily waived the requirement for licensure for nonresidents who qualify for a license in that state where he or she wishes to temporarily practice. Also, 12 states have temporarily waived the requirements for licensure for a nonresident who either holds an ASHA certificate, or

a license from a state with equivalent standards. However, the qualified nonresident can only practice for a maximum number of days, generally ranging from 5–60 days. Further, 10 states require the qualified nonresident to practice in cooperation with, or supervised by, a licensed audiologist. For instance, an exemption provision in the Delaware licensure act states the following:

> The performance of speech pathology or audiology services in this State by any person not a resident of this State who is not licensed under this chapter if such services are performed for no more than 5 *days* in any calendar year and in cooperation with a speech pathologist or audiologist licensed under this chapter, and if such person meets the qualifications and requirements for application for licensure. . . However, a person not a resident of this State who is not licensed under the law of another state which has established licensure requirements at least equivalent to those established (by this chapter), or who is the holder of the Certificate of Clinical Competence of the American Speech and Hearing Association (sic) in Speech Pathology or Audiology or its equivalent, may offer speech pathology or audiology services in the State for no more than 30 *days* in any calendar year, if such services are performed in cooperation with a speech pathologist or audiologist licensed under this chapter (9) (emphasis added).

Once again, when an audiologist who is licensed or based in one state provides HCP services in another state, it would be necessary to establish what statutory or regulatory restrictions exist. Failure to do so may result in the state's Attorney General issuing an order to cease the questioned activity. If this order is ignored, the state has the discretion to levy substantial penalties, both fines and imprisonment.

Interim Practice

According to Table 12.4, 24 states allow a qualified person, or a person licensed in another state, to practice following the application for license. However, a majority of these states permit an interim practice only between the person's application and the licensure board's action on their

Table 12.3.
Residency exemption

Time period	Licensure qualified nonresident	Equivalent certificate or license
Five days	Arkansas[a], Connecticut, Delaware[a], Hawaii[a], Indiana[a], Kentucky, Maine[a], Mississippi[a], Montana[a], Texas, N Dakota[a], Wyoming	
Seven days	Alabama[a]	
Thirty days	Nebraska[a], New York	Alabama, Arkansas, Connecticut, Delaware, Hawaii, Indiana, Kentucky, Mississippi, Montana, N Dakota
Sixty days		Maine
Unspecified	Oregon	Oregon

[a] Can practice, but *only* with cooperation or supervision of licensed audiologist.

Table 12.4.
Temporary license

Period	Interim practice
Between application and board action	Alabama, Arkansas, Delaware, Kentucky, Maine, Maryland, Mississippi, Montana, Nebraska, Nevada, Ohio, Oregon, S Carolina, Tennessee, Virginia
Two months beyond examination	N Carolina, Texas
One year	Georgia, N Dakota, New Jersey
Ninety days	California, Hawaii, New Mexico
Three months	Iowa

license. Whereas, North Carolina and Texas permits an interim practice only 2 months following the applicant's examination period. The remainder of the licensing states permit a qualified person to practice, from 3 months to 1 yr, from the date of the application, independent of the examining process.

This temporary license, for the person either licensed in another state or so qualified by the ASHA certificate, easily becomes a permanent license because, 31 of the 35 states, have reciprocal licensing agreements. Thus, only four states, California, New Mexico, New York, and Oklahoma, require *all* individuals who wish to practice speech-language pathology and audiology to take a qualifying examination in order to obtain a permanent license.

PROFESSIONAL LIABILITY

All the licensure acts provide for penalties if certain provisions of the licensure act are violated. The penalties may be a fine, imprisonment, or both. For example, the penalty provision of the Texas licensure act is as follows:

(a) A person who violates any of the provisions of this Act is guilty of a Class B misdemeanor and on conviction may be punished by confinement in the county jail not exceeding 6 months, by a fine not exceeding $1000, or both.

(b) If a person other than a licensed speech-language pathologist or audiologist has engaged in any act or practice which constitutes an offense under this Act, a district court of any county on application of the committee may issue an injunction or other appropriate order restraining such conduct (10).

Assumption of Liability

However, the above statutory remedies must be sought by the state for violation of the licensure act, because the purpose of licensure is to protect the "public," and not to protect any one particular individual who may be harmed by its violation. Thus, the licensure acts do not provide any compensation for an individual consumer who may have been harmed by the statutory violation. The consumer must rely upon the legal principles of negligence in order to receive compensation. When a person holds himself or herself out to another as having a special expertise with special standards of practice, and then fails to follow these standards, creating an injury, the law allows the injured person to be compensated for this harm.

Professional Malpractice

The increase in professional liability litigation, for speech-language pathologists and audiologists, parallels the growth of private practice. In this respect, private practice, having the advantages of promoting an autonomous profession and public recognition, has the disadvantage of exposing oneself to lawsuit. Thus, for instance, when the audiologist provides professional services, within an HCP, he or she has no choice but to assume the liability for any direct or indirect harm caused by his or her negligent acts of omissions or commissions.

Negligence is within the area of tort law and the remedies, to compensate a harm, are civil and not criminal. Tort law prescribes rules which have been molded by custom and tradition. Frequently, these rules are formalized in statutes. As a rule, society relies upon the judge to interpret the uncodified law and to apply the legal traditions consistently, from case to case. Frequently, these judge-made rules change with the changing social mores.

When a professional embarks to provide services, he or she adopts the standards of the profession, which are separate from the standards of the lay individual. The professional assumes a legal duty to the client to adhere to these standards.

There has been a tremendous increase in the number of professional malpractice lawsuits filed in the last 20 yr. This increase has been primarily in the medical profession. The size of the damage awards has also increased, which has required physicians to either obtain costly malpractice insurance or even to curtail certain areas of their practice.

In one particular case, a patient/plaintiff filed a lawsuit against a defendant orthopaedic surgeon and alleged that the surgeon had failed to recognize and treat circulatory problems which led to the amputation of the plaintiff's leg (11). It is clear that the plaintiff suffered great damages but there remained the question of the defendant's liability. The extent of damages, in a malpractice case, is not as difficult to ascertain as is the issue of liability. A lay jury, and not experts, must decide which facts are relevant when weighing the question of fault. The jury system of justice is placed under great stress when lay jurors are required to assimilate complex medical procedures, about which experts sometimes disagree as to their appropriateness within a given set of circumstances. In this particular case, the jury heard testimony regarding the standards of treatment of the plaintiff's condition as well as testimony regarding the defendant's failure to pass certification examinations administered by the American Board of Orthopaedic Surgeons. Therefore, when a professional is charged with malpractice, the door is opened to public scrutiny of his or her professional practices, as well as training and education.

In order for a plaintiff to be compensated for any harm caused by the professional, or defendant, the following elements of negligence must be established:

1. There must be proof of the existence of the professional relationship which created the duty, or standard of care
2. There must be evidence of a breach of this duty
3. A connection must be made between the breach of the duty and the harm to the client
4. There must be evidence of the harm itself

Each aspect of the negligence formula

must be satisfied before the plaintiff is allowed any recovery.

In the area of professional negligence or malpractice, the standard of care has been described as follows:

1. The law implies that the practitioner represents that he or she possesses the degree of learning and skill ordinarily possessed by practitioners in the locality where he or she practices. Therefore, the requirement is not to possess extraordinary learning and skill but that the practitioner is bound to keep abreast of the times.
2. It is also the duty of the practitioner to use reasonable care and diligence in the exercise of his or her skill. The duty is to provide ordinary and reasonable care and the practitioner is not required to exercise the highest possible degree of care.
3. Finally, the law holds a practitioner liable for an injury to his or her patient resulting from lack of the requisite knowledge and skill, or the omission to exercise reasonable care, or the failure to use his or her best judgment. Therefore, if the practitioner departs from approved methods in general use and so injures the patient, liability is incurred. The liability arises not only from diagnosis and treatment but also from giving instructions to the patient which results in injury (12).

This standard of care is appropriate for the general practitioner and not the specialist. The general practitioner is held to a community standard, which has been referred to as the "locality" rule, whereas the specialist is held to a national standard of care.

This difference in standard has some practical importance in determining whether the plaintiff will be successful. The plaintiff, in a professional malpractice lawsuit, is required to support his or her claim with the testimony of a qualified expert. The expert is needed because the technical aspects of the claim are generally beyond the competence of the lay jurors. If the "locality" rule is appropriate, the plaintiff may have some difficulty obtaining favorable expert testimony. However, if the plaintiff can show that a na-tional standard is appropriate, the plaintiff will not have the potential disadvantage of the professional bias of a community expert, and can seek experts nationally.

The audiologist, as a member of a health profession, will be held to the standard of care similar to that of the physician. The standard will be a national standard of care because the audiologist should be viewed as possessing a special expertise, which does not differ from community to community. Thus, the audiologist must not only possess the necessary training and knowledge, in order to serve the client's hearing health care needs, but also must concentrate on reducing his or her exposure to lawsuit. This limitation of liability occurs through the understanding of the legal aspects of audiological practice, which includes such elements as obtaining malpractice insurance and seeking corporation status (13).

The audiologist who establishes an HCP, assumes the liability for any injury which may occur as a result of this program. Thus, it is critical that the elements of audiological practice are monitored closely in order to minimize the risk of injury to clients. The following techniques and procedures are common elements of audiological practice:

1. Performing tests of audiological assessment
2. Interpreting audiometric tests
3. Counseling patients as to appropriate rehabilitation strategies
4. Developing and implementing such strategies
5. Placing and stabilizing instrumentation on patients
6. Placing patients in an electrical and acoustically treated environments
7. Implementation of appropriate business practices such as to insure that equipment is working properly, to maintain records, to issue consent and medical release of information forms, to induce referrals, and to administer program and personnel (13).

Since the purpose of an HCP is the

prevention and detection of hearing loss, proper interpretation of the audiogram is critical for the success of the program. It should be pointed out that even though an HCP is mandated by the federal government, there is nothing within this federal legislation which eliminates or reduces the liability of the audiologist performing hearing conservation tasks.

The legal liability which may occur as a result of faulty or negligent interpretation of audiograms is entirely dependent upon the quality of harm which is a result of this negligence. The possible harms which can result are as follows:

1. Financial harm to the contractor of the hearing conservation services, which results in the audiometric evaluations having to be repeated by another service
2. Financial harm to the employee, if the employer, based upon the audiologist's interpretation, transfers the employee to a lower paying position
3. Financial harm to the employee for loss of potential Worker's Compensation and Social Security Benefits
4. The potential aggravation of the hearing loss due to the employee being further exposed to noise due to faulty audiometric interpretation
5. The potential damage to the employee's health arising as a consequence of failure of the professional to advise an employer of the need for professional evaluation of the employee's hearing

Malpractice Insurance

Of course, these predictions of harm are speculative. Today, audiologists are not typically being named as defendants in malpractice lawsuits. However, insurance claims have been filed against audiologists alleging acts of malpractice. Such claims have included allegations of negligence in applying electric shocks during an electrodermal response audiometric procedure, negligence in not informing a treating physician of the results of an audiometric exam, negligence in performing a hearing aid evaluation which led to a further hearing loss, and negligence as part of the team involved in the diagnosis and treatment of an acoustic neurinoma,

which resulted in the death of the patient (13).

It is clear that the audiologist, in private practice, should obtain malpractice insurance. Although the majority of lawsuits are settled and do not go to trial, when a claim is made, the insurance carrier has the duty to defend, assuming that the alleged act of malpractice was within the scope of the insurance agreement between the carrier and the audiologist.

The typical malpractice insurance policy is a "Claims-Made" policy. The insurer or carrier agrees to pay off claims which arise from the performance of professional services which are first made against the professional or insured, and reported to the insurer while the policy is in force. Therefore, if a claim is reported to the insurer after the expiration of the policy, even if the alleged acts occurred during the life of the policy, the insurer will not typically honor the claim. This, of course, places the insured at great financial risk if a claim is made after the insured's policy has expired. Other aspects of a typical malpractice policy include provisions: detailing the coverage for liability, including the insurer's duty to defend; stating when the policy does not apply or the exclusions; describing the limits of liability; and outlining the steps the insured should take if a legal claim is made against him or her.

The insured must read over the policy very carefully because it should be remembered that the insurance company is selling insurance and not giving away protection. The major problem the insured will have, after a claim is filed against him or her, is when the insurer denies that it has a duty to defend the claim. This conflict can possibly be avoided if it is clear to the insured what the exclusions to coverage are, and if the premiums are kept up to date. Also, the insured must strictly adhere to the claims reporting procedures. If the insurer refuses to defend the insured, the insured is faced with two lawsuits, one lawsuit as the defendant in a malpractice claim, and the other as a plaintiff in a claim against the insurance company for refusing to defend the first lawsuit. Therefore, even though the value of malpractice insurance cannot be overstated, there are some pitfalls of which the audiologist should be made aware. Notwithstanding the relative probability of being named as a defendant in a lawsuit, the audiologist must appreciate his or her legal responsibilities and promote proper risk management procedures in order to eliminate or reduce the exposure to liability and of successful litigation.

Supportive Personnel Liability

The licensure acts clearly state that while supportive personnel are exempted from licensure, they must be supervised by licensed professionals. While supportive personnel are still responsible for their own acts of negligence, the licensed audiologist, who employs industrial audiometric technicians, for instance, also incurs liability for their negligence. In an employer/employee relationship, the law recognizes the fact that the employer controls the acts of the employee, by establishing the place of employment, the time period of employment, procedures and practices for the delivery of services and the use of equipment, and the payment of wages and benefits. Thus, the employer is liable for any negligent act of his or her employee, assuming that the employee was acting within the scope of the employment agreement.

Employer liability means that if a lawsuit is filed against the industrial technician, the audiologist/employer will also be named as a defendant to the lawsuit. It is possible that the audiologist could pay the entire judgment or settlement if the employee does not have the means to pay, or if the employee cannot be found. Thus, it is critical that the licensed professional has established policies and procedures for their employees.

Subcontractor Liability

A subcontractor, or independent contractor, does not have the above employer/employee relationship. It is possible that an HCP, in certain situations, is more effective when licensed professionals establish a contractor/subcontractor relationship. For instance, the contractor, an audiologist, may have established mobile audiological services and, because of efficiency, subcontracts the interpretation of the audiograms to another qualified audiologist.

Generally, the contractor is not liable for the negligent acts of its subcontractors. However, the contractor should clearly limit its liability to its own acts, and not of the subcontractor's, by incorporating this following clause in the contract outlining the relationship between the contractor and subcontractor:

> The subcontractor shall hold the contractor harmless from any penalties or other liability arising from performance by the subcontractor of this agreement

Establishing Business Practices

Until recently, there appears to have been a general reluctance for speech-language pathologist and audiologists to enter private practice because of financial and professional uncertainties of success. However, with the new Federal Hearing Conservation Amendment, new opportunities have been created for private practice.

The most effective and efficient means of reducing the exposure to liability is by establishing business practices. There are many pragmatic aspects of business to consider, such as a business name and its registration with local and state governments; a business bank account, and the identifying federal employee tax number; a business location, including specifications for office space, furniture and equipment; how to obtain small business loans; the need to consider the evaluation, salaries and fringe benefits for personnel; establishing business forms; accounting practices, and fees and billing; advertising; and client relations. Further, establishing a business identity requires knowledge of basic legal relations including the understanding of third-party insurance, business contracts, the advantages and disadvantages of incorporation, and the need to obtain professional malpractice insurance.

Contract Negotiations

The most important business contracts are those which establish and expand the business practice itself. A contract is a legally enforceable agreement to do, or not to do, a specific thing. Since a contract can either be expressed, in writing or orally, or implied, they impose inherent dangers when parties interact within a business environment. These dangers include:

1. Agreements claimed by one party to be a contract where the other party disagrees
2. Contracts so unclear as to be interpreted contrary to what one party intended
3. Contracts neglecting to cover one or more of the main points
4. Contracts impossible of performance because of external impediments

There are at least four stages in transactions involving business contracts: negotiation of the terms; drafting documents reflecting these terms; the administration of contracts; and the possible litigation to either enforce, avoid or to find out their meaning. A valid contract is created when it is based upon a lawful objective; when there are legally competent parties who are at the age of majority and are mentally competent; when there is a mutual agreement as to its purpose and terms, with evidence of an offer by one party and an acceptance by the other; when each party gives consideration to the other in order to support the agreement, such as a promise to do something or to forbear from doing something, in exchange for a promise or money.

Negotiating a contract requires the following elements:

1. One should be fully prepared before entering an agreement, and should learn all that is possible about the contemplated transaction
2. The essential points, or terms, of the contract should be established such as, the parties, the duration of the contract, how the contract should be performed, the payment and how it is to be made, any representations or warranties, and any waivers of liability
3. There should be an analysis of the risks and benefits of the transaction throughout the contract negotiation
4. There should be a measure of flexibility because a perfect agreement is not realistically attainable

Professional Service Contract

One of the most important contractual negotiations in which an industrial audiologist can engage in is the contract for the professional services themselves. Figure 12.1 is an example of a contract to provide professional audiological services within an HCP.

According to Figure 12.1, the industrial audiologist should secure an exclusive right to provide hearing conservation services. The terms and conditions of the professional service contract will vary according to any special needs the parties may have. However, such terms as the time period of contracting, the type of services rendered, pricing and mode of payment are the basic terms which should be included in any agreement. Also included within the agreement should be any requirements as to space, power and similar matters for which the client would be responsible.

FORENSICS

One measure of the autonomy of a profession is the establishment of its legal identity in the judicial system as experts to be employed in the resolution of legal disputes. The application of audiological data for legal purposes is within the area of forensic audiology.

HCP, Inc. a Michigan corporation, having its offices at 1000 White Road, Detroit, Michigan, (hereinafter called HCP) as exclusive licensee for the providing a hearing conservation program, and _____ (specify company), corporation having offices _____ (specify place of incorporation), (hereinafter called "Client") hereby make this agreement for the purpose of performing audiometric tests on Client's employees, and evaluating Client employee audiograms. For this purpose the parties agree as follows:

1. Hearing Conservation Services

   a. Client grants to HCP for the period of this agreement and subject to the terms and conditions thereof the exclusive right to perform audiometric tests on the premises of Client's property, in an area mutually agreed upon by the parties.

   b. Client grants to HCP for the period of this agreement and subject to the terms and conditions thereof the exclusive right to evaluate said audiometric tests.

   c. HCP agrees to provide its own audiometric equipment and shall be responsible for its maintenance and repair.

2. Terms

The initial terms of this Agreement shall be _____ year(s) commencing _____. At the end of the _____ year period, the Agreement shall automatically be renewed for additional _____ periods unless one party hereto notifies the other of its intention to terminate the Agreement at the end of the current period by notice in writing delivered before the expiration of such period. Client agrees that during each year of this Agreement at least _____ (number of employees) Client employees will be audiometrically tested and at least _____ audiograms will be available for evaluation.

3. Cost of Services

   The cost of audiometric testing per each Client employee is _____. Such cost includes the evaluation of each employee's audiogram. The cost of the audiogram evaluation only is _____ per audiogram. Changes in said costs shall be effective upon mailing of notice thereof by HCP to Client.

4. Payments

   Client will agree to compensate HCP for its services by check within (10) days after receipt of audiometric data or evaluations of said data.

5. Applicable Law

   This Agreement shall be governed in all respects by the laws of the State of Michigan.

6. Additional Terms

   All other additional terms and conditions relating to this Agreement shall be subsequently agreed upon between the parties hereto in writing.

IN WITNESS WHEREOF, the parties hereto have executed this Agreement the day and year first above mentioned.

IN THE PRESENCE OF:

_____

_____
HCP, President

_____
CLIENT, President

Figure 12.1 Sample professional service contract

Application of Audiological Data to the Law

Audiological data can be employed within the legal system to establish the following:

1. Evidence of the effects of otolytic agents, such as, trauma, drugs, disease, age, hereditary effects, and noise, to be employed by the plaintiff or defendant in personal injury claims
2. Evidence of social disability, to be employed to support a claim for Social Security Disability benefits, as regulated by the Federal Social Security Act
3. Evidence of employment disability, to be employed to support a claim for state Worker's Compensation Benefits
4. Evidence of a handicapping condition, to be employed to support special educational and rehabilitative services, as provided for by such federal legislation as the Rehabilitation Act of 1973, and the Education for All Handicapped Children Act of 1975 (14).

Testifying in Medico-Legal Matters

Typically, the audiologist would testify to provide evidence for the purposes of resolving workers's compensation and personal injury claims. The legal system is replete with its own special rules and procedures which the audiologist, as an expert, should be familiar with.

What the Professional Should Know

The most complicated procedures are the rules of evidence, in both the state and federal court systems. The type of evidence an expert gives is called opinion evidence and is obtained during the "discovery" process prior to trial. Typically, this evidence is taken in a deposition. "Discovery" is that time period specifically allowed for the litigating parties to discover the facts upon which the claim is based. In this period, the expert may be asked to either voluntarily give sworn testimony, in the form of an oral deposition, or will be subpoenaed by the court to provide such testimony. A deposition is the taking of oral testimony, under oath, prior to the trial. It is a potent tool of "discovery" which attorneys employ to prepare for trial or for a settlement.

A lay person is prohibited from giving opinion evidence at a deposition, or at trial, and is generally restricted to giving evidence strictly within his or her knowledge. However, the purpose of expert testimony is to give an opinion, based upon the expert's knowledge, experience, or training. The basis for expert testimony is on the facts of the particular case and not upon mere conjecture. Further, the opinion must not be based on evidence consisting of the opinions inferences or conclusions of other witnesses.

An expert has a "property right" in his or her opinion. This means that the expert cannot be compelled by a subpoena to give an opinion. On the other hand, if the expert knows of relevant facts of the case, he or she can be compelled by a subpoena to testify. Since the expert's opinion is a "property right," if the opposing party takes the deposition of the expert, the court may order the expert to be paid.

The technique in providing expert testimony will vary, as a function of the expert's personality, experience and the level of preparation of the individual questioning the expert. Expert testimony is not only used to describe the actual events involving the claim, but to have the expert make certain predictions, in the form of hypothetical questions. The hypothetical question is an artful device employed to clarify the salient issues of the claim.

The audiologist, as expert, should never give sworn testimony without a full understanding of the facts of the claim, and until there has been an opportunity to fully discuss the purpose of his or her testimony with the employing party. It should always be remembered that the sworn testimony creates a public record. This public record can be referred to in cases other than the case it was intended. Thus, the effectiveness of the expert, for future cases, may very well be compromised if there is a past public record of uncomplimentary testimony.

Proper preparation, prior to giving expert testimony, is critical because the legal setting is adversarial. It does not matter if the particular audiologist, as expert, has good intentions and is providing honest testimony if he or she appears to lack credibility. The purpose of cross-examination is to weaken favorable testimony. The opposing side will attempt to chip away at the testimony of the audiological expert by seeking to limit or expose, as inadequate, this expertise.

This potential weakening of valuable expert testimony can be avoided if the following aspects of the examination process are understood:

1. The witness is entitled to a clear, simple and understandable question. The question should not be answered unless it is 100% understood. Always ask to have the question repeated
2. If possible, always answer the question with a simple "yes" or "no." Such an answer, obviously, leaves little room for misinterpretation
3. Only respond to what the question requires and do not volunteer any extra information. You may be opening up areas which may weaken your testimony
4. Do not rush to answer the question
5. Do not let an overzealous questioner anger you. This results in loss of concentration and your testimony may appear less credible before a jury
6. You are allowed to refresh your memory with any relevant record or document

Qualifying the Expert

Prior to being sworn to give testimony at the deposition or trial, the audiologist will have to be "qualified" as an individual who can provide expert testimony. One is qualified as an expert if he or she provides evidence of the requisite education, training or experience. In order to save time and embarrassment, the audiologist, as expert, should inquire as to whether he or she has the proper qualifi-

cations to provide the testimony desired by the employing party.

SUMMARY

Hearing conservation programs offer the audiologist the opportunity to pursue private practice. Private practice requires more effort and commitment to professional excellence due to the added responsibilities of maintaining a business. Therefore, the industrial audiologist, as a private practitioner, must be knowledgeable in the area of state licensure laws and regulations; the legal aspects of professional negligence; business practices, including contracting and liability insurance; and forensic audiology.

As seen from the review of state licensure, there are states that are restrictive on the practice of audiology and do not have provisions for temporary licenses, residency exemptions, supportive personnel, and reciprocity. Therefore, it cannot be assumed that the state licensure laws are uniform. Further, since there has been a striking increase in professional malpractice lawsuits, the audiologist should become litigation minded and strictly adhere to a national standard of audiological practice. While professional autonomy appears, at first glance, to be a very attractive alternative to an employer/employee relationship, it can prove to be a professional and personal disaster if the audiologist does not seriously consider its pitfalls. It is hoped that this chapter will provide some guidance in this particular area.

References

1. Webster's New World Dictionary, 2nd College Edition, Guralnik DB (ed). New York, World Publishing, 1976.
2. Waltz J, Inbau F: Medical Jurisprudence. New York, MacMillan 1971, p 17.
3. Dolan AK: Occupational licensure and obstruction of change in the health care delivery system: some recent developments. In Blair RD, Rubin S (eds): Regulating the Professions. Lexington, Mass, Lexington Books, 1980.
4. Weekly Compilation of Presidential Documents, vol 16, no 21, pp 25–65, Monday, January 14, 1980.
5. Doefler L: A short history of audiology and aural rehabilitation. ASHA, 23:858, 1981.

6. Williams P: *State Requirements for Supportive Personnel, Technicians, and Audiologists.* (Unpublished paper presented at the National Hearing Conservation Assoc. (6th Annual Meeting), Feb. 18, 1982; State Legislation for Speech-Language Pathology and Audiology, American Speech-Language-Hearing Association, 1979.

7. Committee on Supportive Personnel: Guidelines for the employment and utilization of supportive personnel. *ASHA*, 23:165–169, 1981.

8. State of North Dakota, Attorney General's Opinion 81-17, February 26, 1981.

9. Delaware Code Annotated 24 §3701 et seq. at §7044(6).

10. Vernon's Texas Civil Statute, Art. 4512, Sec. 18.

11. *Belobradich v Sarnethsiri*, Michigan Court of Appeals, No. 64573 (1984).

12. *Pike v Honsinger*, 155 NY 201, 1898.

13. Muraski A: Legal aspects of audiological practice. In Kramer MB, Armbruster JM (eds): *Forensic Audiology* Baltimore, University Park Press, 1982.

14. Muraski, A: Forensic audiology. *Audiol: A J Cont Ed* 7(10), 1982.

CHAPTER 13

Marketing Hearing Conservation Services to Industry

JEFFREY C. MORRILL and JEFFREY E. COPELAND

MARKETING CONCEPT

Any business organization must sell products or services to survive and ultimately prosper. Growth of the business depends upon various intertwined activities leading to the successful completion of a sale. Often the most important activity in the organization is marketing. Marketing activities directly or indirectly help to sell the products or services.

Selling established products or services is primary to the marketing effort. The financial rewards generated by sales can be used to develop other related product lines or services to fill the needs of the market. In so doing, the business enterprise is able to adapt to changing needs, and therefore, to better satisfy the customers. Generation of additional profits is attained, which is the end result of any successful business whether it is a small grocery store, a large multinational manufacturing firm or an industrial hearing conservation service. Remarkably, each has marketing as the common denominator to achieve the organization's goal: profit.

The importance of marketing in any business organization is easily understood. But, what is marketing? Since marketing consists of a multitude of activities, a definition is difficult to commit to a single sentence. Marketing textbooks have struggled at length, often creating paragraphs of definitions encompassing all facets of marketing activities. Sales and the buy decision rest with the decision of humans. Therefore, our definition of marketing encompasses one fostered in human behavior. "Marketing is human activity directed towards satisfying needs and wants through any exchange process" (1).

Marketing as a business discipline originates in human needs and wants. Humans need oxygen, food, water, clothing, safety, and shelter to survive, but humans want education, recreation, power, family, and luxuries to live comfortably. A human need is not created by society nor by marketing, but does exist as a result of human biology. Wants consist of desires for specific satisfaction of needs. An individual needs food, but wants lobster; needs clothing, but wants a suit for every day of the week; and needs shelter, but buys a house with a large mortgage.

These distinctions help dispel the frequent societal claim that marketing creates needs or that marketing prompts people to buy things they really don't need. Needs are not created by marketing, needs exist before marketing. Marketing, with the assistance of other influential individuals in our society, specifically influences wants. It effectively illuminates in the human mind how a particular product or service would satisfy the stated need. Marketing must influence an individual's intention to buy by making the product or service affordable, attractive and readily available.

Marketing of Products and Services

The broad category of products are prompted and developed from the existence of human needs and wants. A product is something capable of satisfying a need or want. Products are comprised of objects, services, places, ideas and organizations. Needs and wants do not define marketing alone. A third element must be added. This element is the process of exchange (1).

The exchange process requires two parties and each party has something mutually valuable. Secondly, each party must have open communication and something of value available. Last, each party must be free to accept or reject the offer. If, upon examination of the above conditions, both parties are better off or at least no worse off than before, exchange is possible.

A product, as stated earlier, can be a good, a service or an idea. A physical object is a good, while a service results from the human and mechanical effort to satisfy societal want.

Industrial hearing conservation is a marketing service employing physical products with technical knowledge. The marketing of this service must be viewed with the same philosophy as marketing a physical instrument. The challenge rests in marketing the abilities of the industrial hearing conservation firm in terms of technical expertise, experience in professional review of audiograms, consultation experience for program supervision, etc. The intangibles create the challenge for both the industrial hearing consultant and the client, who looks to the consultant's expertise to satisfy a critical want. The want projected by the client may result from a need to satisfy current governmental regulations, a fear of potential workmen's compensation awards or a genuine interest in providing additional employee health benefits to keep a trained individual on the job, thereby maximizing company profits. Regardless of the client's motive, the marketing of the hearing conservation service must be skillfully targeted to the specified want. The marketing efforts must be directed at creating a service that is appropriate, affordable and readily available.

Human tendency is to avoid risk. All marketing efforts put forth by the industrial hearing conservation firm must alleviate any client doubt that the service offered potentially increases risk.

MARKETING OF SERVICES VS MARKETING OF PHYSICAL PRODUCTS

The marketing and sales of services is much more difficult than the marketing and sales of physical products due to the intangibility of services compared to products. It is hard for management to visualize differences in expertise, dedication, training, skill, and ability—all of which are key concepts in selling a service. These are intangibles, therefore, the sales effort must be extremely creative in order to illuminate only the most salient and exemplary facts. The service must be presented as a product and defined in terms of quality, workmanship, technology, and dependability.

Products are most often sold on demonstration, where the buyer can experience and observe the features of the device. It would be difficult to sell an automobile or a copy machine on a verbal presentation alone. Services must be sold in the same manner. Many "tools of the trade" can be carried to sales meetings for demonstration. For example, a representative of an industrial hearing conservation firm would carry otoscopes, ear protectors, audiograms, computer reports, training materials, and noise measuring equipment. Photographs or illustrations (preferably in professionally prepared brochures) representing all phases of each program component are essential to communicate the realism of the service and bridge the gap of intangibility.

Presentation materials should be informative, factual and well documented in order to add substance and "feel" to the sales presentation. For example, a high-lighted copy of the OSHA regulation will quickly resolve any questions relative to requirements. If otoscopics are being discussed, a few photographs of otoscopically observed ear problems and OSHA's recommendations on otoscopics will quickly validate the importance of performing them (2). Any discussion on workers compensation should be accompanied by copies of the state's compensation laws on hearing loss, which illuminate potential loss liability, and a comparison of other states with greater dollar values to show trends. This approach gives credence to the presentation, leaves little doubt that the salesperson knows the technical aspects of the business, and helps establish the importance of the program concept.

MOTIVATING FACTORS IN ESTABLISHING A HEARING CONSERVATION PROGRAM

Historically, the market for hearing conservation services in industry is stimulated by the threat of workers compensation claims from occupationally induced hearing loss and from federal or state regulations mandating programs to protect workers. These continue to be the moving forces behind management's consideration in developing and maintaining industrial hearing conservation programs. American business is now motivated to implement appropriate hearing conservation programs to minimize potential liabilities and protect the bottom line profits.

Ideally, hearing conservation should be offered as a component of an employee benefit program in order to emphasize the importance of hearing in our daily lives. Unfortunately, the insidious nature of hearing loss stimulates little interest toward developing voluntary preventive programs. Other preventive programs such as safety glasses, hard hats, safety shoes, and machine guards are easier to sell to management as the resulting injuries from lack of these programs are immediately apparent. In addition, these discrete accidents create lost work time, damage the corporate image, and commonly result in payment of workers compensation benefits.

In contrast to these visibly catastrophic accidents, the damage from noise exposure is invisible and, except for the deafened person, goes unnoticed. Although millions of workers are affected by noise exposure, hearing loss due to noise seldom causes lost work time and rarely results in workers compensation claims in relation to the potential compensable claims that exist. Therefore, the sense of urgency to implement hearing conservation programs simply has never emerged.

While the OSHA noise regulation has enhanced industry's awareness of the need, it has done little to stimulate management enthusiasm to support hearing conservation programs. Hearing conservation programs are often viewed as an expense rather than an investment by most of American industry. By comparison, other more traditional preventive programs, such as those mentioned earlier, have complete management support, interest and participation. For example, no one is allowed to enter a designated area in a factory without safety glasses or hard hats, but entry into a hazardous noise area without ear protection is the rule rather than the exception.

DEVELOPING COMPLIANCE WITH HEARING CONSERVATION PROGRAMS

It is easy to legislate the requirements to conduct these programs, but it is impossible to enforce the actual day-to-day implementation of them through regulation alone. Effective compliance must come from management's interest and support, and the worker's desire to voluntarily participate. Management is stimulated by a fear of profit reduction due to potential compensation claims, while employee support must be generated through education.

The changes in awareness and attitudes

must transcend the entire spectrum of those involved: employee, employer, institutions, and OSHA itself, in order to generate a more total acceptance of hearing conservation. Hearing conservation may appear to be a program with no apparent benefits. In fact, it often creates employee complaints, slows production during implementation, and, although infrequently, may stimulate some initial workers compensation claims. Often management is very reluctant to "open Pandora's box" and, without good reason to do otherwise, still do little more than is necessary to meet federal requirements.

NECESSITY FOR CONSULTATIVE ASSISTANCE

With the exception of the larger corporate entities, very few companies possess the internal capabilities to perform many of the required technical aspects to achieve effective hearing conservation programs. In fact, nearly all companies are in need of at least some outside professional services to develop or maintain their hearing conservation programs.

The various program components which may be considered needs and wants by American business and available for exchange include:

1. Noise measurement and analysis
2. Noise engineering and control
3. Audiometric testing
4. Technician training and certification
5. Professional review of audiograms
6. Computerized data management systems and record analysis
7. Employee education and training
8. Selection and training in the use of personal ear protection
9. Medical/legal evaluation and expert witness
10. Employee counseling and referral

However, the one program component which must be developed in-house is the day-to-day supervision and administration of ear protection utilization. The above services definitely illuminate the diverse marketing complexities and opportunities afforded the industrial hearing conservation firm.

In today's litigious business atmosphere, it is probable that outside providers of service can bear contingent liability for program problems. Therefore, the services to be offered should be limited to those where expertise and modern technology can be assured. The industrial hearing conservation firm must make certain that its abilities and expertise allow for the successful avoidance of industrial hearing conservation program pitfalls. This is essential before accepting responsibility for any program component.

MARKET STRATEGY DEVELOPMENT

The industrial market for hearing conservation services has been outlined. How should the hearing conservation firm approach fulfilling these needs? The key to successful marketing rests upon an educated marketing strategy. A marketing strategy forms the foundation of a successful marketing plan. It outlines the plan of action. The marketing strategy must answer the question: how best shall we use the strengths and resources of our organization to meet its own objectives and best meet the needs and wants of our target market (3)?

A target market consists of companies for whom the industrial hearing conservation firm creates and maintains the marketing mix that specifically fits the needs and preferences of that group. A marekting mix consists of four essential elements: product, place, price, and promotion (4).

Obviously, a marketing mix must be in place before marketing efforts begin. Let's look at each component.

Product

The product line can only be as diverse as the expertise of the firm. The wide array of potential hearing conservation services to be marketed has already been outlined. Most industries will need a combination of those services; few will need all. The realistic and honest investigation of the industrial hearing conservation firm's strengths will clearly illuminate those hearing conservation services which the firm can successfully offer the industrial client. Weaknesses will preclude offering the full range unless proper steps are taken to alleviate those weaknesses. A jack of all trades, but a master of none has no room in the professional hearing conservation consultant area.

Place

Place encompasses the marketing geographical area serviced. The resources of the hearing consultant firm will be the limiting factor. Money and people are two key resources. A critical inventory of the resources will outline the geographic market one serves. By successfully marketing the hearing conservation service in the area governed by current resources, profitability will beget growth and growth will beget resources. Resources allow for the controlled geographic expansion to address the needs of incremental businesses. Geographic limitations should be defined based upon current resources.

Price

Resources cost dollars. The service provided must be exchanged at a price level to assure profitability and insure that the industrial client is better off with the affordable service than without the service. It is important to remember that selling at a loss is a precursor to bankruptcy. A potential client always wishes to reduce risk. Assuring your business is profitable reduces the client's risk immensely, as your firm demonstrates it will be around next year to service the everchanging needs and wants of the client.

Promotion

Effective communication is critical to the marketing exchange process. Earlier, the importance and relevance of brochures, pictures and other sales aides to put industrial hearing conservation service in terms of a product were explained. The desired end result must be effective promotion, i.e., effective communication (5).

WHO IS THE CLIENT?

Once the marketing mix has been put in place, identification of those companies with the needs and wants of your specific service is necessary. The current legislative environment governed by the March 8, 1983 OSHA regulation (see Appendix I) specifically highlights all industry subjected to 85 dB time-weighted average (TWA) for 8 hr requiring a hearing conservation program (6). These companies must then be identified and approached. Their specific wants or preferences must be satisfied by offering a service that leaves both parties better off than if neither had met. Exchange will be impossible unless this marketing phenomena occurs.

Industry varies in size and scope. Employees in small industries often wear many hats, whereas large industries maintain specific departments employing specialists. The industrial hearing conservation consultant or marketer must be well prepared to speak with plant managers, personnel managers, safety directors, occupational health nurses and physicians, industrial hygienists, audiologists or, perhaps, the president of the company.

Recognition of the target customer and the management team within is primary in identifying the decision maker. The marketer must be prepared to assist anyone in the company to discuss the hearing conservation needs of that company relative to the satisfaction of those needs by the hearing conservation firm's services.

FOCUS ON THE BENEFITS DERIVED FROM A PROGRAM

Recognition of the need for a hearing conservation program is often clear. However, it may be perceived to be less important than other safety programs to the prospective purchaser of services. It is essential that the client be made aware of the short-term and long-term value of the purchase. Thus, the presentation must center around benefits to the employer and how the various services will allow for a return on the investment.

For example, touting professional credentials will have little importance unless they can be translated to some actual benefit to the buyer. Without a knowledge of what an audiologist's training actually is, there is little point in discussing academic credentials. What is important is that a program requirement for a supervising audiologist exists and the consultant or the client firm possesses those credentials. Otherwise, valuable sales time will be spent in educating the person on what an audiologist is, or convincing the client that one consultant's expertise is greater than another. That only creates insecurity and potential animosity. Of course, professional credentials can be rather important in compensation or OSHA litigation. However, care must be exercised in discussing these potential consequences to avoid "scare tactic" selling.

Any program aspects that cannot be directly attributed to the outcome of a successful program should not be discussed in a sales meeting. The prospective buyer may perceive extras as frills that result in expenses that are being paid for, but not really needed. A summary of some benefits which a comprehensive approach to hearing conservation will offer are listed in the following objectives of a hearing conservation program:

Hearing Conservation Program Objectives

1. Protection of the employee against hearing loss and ear disease
2. Protection of the employer against a loss of image and profits which result from medico-legal situations such as:
   Lawsuits
   Workers' compensation claims
   OSHA citations
   Loss of employee productivity
   Hearing or noise-related accidents
   Potential union problems

3. Compliance with all federal (OSHA) and state regulations that insure the maximum protection for both employee and employer

It is essential that the sales presentation and materials address how each of these objectives will be met through the various program aspects being presented for purchase or, alternately, how they will not be met in a partial program or simplified approach. Hearing conservation is a sound investment for industry, if done properly. It is only an expense if approached unprofessionally.

HEARING PROFESSIONAL AS A MARKETING PERSON

The marketing and sales of professional services by hearing professionals (i.e. audiologists, physicians and otolaryngologists) presents a very unique, and often frustrating, situation. The individual who is best qualified to represent the service is perhaps the least capable of selling it. Unless that individual has had prior sales experience, or has had the opportunity to receive formal sales training, the road to success may be difficult. If all people selling hearing conservation services were hearing professionals, it would be less of a problem for both industry and the seller. However, the hearing conservation industry has become extremely competitive and, in addition to the hearing professional, experienced professional sales people have also been attracted to the market place. It would be ideal if those sales people were matched with programs conducted by hearing professionals offering a comprehensive approach to hearing conservation.

The hearing professional must begin to respond like a professional salesperson or otherwise accept the frequent consequence of losing a contract because of differences in presentation rather than differences in program. In fact, the professional salesperson may obtain the sale with an inferior service and less real program capabilities. There may also be a lack of knowledge and understanding of the actual program needs and future consequences for the client.

Hearing professionals generally have a strong tendency to illuminate the details of what will happen to employees in the presence of noise and the problems associated in controlling the various program aspects, such as workers compensation cases. That may be the reality of the situation and it may be professionally accurate and appropriate; however, these truths raise issues which illustrate the problems rather than the benefits of achieving the controls necessary to prevent potential employee noise-induced hearing loss.

The employer needs an effective hearing conservation program. The consultant must market the tools necessary for the employees to accept and bless the program. For example, the experienced professional knows the necessity for detailed employee education on all aspects of noise, hearing conservation, human aspects and ear protection utilization in order to achieve voluntary compliance in the hearing conservation program and to avoid employee compensation claims. The professional understands the importance of instructing the client's employees in a formal setting separate from the hearing test. This critical program aspect is a tool that must be communicated to the employer.

To further illustrate the sales problem, consider the situation of two diverse sales approaches on this issue. The hearing professional presents the situation as described above. It is comprehensive and professional, but it is also complex and expensive. Contrast this to the salesperson who may present quite a different solution to the problem. This approach suggests that employee education can, in fact, be accomplished in a few minutes at the same time the test is being conducted and that this will fulfill all OSHA obligations for training, and the employer need not incur added expenses for the more lengthy training program. This approach

will thus save hours of employee lost work time and that converts to real cost differences in the two program approaches. Has the sales person misrepresented the product or is the approach unethical? Probably not, since OSHA compliance was the only thing being sold, not employer/employee protection against future hearing loss.

This represents only one issue in the sale of hearing conservation programs, but, point by point, the successful salesperson will sell simplicity, low cost and compliance, which is precisely what the prospective purchaser wants and often buys. The successful hearing professional or marketer must meet the challenge by selling the value of real cost savings in controlling hearing loss due to noise and eliminating future compensation claims by motivating workers to want to help themselves.

In a market place dictated by cost and lack of internal expertise about hearing conservation in industry, the buyer may be inclined to purchase the program which will be the least expensive, yet is said to comply with the OSHA regulation. It is simply not understood by the prospective client that such an oversimplified approach may not meet the objectives set fourth in achieving effective hearing conservation.

The importance of quality assurance, the problems associated with implementing a more complex program and the unknown variables of the consultant's capabilities can cause uncertainty if not treated properly. These can create barriers for the hearing professional as a marketer. In fact, the red flags which are raised when illustrating what measures should be implemented may actually pave the road for an easy sale for the salesperson presenting a simpler, low cost approach. Yes, the hearing professional's complex sales effort can actually be counter productive if it is too detailed and is problem rather than solution oriented. The presentation must be well organized and documented to illuminate how each program component will present a means to solve each program objective and achieve a return on investment for the client.

ETHICS AND MARKETING

There are four basic principles that should be considered in any marketing presentation: (a) a business philosophy; (b) professional ethics; (c) professional and personal liability; and, (d) reputation.

The first consideration, *business philosophy*, deals with the direction of the individual or the company's concept of business growth, goals, objectives, and the designed formal business plan. These must be decided upon and reviewed periodically to determine if the sales approach meets the business expectations set out in the business plan. For example, if a decision has been made to achieve both rapid growth and an expanded market place, then a decision to offer less complicated services may prevail to produce more immediate sales success. A formal business plan or a marketing strategy is a must. When this is properly implemented and controlled, achieving the organization's goals can be assured.

The second consideration, *professional ethics*, will be somewhat infuenced by the professional associations to which the individual or organization belongs. However, ethics is a highly personal matter and is undoubtedly more a function of the individual's level of expertise and knowledge than simply adherence to a set of guidelines established by a professional association. In sales, the question of ethics is really a matter of how one sells the service, product or concept. In other words, does one sell only what he or she believes is needed, or what the prospective buyer perceives to be adequate? A thorough explanation of the professional's viewpoints and rationale on the differences between the more complex and perceived program's needs will probably satisfy the ethical question. then the salesperson need only address a second ethical

question: if the prospective buyer wants something less than what is believed to be needed, is the seller willing to provide it?

The third consideration, *professional and personal liability*, is a matter of growing concern due to the ever-increasing problem of malpractice and third party liability litigation. In general, insurance accommodates the devastating effects of liability lawsuits; however, the cost of insurance is also escalating and one's exposure could conceivably be more than the limits of typical liability and malpractice coverage. In providing a service, the results are often as intangible as the concept of the service itself. Therefore, it becomes even more important to offer every possible aspect of quality assurance, modern technology and knowledge available to guard against contingent liability problems. Of course, adequate insurance coverage is essential.

In a liability situation, the question may become one of whether the hearing professional provided a level of service which was adequate to control the employee's noise exposure problems. This could be aggravated by establishing that one, in fact, had knowledge of added program parameters that should have been implemented but were not presented strongly enough to the client. In addition, the client may deny any recollection of those recommended program components.

If a decision is made to provide minimal services to acquire the sale, which are less than those recommended by the hearing professional, it is advisable to seek proper legal advice for the inclusion of contract clauses to cover waiver of liability, no guarantees implied and other protective aspects may be appropriate. The legal contract should perhaps be supported by written recommendations detailing the added program aspects which the hearing professional recommends to achieve an effective program.

While this may sound more like the

legal aspects of hearing conservation, it is actually a form of sales essential to business longevity. Certainly any prospect who is properly appraised of the probable pitfalls of a partial program will be forced to reconsider the decision or at least consider strengthening the program in the future.

The final consideration in the marketing and sales decision-making process is *reputation*, which is strictly a personal matter. In fact, the order of presentation of these four basic considerations could undoubtedly be arranged in various arrays of priority. This ranking, hopefully, will be dictated more by the regard for reputation than any other consideration discussed herein. In the professional and industrial environment, reputation is everything.

The situation of program complexity and cost creates a very challenging sales problem. The problem is one of selling the differences through educating the prospective client of valid needs. In the process, one must make early decisions if this educational effort will destroy the sale, and whether or not the program could be "upgraded" through continued sales and demonstration efforts. All other considerations aside, the employees will probably be better served in even a simple program conducted by an experienced hearing professional with comprehensive program capabilities.

Hopefully, the importance of implementing a comprehensive program can be communicated and sold initially. Then competition will exist only among the available comprehensive programs. Competition is absolutely essential to any industry—without it, few technological advances would occur. In an "apples-to-apples" comparison, the client is then assured that the needs will be best served by the dedicated industrial hearing consultant. The exchange process completes the ideal marketing goal—both parties will be better off than if the exchange had not occurred.

A hearing professional selling hearing conservation services must become a professional sales person in order to achieve success. Tenacity, perseverance, personality, and an unflagging commitment to be of service to the client are a few sales qualities that assure success.

One thing is certain among all industries—nothing happens until something is sold, then it's only a matter of keeping promises. Keeping promises is both a personal commitment and a business obligation, which is all-important in satisfying business and retaining customers. There exists a great deal of initial expense in selling and implementing a hearing conservation program. Therefore, the initial opportunity for profit is ordinarily much less than one can expect in future years as the consultant-customer relationship matures. Regardless of the cost involved, the consultant must insure a successful program implementation or the opportunity for future business will be unlikely.

COST OF SALES

Keeping promises is largely tied to cost and cost is often the most difficult aspect of sales. In other words, it is not likely that promises will be kept and proper service provided if there is not sufficient income to cover all expenses and a margin for profit. Personal commitment is one thing and reputation is important, but no one is willing to work without income.

It is essential that a detailed cost analysis be conducted to establish precise costs for direct services and follow-up, sales and marketing, administrative functions, depreciation, taxes, overhead (lights, rent, etc.), and profit. Without establishing cost, the marketing function may be short lived. No organization can afford to sell products or services at a loss forever. It is better to calculate cost from the outset than realize the failure of the business due to lack of profit. When costs have been established, the consultant will know what minimum fees must be applied to each service. If reputation is important, then selling those services for less will be detrimental to the emerging hearing conservation industry and the consultant's business.

When the precise costs to comfortably deliver services are known, it is much easier to present the product and respective prices to the prospective client. When an apples-to-apples comparison is being made and there exists broad cost differences, the cheaper services probably represent a financial loss and the consequences of that are evident; both the consultant and the client become disenchanted and ultimately the more comprehensive program with more realistically priced services will be considered. However, if the client was undersold initially, the desire to continue to do business with the same provider is not great. Remember, successful marketing must reduce risk for the client.

Some of the more common oversights which are made in projecting costs are the expense of interest, state and federal taxes, insurance, employee benefits, equipment repair and replacement, travel and sales expense, profit, and, perhaps most important, client follow-up services. It is better to overestimate expense and sell client service than lose money and be unable to provide it.

SUMMARY

In the process of selling professional services, it is essential to highlight program objectives and how each program aspect will provide an eventual benefit to the employer. In concept, the sales approach must be similar to selling insurance, although the pay-off is of a positive nature. Hearing conservation provides a pay-off of insurance against losses rather than reimbursement for losses incurred.

If the sales approach follows an outline of meeting predetermined objectives, and pathways to understanding those goals are offered, then the decision of implementing a more complex, more expensive, but effective program will be easier.

Formal training as a salesperson may have some benefits, however, the organization of program materials which will educate management to appreciate the differences in quality, expertise and commitment are probably far more important. It is essential to illuminate what may happen if the employer does not implement an effective program rather than what may happen if he does.

Basically, the determination of what will be offered for sale and how it will be sold can be organized with a formal business plan or marketing strategy and a corresponding business philosophy. Professional ethics will have some effect on what is sold and personal liability may partially determine how it is sold. Of utmost importance is reputation and that can be seriously influenced by the cost at which the service is offered.

The unique situation of selling an intangible product in a competitive sales environment demands creativity and perseverance, but most of all, it demands an in-depth understanding of why each program aspect should be implemented, what results can be expected and how to demonstrate and display program results in a manner that the nonprofessional business person can understand. Then the sales task and consultant-client relationship will be a constant, maturing process.

References

1. Kotler P: *Marketing Management*, ed 3. Englewood Cliffs, NJ, Prentice Hall, 1976, p 5, 6.
2. Occupational Safety and Health Administration: Occupational noise exposure; hearing conservation amendment; *Federal Register* 46:11, 4078–4179, January 16, 1981.
3. Ferrell C and Pride W: *Marketing*. ed 3. Boston, Houghton Mifflin, 1983, p 34.
4. Eckhouse RH, et al.: *Business Policy: A Framework for Analysis*, ed 3. Columbus, OH, Grid Publishing, 1980, p 147.
5. Micali PJ: *Success Handbook for Salespeople*, Boston, CBI Publishing Company, 1981, p 35.
6. Occupational Safety and Health Administration: Occupational noise exposure; hearing conservation amendment; final rule. *Federal Register* 48:46, 9738–9785, March 9, 1983.

Department of Labor Occupational Noise Exposure Standard

(Code of Federal Regulations, Title 29, Chapter XVII, Part 1910, Subpart G, 36 FR 10466, May 29, 1971; Amended by 46 FR 4161, January 16, 1981; Amended by 48 FR 9776, March 8, 1983)

§ 1910.95 Occupational noise exposure.

(a) Protection against the effects of noise exposure shall be provided when the sound levels exceed those shown in Table G-16a when measured on the A scale of a standard sound level meter at slow response. When noise levels are determined by octave band analysis, the equivalent A-weighted sound level may be determined as follows:

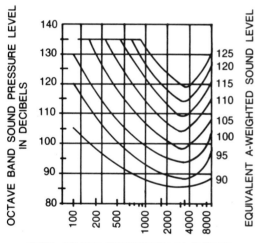

BAND CENTER FREQUENCY IN CYCLES PER SECOND

Figure G.9. Equivalent sound level contours. Octave band sound pressure levels may be converted to the equivalent A-weighted sound level by plotting them on this graph and noting the A-weighted sound level corresponding to the point of highest penetration into the sound level contours. This equivalent A-weighted sound level, which may differ from the actual A-weighted sound level of the noise, is used to determine exposure limits from Table G-16a.

(b)(1) When employees are subjected to sound exceeding those listed in Table G–16a, feasible administrative or engineering controls shall be utilized. If such controls fail to reduce sound levels within the levels of Table G–16a, personal protective equipment shall be provided and used to reduce sound levels within the levels of the table.

(2) If the variations in noise level involve maxima at intervals of 1 second or less, it is to be considered continuous.

(c) *Hearing conservation program.* (1) The employer shall administer a continuing, effective hearing conservation program, as described in paragraphs (c) through (o) of this section, whenever employee noise exposures equal or exceed an 8-hour time-weighted average sound level (TWA) of 85 decibels measured on the A scale (slow response) or, equivalently, a dose of fifty percent. For purposes of the hearing conservation program, employee noise exposures shall be computed in accordance with Appendix A and Table G–16a, and without regard to any attenuation provided by the use of personal protective equipment.

(2) For purposes of paragraph (c) through (n) of this section, an 8-hour time-weighted average of 85 decibels or a dose of fifty percent shall also be referred to as the action level.

(d) *Monitoring.* (1) When information indicates that any employee's exposure may equal or exceed an 8-hour time-weighted average of 85 decibels, the employer shall develop and implement a monitoring program. (i) The sampling strategy shall be designed to identify employees for inclusion in the hearing conservation program and to enable the proper selection of hearing protectors.

(ii) Where circumstances such as high worker mobility, significant variations in sound level, or a significant component of impulse noise make area monitoring generally inappropriate, the employer shall use representative personal sampling to comply with the monitoring requirements of this paragraph unless the employer can show that area sampling produces equivalent results.

(2)(i) All continuous, intermittent and impulsive sound levels from 80 decibels to 130 decibels shall be integrated into the noise measurements.

(ii) Instruments used to measure employee

noise exposure shall be calibrated to ensure measurement accuracy.

(3) Monitoring shall be repeated whenever a change in production, process, equipment or controls increases noise exposures to the extent that:

(i) Additional employees may be exposed at or above the action level; or

(ii) The attenuation provided by hearing protectors being used by employees may be rendered inadequate to meet the requirements of paragraph (j) of this section.

(e) *Employee notification.* The employer shall notify each employee exposed at or above an 8-hour time-weighted average of 85 decibels of the results of the monitoring.

(f) *Observation of monitoring.* The employer shall provide affected employees or their representatives with an opportunity to observe any noise measurements conducted pursuant to this section.

(g) *Audiometric testing program.* (1) The employer shall establish and maintain an audiometric testing program as provided in this paragraph by making audiometric testing available to all employees whose exposures equal or exceed an 8-hour time-weighted average of 85 decibels.

(2) The program shall be provided at no cost to employees.

(3) Audiometric tests shall be performed by a licensed or certified audiologist, otolaryngologist, or other physician, or by a technician who is certified by the Council of Accreditation in Occupational Hearing Conservation, or who has satisfactorily demonstrated competence in administering audiometric examinations, obtaining valid audiograms, and properly using, maintaining and checking calibration and proper functioning of the audiometers being used. A technician who operates microprocessor audiometers does not need to be certified. A technician who performs audiometric tests must be responsible to an audiologist, otolaryngologist or physician.

(4) All audiograms obtained pursuant to this section shall meet the requirements of Appendix C: *Audiometric Measuring Instruments.*

(5) *Baseline audiogram.* (i) Within 6 months of an employee's first exposure at or above the action level, the employer shall establish a valid baseline audiogram against which subsequent audiograms can be compared.

(ii) *Mobile test van exception.* Where mobile test vans are used to meet the audiometric testing obligation, the employer shall obtain a valid baseline audiogram within 1 year of an employee's first exposure at or above the action level. Where baseline audiograms are obtained more than 6 months after the employee's first exposure at or above the action level, employees shall wear hearing protectors for any period exceeding 6 months after first exposure until the baseline audiogram is obtained.

(iii) Testing to establish a baseline audiogram shall be preceded by at least 14 hours without exposure to workplace noise. Hearing protectors may be used as a substitute for the requirement that baseline audiograms be preceded by 14 hours without exposure to workplace noise.

(iv) The employer shall notify employees of the need to avoid high levels of non-occupational noise exposure during the 14-hour period immediately preceding the audiometric examination.

(6) *Annual audiogram.* At least annually after obtaining the baseline audiogram, the employer shall obtain a new audiogram for each employee exposed at or above an 8-hour time-weighted average of 85 decibels.

(7) *Evaluation of audiogram.* (i) Each employee's annual audiogram shall be compared to that employee's baseline audiogram to determine if the audiogram is valid and if a standard threshold shift as defined in paragaph (g)(10) of this section has occurred. This comparison may be done by a technician.

(ii) If the annual audiogram shows that an employee has suffered a standard threshold shift, the employer may obtain a retest within 30 days and consider the results of the retest as the annual audiogram.

(iii) The audiologist, otolaryngologist, or physician shall review problem audiograms and shall determine whether there is a need for further evaluation. The employer shall provide to the person performing this evaluation the following information:

(A) A copy of the requirements for hearing conservation as set forth in paragraphs (c) through (n) of this section;

(B) The baseline audiogram and most recent audiogram of the employee to be evaluated;

(C) Measurements of background sound pressure levels in the audiometric test room as required in Appendix D: Audiometric Test Rooms.

(D) Records of audiometer calibrations required by paragraph (h)(5) of this section.

(8) *Follow-up procedures.* (i) If a comparison of the annual audiogram to the baseline audiogram indicates a standard threshold shift as defined in paragraph (g)(10) of this section has occurred, the employee shall be informed of this fact in writing, within 21 days of the determination.

(ii) Unless a physician determines that the

standard threshold shift is not work related or aggravated by occupational noise exposure, the employer shall ensure that the following steps are taken when a standard threshold shift occurs:

(A) Employees not using hearing protectors shall be fitted with hearing protectors, trained in their use and care, and required to use them.

(B) Employees already using hearing protectors shall be refitted and retained in the use of hearing protectors and provided with hearing protectors offering a greater attenuation if necessary.

(C) The employee shall be referred for a clinical audiological evaluation or an otological examination, as appropriate, if additional testing is necessary or if the employer suspects that a medical pathology of the ear is caused or aggravated by the wearing of hearing protectors.

(D) The employee is informed of the need for an otological examination if a medical pathology of the ear that is unrelated to the use of hearing protectors is suspected.

(iii) If subsequent audiometric testing of an employee whose exposure to noise is less than an 8-hour TWA of 90 decibels indicates that a standard threshold shift is not persistent, the employer:

(A) Shall inform the employee of the new audiometric interpretation; and

(B) May discontinue the required use of hearing protectors for that employee.

(9) *Revised baseline.* An annual audiogram may be substituted for the baseline audiogram when, in the judgment of the audiologist, otolaryngologist or physician who is evaluating the audiogram:

(i) The standard threshold shift revealed by the audiogram is persistent; or

(ii) The hearing threshold shown in the annual audiogram indicates significant improvement over the baseline audiogram.

(10) *Standard threshold shift.* (1) As used in this section, a standard threshold shift is a change in hearing threshold relative to the baseline audiogram of an average of 10 dB or more at 2000, 3000, and 4000 Hz in either ear.

(ii) In determining whether a standard threshold shift has occurred, allowance may be made for the contribution of aging (presbycusis) to the change in hearing level by correcting the annual audiogram according to the procedure described in Appendix F: *Calculation and Application of Age Correction to Audiograms.*

(h) *Audiometric test requirements.* (1) Audiometric tests shall be pure tone, air conduction, hearing threshold examinations, with test frequencies including as a minimum 500, 1000, 2000, 3000, 4000, and 6000 Hz. Tests at each frequency shall be taken separately for each ear.

(2) Audiometric tests shall be conducted with audiometers (including microprocessor audiometers) that meet the specifications of, and are maintained and used in accordance with, American National Standard Specification for Audiometers, S3.6–1969.

(3) Pulsed-tone and self-recording audiometers, if used, shall meet the requirements specified in Appendix C: *Audiometric Measuring Instruments.*

(4) Audiometric examinations shall be administered in a room meeting the requirements listed in Appendix D: *Audiometric Test Rooms.*

(5) *Audiometer calibration.* (i) The functional operation of the audiometer shall be checked before each day's use by testing a person with known, stable hearing thresholds, and by listening to the audiometer's output to make sure that the output is free from distorted or unwanted sounds. Deviations of 10 decibels or greater require an acoustic calibration.

(ii) Audiometer calibration shall be checked acoustically at least annually in accordance with Appendix E: *Acoustic Calibration of Audiometers.* Test frequencies below 500 Hz and above 6000 Hz may be omitted from this check. Deviations of 15 decibels or greater require an exhaustive calibration.

(iii) An exhaustive calibration shall be performed at least every two years in accordance with sections 4.1.2; 4.1.3; 4.1.4.3; 4.2; 4.4.1; 4.4.2; 4.4.3; and 4.5 of the American National Standard Specification for Audiometers, S3.6–1969. Test frequencies below 500 Hz and above 6000 Hz may be omitted from this calibration.

(i) *Hearing protectors.* (1) Employers shall make hearing protectors available to all employees exposed to an 8-hour time-weighted average of 85 decibels or greater at no cost to the employees. Hearing protectors shall be replaced as necessary.

(2) Employers shall ensure that hearing protectors are worn:

(i) By an employee who is required by paragraph (b)(1) of this section to wear personal protective equipment; and

(ii) By any employee who is exposed to an 8-hour time-weighted average of 85 decibels or greater, and who:

(A) Has not yet had a baseline audiogram established pursuant to paragraph (g)(5)(ii); or

(B) Has experienced a standard threshold shift.

(3) Employees shall be given the opportu-

nity to select their hearing protectors from a variety of suitable hearing protectors provided by the employer.

(4) The employer shall provide training in the use and care of all hearing protectors provided to employees.

(5) The employer shall ensure proper initial fitting and supervise the correct use of all hearing protectors.

(j) *Hearing protector attenuation.* (1) The employer shall evaluate hearing protector attenuation for the specific noise environments in which the protector will be used. The employer shall use one of the evaluation methods described in Appendix B: *Methods for Estimating the Adequacy of Hearing Protection Attenuation.*

(2) Hearing protectors must attenuate employee exposure at least to an 8-hour time-weighted average of 90 decibels as required by paragraph (b) of this section.

(3) For employees who have experienced a standard threshold shift, hearing protectors must attenuate employee exposure to an 8-hour time-weighted average of 85 decibels or below.

(4) The adequacy of hearing protector attenuation shall be re-evaluated whenever employee noise exposures increase to the extent that the hearing protectors provided may no longer provide adequate attenuation. The employee shall provide more effective hearing protectors where necessary.

(k) *Training program.* (1) The employer shall institute a training program for all employees who are exposed to noise at or above an 8-hour time-weighted average of 85 decibels, and shall ensure employee participation in such program.

(2) The training program shall be repeated annually for each employee included in the hearing conservation program. Information provided in the training program shall be updated to be consistent with changes in protective equipment and work processes.

(3) The employer shall ensure that each employee is informed of the following:

(i) The effects of noise on hearing;

(ii) The purpose of hearing protectors, the advantages, disadvantages, and attenuation of various types, and instructions on selection, fitting, use, and care; and

(iii) The purpose of audiometric testing, and an explanation of the test procedures.

(l) *Access to information and training materials.* (1) The employer shall make available to affected employees or their representatives copies of this standard and shall also post a copy in the workplace.

(2) The employer shall provide to affected employees any informational materials pertaining to the standard that are supplied to the employer by the Assistant Secretary.

(3) The employer shall provide, upon request, all materials related to the employer's training and education program pertaining to this standard to the Assistant Secretary and the Director.

(m) *Recordkeeping.*—(1) *Exposure measurements.* The employer shall maintain an accurate record of all employee exposure measurements required by paragraph (d) of this section.

(2) *Audiometric tests.* (i) The employer shall retain all employee audiometric test records obtained pursuant to paragraph (g) of this section:

(ii) This record shall include:

(A) Name and job classification of the employee;

(B) Date of the audiogram;

(C) The examiner's name;

(D) Date of the last acoustic or exhaustive calibration of the audiometer; and

(E) Employee's most recent noise exposure assessment.

(F) The employer shall maintain accurate records of the measurements of the background sound pressure levels in audiometric test rooms.

(3) *Record retention.* The employer shall retain records required in this paragraph (m) for at least the following periods.

(i) Noise exposure measurement records shall be retained for two years.

(ii) Audiometric test records shall be retained for the duration of the affected employee's employment.

(4) *Access to records.* All records required by this section shall be provided upon request to employees, former employees, representatives designated by the individual employee, and the Assistant Secretary. The provisions of 29 CFR 1910.20 (a)–(e) and (g)–(i) apply to access to records under this section.

(5) *Transfer of records.* If the employer ceases to do business, the employer shall transfer to the successor employer all records required to be maintained by this section, and the successor employer shall retain them for the remainder of the period prescribed in paragraph (m) (3) of this section.

(n) *Appendices.* (1) Appendices A, B, C, D, and E to this section are incorporated as part of this section and the contents of these Appendices are mandatory.

(2) Appendices F and G to this section are informational and are not intended to create any additional obligations not otherwise im-

posed or to detract from any existing obligations.

(o) *Exemptions.* Paragraphs (c) through (n) of this section shall not apply to employers engaged in oil and gas well drilling and servicing operations.

(n) *Startup date.* Baseline audiograms required by paragraph (g) of this section shall be completed by March 1, 1984.

*   *   *   *   *

Appendix A: Noise Expsoure Computation

This Appendix is Mandatory

I. Computation of Employee Noise Exposure

(1) Noise dose is computed using Table G–16a as follows:

(i) When the sound level, L, is constant over the entire work shift, the noise dose, D, in percent, is given by: D = 100 C/T where C is the total length of the work day, in hours, and T is the reference duration corresponding to the measured sound level, L, as given in Table G–16a or by the formula shown as a footnote to that table.

(ii) When the workshift noise exposure is composed of two or more periods of noise at different levels, the total noise dose over the work day is given by:

$$D = 100 \ (C_1/T_1 + C_2/T_2 + \cdots + C_n/T_n),$$

where C_n indicates the total time of exposure at a specific noise level, and T_n indicates the reference duration for that level as given by Table G–16a.

(2) The eight-hour time-weighted average sound level (TWA), in decibels, may be computed from the dose, in percent, by means of the formula: TWA = 16.61 $\log_{10}$ (D/100) + 90. For an eight-hour workshift with the noise level constant over the entire shift, the TWA is equal to the measured sound level.

(3) A table relating dose and TWA is given in Section II.

TABLE G–16a

A-weighted sound level, L (decibel)	Reference duration, T (hour)
80	32
81	27.9
82	24.3
83	21.1
84	16.4
85	16
86	13.9
87	12.1
88	10.6
89	9.2
90	8
91	7.0

TABLE G–16a—Continued

A-weighted sound level, L (decibel)	Reference duration, T (hour)
92	6.1
93	5.3
94	4.6
95	4
96	3.5
97	3.0
98	2.6
99	2.3
100	2
101	1.7
102	1.5
103	1.3
104	1.1
105	1
106	0.87
107	0.76
108	0.66
109	0.57
110	0.5
111	0.44
112	0.38
113	0.33
114	0.29
115	0.25
116	0.22
117	0.19
118	0.16
119	0.14
120	0.125
121	0.11
122	0.095
123	0.082
124	0.072
125	0.063
126	0.054
127	0.047
128	0.041
129	0.036
130	0.031

In the above table the reference duration, T, is computed by

$$T = \frac{8}{2^{(L-90)/5}}$$

where L is the measured A-weighted sound level.

II. Conversion Between "Dose" and "8-Hour Time Weighted Average" Sound Level

Compliance with paragraphs (c)–(r) of this regulation is determined by the amount of exposure to noise in the workplace. The amount of such exposure is usually measured with an audiodosimeter which gives a readout in terms of "dose." In order to better understand the requirements of the amendment, dosimeter readings can be converted to an "8-hour time-weighted average sound level" (TWA).

In order to convert the reading of a dosimeter into TWA, see Table A–1, below. This table applies to dosimeters that are set by the manufacturer to calculate dose or percent exposure according to the relationships in Table G–16a. So, for example, a dose of 91 percent over an eight hour day results in a TWA of 89.3 dB, and, a dose of 50 percent corresponds to a TWA of 85 dB.

If the dose as read on the dosimeter is less than or greater than the values found in Table A–1, the TWA may be calculated by using the formula: $TWA = 16.61 \log_{10}(D/100) + 90$ where TWA = 8-hour time-weighted average sound level and D = accumulated dose in percent exposure.

TABLE A–1.—CONVERSION FROM "PERCENT NOISE EXPOSURE" OR "DOSE" TO "8-HOUR TIME-WEIGHTED AVERAGE SOUND LEVEL" (TWA)

Dose or percent noise exposure	TWA
10	73.4
15	76.3
20	78.4
25	80.0
30	81.3
35	82.4
40	83.4
45	84.2
50	85.0
55	85.7
60	86.3
65	86.9
70	87.4
75	87.9
80	88.4
81	88.5
82	88.6
83	88.7
84	88.7
85	88.8
86	88.9
87	89.0
88	89.1
89	89.2
90	89.2
91	89.3
92	89.4
93	89.5
94	89.6
95	89.6
96	89.7
97	89.8
98	89.9
99	89.9
100	90.0
101	90.1
102	90.1
103	90.2
104	90.3
105	90.4
106	90.4
107	90.5
108	90.6
109	90.6
110	90.7
111	90.8
112	90.8
113	90.9
114	90.9
115	91.1
116	91.1
117	91.1

Table A–1.—Continued

Dose or percent noise exposure	TWA
118	91.2
119	91.3
120	91.3
125	91.6
130	91.9
135	92.2
140	92.4
145	92.7
150	92.9
155	93.2
160	93.4
165	93.6
170	93.8
175	94.0
180	94.2
185	94.4
190	94.6
195	94.8
200	95.0
210	95.4
220	95.7
230	96.0
240	96.3
250	96.6
260	96.9
270	97.2
280	97.4
290	97.7
300	97.9
310	98.2
320	98.4
330	98.6
340	98.8
350	99.0
360	99.2
370	99.4
380	99.6
390	99.8
400	100.0
410	100.2
420	100.4
430	100.5
440	100.7
450	100.8
460	101.0
470	101.2
480	101.3
490	101.5
500	101.6
510	101.8
520	101.9
530	102.0
540	102.2
550	102.3
560	102.4
570	102.6
580	102.7
590	102.8
600	102.9
610	103.0
620	103.2
630	103.3
640	103.4
650	103.5
660	103.6
670	103.7
680	103.8
690	103.9
700	104.0
710	104.1
720	104.2
730	104.3
740	104.4

TABLE A-1.—Continued

Dose or percent noise exposure	TWA
750	104.5
760	104.6
770	104.7
780	104.8
790	104.9
800	105.0
810	105.1
820	105.2
830	105.3
840	105.4
850	105.4
860	105.5
870	105.6
880	105.7
890	105.8
900	105.8
910	105.9
920	106.0
930	106.1
940	106.2
950	106.2
960	106.3
970	106.4
980	106.5
990	106.5
999	106.6

Appendix B: Methods for Estimating the Adequacy of Hearing Protector Attenuation

This Appendix is Mandatory

For employees who have experienced a significant threshold shift, hearing protector attenuation must be sufficient to reduce employee exposure to a TWA of 85 dB. Employers must select one of the following methods by which to estimate the adequacy of hearing protector attenuation.

The most convenient method is the Noise Reduction Rating (NRR) developed by the Environmental Protection Agency (EPA). According to EPA regulation, the NRR must be shown on the hearing protector package. The NRR is then related to an individual worker's noise environment in order to assess the adequacy of the attenuation of a given hearing protector. This Appendix describes four methods of using the NRR to determine whether a particular hearing protector provides adequate protection within a given exposure environment. Selection among the four procedures is dependent upon the employer's noise measuring instruments.

Instead of using the NRR, employers may evaluate the adequacy of hearing protector attenuation by using one of the three methods developed by the National Institute for Occupational Safety and Health (NIOSH), which are described in the "List of Personal Hearing Protectors and Attenuation Data," HEW Publication No. 76–120, 1975, pages 21–37. These methods are known as NIOSH methods #1, #2 and #3. The NRR described below is a simplification of NIOSH method #2. The most complex method is NIOSH method #1, which is probably the most accurate method since it uses the largest amount of spectral information from the individual employee's noise environment. As in the case of the NRR method described below, if one of the NIOSH methods is used, the selected method must be applied to an individual's noise environment to assess the adequacy of the attenuation. Employers should be careful to take a sufficient number of measurements in order to achieve a representative sample for each time segment.

Note.—The employer must remember that calculated attenuation values reflect realistic values only to the extent that the protectors are properly fitted and worn.

When using the NRR to assess hearing protector adequacy, one of the following methods must be used:

(i) When using a dosimeter that is capable of C-weighted measurements:

(A) Obtain the employee's C-weighted dose for the entire workshift, and convert to TWA (see Appendix A, II).

(B) Subtract the NRR from the C-weighted TWA to obtain the estimated A-weighted TWA under the ear protector.

(ii) When using a dosimeter that is not capable of C-weighted measurements, the following method may be used:

(A) Convert the A-weighted dose to TWA (see Appendix A).

(B) Subtract 7 dB from the NRR.

(C) Subtract the remainder from the A-weighted TWA to obtain the estimated A-weighted TWA under the ear protector.

(iii) When using a sound level meter set to the A-weighting network:

(A) Obtain the employee's A-weighted TWA.

(B) Subtract 7 dB from the NRR, and subtract the remainder from the A-weighted TWA to obtain the estimated A-weighted TWA under the ear protector.

(iv) When using a sound level meter set on the C-weighting network:

(A) Obtain a representative sample of the C-weighted sound levels in the employee's environment.

(B) Subtract the NRR from the C-weighted average sound level to obtain the estimated A-weighted TWA under the ear protector.

(v) When using area monitoring procedures and a sound level meter set to the A-weighting network.

(A) Obtain a representative sound level for the area in question.

(B) Subtract 7 dB from the NRR and subtract the remainder from the A-weighted sound level for that area.

(vi) When using area monitoring procedures and a sound level meter set to the C-weighting network:

(A) Obtain a representative sound level for the area in question.

(B) Subtract the NRR from the C-weighted sound level for that area.

Appendix C: Audiometric Measuring Instruments

This Appendix is Mandatory

1. In the event that pulsed-tone audiometers are used, they shall have a tone on-time of at least 200 milliseconds.

2. Self-recording audiometers shall comply with the following requirements:

(A) The chart upon which the audiogram is traced shall have lines at positions corresponding to all multiples of 10 dB hearing level within the intensity range spanned by the audiometer. The lines shall be equally spaced and shall be separated by at least ¼ inch. Additional increments are optional. The audiogram pen tracings shall not exceed 2 dB in width.

(B) It shall be possible to set the stylus manually at the 10-dB increment lines for calibration purposes.

(C) The slewing rate for the audiometer attenuator shall not be more than 6 dB/sec except that an initial slewing rate greater than 6 dB/sec is permitted at the beginning of each new test frequency, but only until the second subject response.

(D) The audiometer shall remain at each required test frequency for 30 seconds (±3 seconds). The audiogram shall be clearly marked at each change of frequency and the actual frequency change of the audiometer shall not deviate from the frequency boundaries marked on the audiogram by more than ±3 seconds.

(E) It must be possible at each test frequency to place a horizontal line segment parallel to the time axis on the audiogram, such that the audiometric tracing crosses the line segment at least six times at that test frequency. At each test frequency the threshold shall be the average of the midpoints of the tracing excursions.

Appendix D: Audiometric Test Rooms

This Appendix is Mandatory

Rooms used for audiometric testing shall not have background sound pressure levels exceeding those in Table D-1 when measured by equipment conforming at least to the Type 2 requirements of American National Standard Specification for Sound Level Meters, S1.4-1971 (R1976), and to the Class II requirements of American National Standard Specification for Octave, Half-Octave, and Third-Octave Band Filter Sets, S1.11-1971 (R1976).

TABLE D-1.—MAXIMUM ALLOWABLE OCTAVE-BAND SOUND PRESSURE LEVELS FOR AUDIOMETRIC TEST ROOMS

Octave-band center frequency (Hz)	500	1000	2000	4000	8000
Sound pressure level (dB)	40	40	47	57	62

Appendix E: Acoustic Calibration of Audiometers

This Appendix is Mandatory

Audiometer calibration shall be checked acoustically, at least annually, according to the procedures described in this Appendix. The equipment necessary to perform these measurements is a sound level meter, octave-band filter set, and a National Bureau of Standards 9A coupler. In making these measurements, the accuracy of the calibrating equipment shall be sufficient to determine that the audiometer is within the tolerances permitted by American Standard Specification for Audiometers, S3.6-1969.

(1) Sound Pressure Output Check

A. Place the earphone coupler over the microphone of the sound level meter and place the earphone on the coupler.

B. Set the audiometer's hearing threshold level (HTL) dial to 70 dB.

C. Measure the sound pressure level of the tones that each test frequency from 500 Hz through 6000 Hz for each earphone.

D. At each frequency the readout on the sound level meter should correspond to the levels in Table E-1 or Table E-2, as appropriate, for the type of earphone, in the column entitled "sound level meter reading."

(2) Linearity Check

A. With the earphone in place, set the frequency to 1000 Hz and the HTL dial on the audiometer to 70 dB.

B. Measure the sound levels in the coupler at each 10-dB decrement from 70 dB to 10 dB, noting the sound level meter reading at each setting.

C. For each 10-dB decrement on the audiometer the sound level meter should indicate a corresponding 10 dB decrease.

D. This measurement may be made electrically with a voltmeter connected to the earphone terminals.

(3) Tolerances

When any of the measured sound levels deviate from the levels in Table E-1 or Table

E–2 by ±3 dB at any test frequency between 500 and 3000 Hz, 4 dB at 4000 Hz, or 5 dB at 6000 Hz, an exhaustive calibration is advised. An exhaustive calibration is required if the deviations are greater than 10 dB at any test frequency.

TABLE E–1.—REFERENCE THRESHOLD LEVELS FOR TELEPHONICS—TDH–39 EARPHONES

Frequency, Hz	Reference threshold level for TDH–39 earphones, dB	Sound level meter reading, dB
500	11.5	81.5
1000	7	77
2000	9	79
3000	10	80
4000	9.5	79.5
6000	15.5	85.5

TABLE E–2.—REFERENCE THRESHOLD LEVELS FOR TELEPHONICS—TDH–49 EARPHONES

Frequency, Hz	Reference threshold level for TDH–49 earphones, dB	Sound level meter reading, dB
500	13.5	83.5
1000	7.5	77.5
2000	11	81.0
3000	9.5	79.5
4000	10.5	80.5
6000	13.5	83.5

Appendix F: Calculations and Application of Age Corrections to Audiograms

This Appendix Is Non-Mandatory

In determining whether a standard threshold shift has occurred, allowance may be made for the contribution of aging to the change in hearing level by adjusting the most recent audiogram. If the employer chooses to adjust the audiogram, the employer shall follow the procedure described below. This procedure and the age correction tables were developed by the National Institute for Occupational Safety and Health in the criteria document entitled "Criteria for a Recommended Standard ... Occupational Exposure to Noise," ((HSM)–11001).

For each audiometric test frequency:

(i) Determine from Tables F–1 or F–2 the age correction values for the employee by:

(A) Finding the age at which the most recent audiogram was taken and recording the corresponding values of age corrections at 1000 Hz through 6000 Hz;

(B) Finding the age at which the baseline audiogram was taken and recording the corresponding values of age corrections at 1000 Hz through 6000 Hz.

(ii) Subtract the values found in step (i)(A) from the value found in step (i)(B).

(iii) The differences calculated in step (ii) represented that portion of the change in hearing that may be due to aging.

Example: Employee is a 32-year-old male. The audiometric history for his right ear is shown in decibels below.

Employee's age	Audiometric test frequency (Hz)				
	1000	2000	3000	4000	6000
26	10	5	5	10	5
*27	0	0	0	5	5
28	0	0	0	10	5
29	5	0	5	15	5
30	0	5	10	20	10
31	5	10	20	15	15
*32	5	10	10	25	20

The audiogram at age 27 is considered the baseline since it shows the best hearing threshold levels. Asterisks have been used to identify the baseline and most recent audiogram. A threshold shift of 20 dB exists at 4000 Hz between the audiograms taken at ages 27 and 32.

(The threshold shift is computed by subtracting the hearing threshold at age 27, which was 5, from the hearing threshold at age 32, which is 25). A retest audiogram has confirmed this shift. The contribution of aging to this change in hearing may be estimated in the following manner:

Go to Table F–1 and find the age correction values (in dB) for 4000 Hz at age 27 and age 32.

	Frequency (Hz)				
	1000	2000	3000	4000	6000
Age 32	6	5	7	10	14
Age 27	5	4	6	7	11
Difference	1	1	1	3	3

The difference represents the amount of hearing loss that may be attributed to aging in the time period between the baseline audiogram and the most recent audiogram. In this example, the difference at 4000 Hz is 3 dB. This value is subtracted from the hearing level at 4000 Hz, which in the most recent audiogram is 25, yielding 22 after adjustment. Then the hearing threshold in the baseline audiogram at 4000 Hz (5) is subtracted from the adjusted annual audiogram hearing threshold at 4000 Hz (22). Thus the age-corrected threshold shift would be 17 dB (as opposed to a threshold shift of 20 dB without age correction).

TABLE F-1.—AGE CORRECTION VALUES IN DECIBELS FOR MALES

Years	Audiometric Test Frequencies (Hz)				
	1000	2000	3000	4000	6000
20 or younger	5	3	4	5	8
21	5	3	4	5	8
22	5	3	4	5	8
23	5	3	4	6	9
24	5	3	5	6	9
25	5	3	5	7	10
26	5	4	5	7	10
27	5	4	6	7	11
28	6	4	6	8	11
29	6	4	6	8	12
30	6	4	6	9	12
31	6	4	7	9	13
32	6	5	7	10	14
33	6	5	7	10	14
34	6	5	8	11	15
35	7	5	8	11	15
36	7	5	9	12	16
37	7	6	9	12	17
38	7	6	9	13	17
39	7	6	10	14	18
40	7	6	10	14	19
41	7	6	10	14	20
42	6	7	11	16	20
43	8	7	12	16	21
44	8	7	12	17	22
45	8	7	13	18	23
46	8	8	13	19	24
47	8	8	14	19	24
48	9	8	14	20	25
49	9	9	15	21	26
50	9	9	16	22	27
51	9	9	16	23	28
52	9	10	17	24	29
53	9	10	18	25	30
54	10	10	18	26	31
55	10	11	19	27	32
56	10	11	20	28	34
57	10	11	21	29	35
58	10	12	22	31	36
59	11	12	22	32	37
60 or older	11	13	23	33	38

TABLE F-2.—AGE CORRECTION VALUES IN DECIBELS FOR FEMALES

Years	Audiometric Test Frequencies (Hz)				
	1000	2000	3000	4000	6000
20 or younger	7	4	3	3	6
21	7	4	4	3	6
22	7	4	4	4	6
23	7	5	4	4	7
24	7	5	4	4	7
25	8	5	4	4	7
26	8	5	5	4	8
27	8	5	5	5	8
28	8	5	5	5	8
29	8	5	5	5	9
30	8	6	5	5	9
31	8	6	6	5	9
32	9	6	6	6	10
33	9	6	6	6	10
34	9	6	6	6	10
35	9	6	7	7	11
36	9	7	7	7	11
37	9	7	7	7	12
38	10	7	7	7	12
39	10	7	8	8	12
40	10	7	8	8	13
41	10	8	8	8	13
42	10	8	9	9	13
43	11	8	9	9	14
44	11	8	9	9	14
45	11	8	10	10	15
46	11	9	10	10	15
47	11	9	10	11	16
48	12	9	11	11	16
49	12	9	11	11	16
50	12	10	11	12	17
51	12	10	12	12	17
52	12	10	12	13	18
53	13	10	13	13	18
54	13	11	13	14	19
55	13	11	14	14	19
56	13	11	14	15	20
57	13	11	15	15	20
58	14	12	15	16	21
59	14	12	16	16	21
60 or older	14	12	16	17	22

Appendix G: Monitoring Noise Levels
Non-Mandatory Informational Appendix

This appendix provides information to help employers comply with the noise monitoring obligations that are part of the hearing conservation amendment.

What is the purpose of noise monitoring?

This revised amendment requires that employees be placed in a hearing conservation program if they are exposed to average noise levels of 85 dB or greater during an 8 hour workday. In order to determine if exposures are at or above this level, it may be necessary to measure or monitor the actual noise levels in the workplace and to estimate the noise exposure or "dose" received by employees during the workday.

When is it necessary to implement a noise monitoring program?

It is not necessary for every employer to measure workplace noise. Noise monitoring or measuring must be conducted only when exposures are at or above 85 dB. Factors which suggest that noise exposures in the workplace may be at this level include employee complaints about the loudness of noise, indications that employees are losing their hearing, or noisy conditions which make normal conversation difficult. The employer should also consider any information available regarding noise emitted from specific machines. In addition, actual workplace noise measurements can suggest whether or not a monitoring program should be initiated.

How is noise measured?

Basically, there are two different instruments to measure noise exposures: the sound level meter and the dosimeter. A sound level meter is a device that measures the intensity of sound at a given moment. Since sound level meters provide a measure of sound intensity at only one point in time, it is generally necessary to take a number of measurements at different times during the day to estimate noise exposure over a workday. If noise levels fluctuate, the amount of time noise remains at each of the various measured levels must be determined.

To estimate employee noise exposures with a sound level meter it is also generally necessary to take several measurements at different locations within the workplace. After appropriate sound level meter readings are obtained, people sometimes draw "maps" of the sound levels within different areas of the workplace. By using a sound level "map" and information on employee locations throughout the day, estimates of individual exposure levels can be developed. This measurement method is generally referred to as *area* noise monitoring.

A dosimeter is like a sound level meter except that it stores sound level measurements and integrates these measurements over time, providing an average noise exposure reading for a given period of time, such as an 8-hour workday. With a dosimeter, a microphone is attached to the employee's clothing and the exposure measurement is simply read at the end of the desired time period. A reader may be used to read-out the dosimeter's measurements. Since the dosimeter is worn by the employee, it measures noise levels in those locations in which the employee travels. A sound level meter can also be positioned within the immediate vicinity of the exposed worker to obtain an individual exposure estimate. Such procedures are generally referred to as *personal* noise monitoring.

Area monitoring can be used to estimate noise exposure when the noise levels are relatively constant and employees are not mobile. In workplaces where employees move about in different areas or where the noise intensity tends to fluctuate over time, noise exposure is generally more accurately estimated by the personal monitoring approach.

In situations where personal monitoring is appropriate, proper positioning of the microphone is necessary to obtain accurate measurements. With a dosimeter, the microphone is generally located on the shoulder and remains in that position for the entire workday. With a sound level meter, the microphone is stationed near the employee's head, and the instrument is usually held by an individual who follows the employee as he or she moves about.

Manufacturer's instructions, contained in dosimeter and sound level meter operating manuals, should be followed for calibration and maintenance. To ensure accurate results, it is considered good professional practice to calibrate instruments before and after each use.

How often is it necessary to monitor noise levels?

The amendment requires that when there are significant changes in machinery or production processes that may result in increased noise levels, remonitoring must be conducted to determine whether additional employees need to be included in the hearing conservation program. Many companies choose to remonitor periodically (once every year or two) to ensure that all exposed employees are included in their hearing conservation programs.

Selected Standards Related to Noise Measurements

A. American National Standards Institute and Acoustical Society of America, New York: ANSI and ASA Standards

1. ANSI S1.2-1960: *Physical Measurement of Sound.*
2. ANSI S1.4-1983: *American National Standard Specification for Sound Level Meters.*
3. ANSI S1.8-1969 (R1974): *American National Standard Preferred Reference Quantities for Acoustical Levels.*
4. ANSI S1.10-1966 (R1976): *American National Standard Method for the Calibration of Microphones.*
5. ANSI S1.13-1971 (R1976): *American National Standard Methods for the Measurement of Sound Pressure Levels.*
6. ANSI S1.21-1972: *Sound Power Levels of Small Sources in Reverberation Rooms.*
7. ANSI 21.23-1976: *American National Standard Method for the Designation of Sound Power Emitted by Machinery and Equipment.*
8. ANSI S1.25-1978: *American National Standard Specification for Personal Noise Dosimeters.*
9. ANSI S1.27-Draft-1978: *E-Weighting Network for Noise Measurement.*
10. ANSI S1.29-1979: *American National Standard Method for the Measurement and Designation of Noise Emitted by Computer and Business Equipment.*
11. ANSI S1.30-1979: *American National Standard Guidelines for the Use of Sound Power Standards and for the Preparation of Noise Test Codes.*
12. ANSI S1.31-1980: *American National Standard Precision Methods for the Determination of Sound Power Levels of Broad-Band Noise Sources in Reverberation Rooms.*
13. ANSI S1.32-1980: *American National Standard Precision Methods for the Determination of Sound Power Levels of Discrete-Frequency and Narrow-Band Noise Sources in Reverberation Rooms.*
14. ANSI S1.33-1982: *Engineering Methods for the Determination of Sound Power Levels of Noise Sources in a Special Reverberation Test Room.*
15. ANSI S1.34-1980: *American National Standard Engineering Methods for the Determination of Sound Power Levels of Noise Sources for Essentially Free-Field Conditions over a Reflecting Plane.*
16. ANSI S1.35-1979: *American National Standard Precision Methods for the Determination of Sound Power Levels of Noise Sources in Anechoic and Hemi-Anechoic Rooms.*
17. ANSI S1.36-1979: *American National Standard*

Survey Methods for the Determination of Sound Power Levels of Noise Sources.
18. ANSI S2.2-1959 (R1982): *American National Standard Methods for the Calibrations of Shock and Vibration Pickups.*
19. ANSI S2.4-1976 (R1982): *American National Standard Method for Specifying the Characteristics of Auxiliary Enalog Equipment for Shock and Vibration Measurements.*
20. ANSI S2.8-1972 (R1978): *American National Standard Guide for Describing the Characteristics of Resilient Mountings.*
21. ANSI S2.9-1976 (R1982): *American National Standard Nomenclature for Specifying Damping Properties of Materials.*
22. ANSI S2.10-1971 (R1982): *American National Standard Methods for Analysis and Presentation of Shock and Vibration Data.*
23. ANSI S2.11-1969 (R1978): *American National Standard for the Selection of Calibrations and Tests for Electrical Transducers used for Measuring Shock and Vibration.*
24. ANSI S2.17-1980: *American National Standard Techniques of Machinery Vibration Measurement.*
25. ANSI S2.38-1982: *American National Standard Field Balancing Equipment-Description and Evaluation.*
26. ANSI S2.42-1982: *American National Standard Procedures for Balancing Flexible Rotors.*
27. ANSI S3.4-1980: *American National Standard Procedure for the Computation of Loudness of Noise.*
28. ANSI S3.14-1977: *American National Standard for Rating Noise with Respect to Speech Interference.*
29. ANSI S3.17-1975 (R1980): *American National Standard Method for Rating the Sound Power Spectra of Small Stationary Noise Sources.*
30. ANSI S3.18-1979: *American National Standard Guide for the Evaluation of Human Exposure to Whole-Body Vibration.*
31. ANSI S3.23-1980: *American National Standard Sound Level Descriptors for Determination of Compatible Land Use.*
32. ANSI S3.29-1983: *American National Standard Guide to the Evaluation of Human Exposure to Vibration in Buildings.*
33. ANSI S12.1-1983: *American National Standard Guidelines for the Preparation of Standard Procedures for the Determination of Noise Emission from Sources.*
34. ANSI Z24.21-1957 (R1978): *American National Standard Method for Specifying the Character-*

istics of Pickups for Chock and Vibration Measurement.
35. ASA STD 3-1975: Test-Site Measurement of Maximum Noise Emitted by Engine-Powered Equipment.

B. International Electrotechnical Commission, Geneva, Switzerland: IEC

1. IEC/184 (1965): Specifying the Characteristics of Electromechanical Transducers for Shock and Vibration Measurements.
2. IEC/222 (1966): Specifying the Characteristics of Auxiliary Equipment for Shock and Vibration Measurement.
3. IEC/327 (1971): Precision Method for Pressure Calibration of One-inch Standard Condenser Microphones by the Reciprocity Technique.
4. IEC/486 (1974): Precision Method for the Free-Field Calibration of One-inch Condenser Microphones by the Reciprocity Technique.
5. IEC/537 (1976): Frequency Weighting for the Measurement of Aircraft noise (D weighting).
6. IEC/651 (1979): Sound Level Meters.

C. Internal Organization for Standardization, Geneva, Switzerland: ISO

1. ISO/R131-1959: Expression of the Physical and Subjective Magnitudes of Sound or Noise.
2. ISO/R140-1960: Field and Laboratory Measurements of Airborne and Impact Sound Transmission.
3. ISO/R243-1963: Measurement of Absorption Coefficients in a Reverberation Room.
4. ISO/R357-1963: Power and Intensity Levels of Sound or Noise.
5. ISO/R362-1964: Measurement of Noise Emitted by Vehicles.
6. ISO/R495-1966: Preparation of Test Codes for Measuring the Noise Emitted by Machines.
7. ISO/R507-1970: Describing Aircraft Noise around a Airport.
8. ISO/532-1975: Calculating Loudness Level.
9. ISO/R717-1968: Rating of Sound Insulation for Dwellings.
10. ISO/R1680-1970: Test Code for the Measurement of the Airborne Noise Emitted by Roting Electrical Machinery.
11. ISO/R1761-1970: Monitoring Aircraft Noise Around an Airport.
12. ISO/R1996-1971: Acoustics—Assessment of Noise with Respect to Community Response.
13. ISO/R1999-1975: Acoustics—Assessment of Occupational Noise Exposure for Hearing Conservation Purposes.
14. ISO/2041-1975: Mechanical Vibration and Shock—Vocabulary.
15. ISO/R2151-1972: Measurement of Airborne Noise Emitted by Compressor/Primemover Units Intended for Outdoor Use.
16. ISO/R2204-1973: Guide to the Measurement of Acoustical Noise and Evaluation of its Effect on Man.
17. ISO/2249-1973. Acoustics—Description and Measurement of Physical Properties of Sonic Booms.
18. ISO/2922-1975: Acoustics—Measurements of Noise Emitted by Vessels on Inland-Water-Ways and Harbours.
19. ISO/2923-1975: Acoustics—Measurement of Noise on Board Vessels.
20. ISO/3095-1975: Acoustics—Measurement of Noise Emitted by Railbound Vehicles.
21. ISO/TR 3352-1974. Acoustics—Assessment of Noise with Respect to its Effect on the Intelligibility of Speech.
22. ISO 3381-1976. Acoustics—Measurement of Noise Inside Railbound Vehicles.
23. ISO 3740-1978. Acoustics—Determination of Sound Power Levels of Noise Sources—Guidelines for the Use of Basic Standards and for the Preparation of Noise Test Codes.
24. ISO 3741-1975. Acoustics—Determination of Sound Power Levels of Noise Sources—Precision Methods for Broad-Band Sources in Reverberation Rooms.
25. ISO 3742-1975. Acoustics—Determination of Sound Power Levels of Noise Sources—Precision Methods for Discrete-Frequency and Narrow-Band Sources in Reverberation Rooms.
26. ISO 3743-1977: Acoustics—Determination of Sound Power Levels of Noise Sources—Engineering Methods for Special Reverberation Test Rooms.
27. ISO 3744-1978: Acoustics—Determination of Sound Power Levels of Noise Sources—Engineering Methods for Free-Field Conditions Over a Reflecting Plane.
28. ISO 3745-1977: Acoustics—Determination of Sound Power Levels of Noise Sources—Precision Methods for Anechoic and Semi-Anechoic Rooms.
29. ISO/3945-1977: Mechanical Vibration of Large Rotating Machines with Speech Range from 10 to 200 revs/s—Measurement and Evaluation of Vibration.
30. ISO 4869: Measurement of Sound Attenuation of Hearing Protectors, Subjective Method (1978.09).
31. ISO 5129: Measurement of Noise Inside Aircraft (1981.04).
32. ISO 5130: Survey Method for the Measurement of Noise Emitted by Stationary Road Vehicles (1977.08).

D. American Society for Testing Materials, Philadelphia: ASTM Standards

1. ASTM—1973 Classification E 413: Determination of sound transmission class.

Index